About the Author

Jean Carper is a well-known authority on health and nutrition. She is a former senior medical correspondent for CNN in Washington and a former radio and TV on-air reporter. She has written fifteen books and is currently preparing *THE FOOD PHARMACY EATER'S GUIDE*

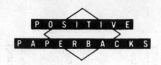

Babies!
A Parent's Guide to Surviving (and Enjoying!) Baby's First Year
Christopher Green

The First Five Minutes
You May Never Get a Second Chance to Make a First Impression
Norman King

The Food Pharmacy
Dramatic New Evidence that Food is Your Best Medicine
Jean Carper

The Good Marriage
A Guide to Getting Wed and Enjoying Marriage in Modern Times
Helen Garlick and Jane Stuart Sheppard

Intangible Evidence
Exploring the Paranormal World and Developing Your Psychic Skills
Bernard Gittelson

Loveshock
How to Recover From a Broken Heart and Love Again
Stephen Gullo Ph.D. and Connie Church

Necessary Losses
**The Loves, Illusions, Dependencies and Impossible Expectations That
All of Us Have to Give Up in Order to Grow**
Judith Viorst

The Power of Your Subconscious Mind
Dr Joseph Murphy

60-Second Shiatzu
How to Energise, Erase Pain and Conquer Tension in One Minute
Eva Shaw

Talk Language
How to Use Conversation for Profit and Pleasure
Allan Pease with Alan Garner

The Tao of Health, Sex and Longevity
A Modern, Practical Approach to the Ancient Way
Daniel Reid

Unlimited Power
Anthony Robbins

Who Needs God
Harold Kushner

The Working Mother's Survival Guide
Jill Black

SELF-HELP FROM SIMON & SCHUSTER

JEAN CARPER

THE
FOOD
PHARMACY

Dramatic New Evidence
That Food Is Your
Best Medicine

SIMON & SCHUSTER

LONDON • SYDNEY • NEW YORK • TOKYO • TORONTO

First published in Great Britain by
Simon & Schuster Ltd in 1989

First published in *Positive Paperbacks* in 1990
Reprinted 1990, 1991, 1992

Simon & Schuster Ltd,
West Garden Place
Kendal Street
London W2 2AQ

Simon & Schuster of Australia Pty Ltd,
Sydney

British Library Cataloguing-in-Publication Data available

ISBN 0-671-71502-X *(Positive Paperback edition)*

Printed and bound in Great Britain by
Butler & Tanner Ltd, Frome and London

ACKNOWLEDGMENTS

Primary thanks must go to the hundreds of physicians and scientists whose interviews, presentations, and published works made this book possible. First among them are the following scientists whose pioneering investigations are chronicled in detail in *The Food Pharmacy:* James Anderson, M.D.; Warren Burger, Ph.D.; Victor Gurewich, M.D.; Dale Hammerschmidt, M.D.; Thomas Kensler, Ph.D.; Jack Konowalchuk, Ph.D.; William Lands, Ph.D.; the late Marilyn Menkes, Ph.D.; Asaf Qureshi, Ph.D.; Khem Shahani, Ph.D.; Anthony Sobota, Ph.D.; Hans Stich, Ph.D.; Walter Troll, Ph.D.; Lee Wattenberg, M.D.; Robert Yolken, M.D.; and Irwin Ziment, M.D.

Also special thanks to Norman Farnsworth, Ph.D., for use of his extensive database on food chemicals, as well as personal interviews, and to James Duke, Ph.D., at the U.S. Department of Agriculture, who also made available his files on the medicinal aspects of foods.

An important person in this book's history is Walter Mertz, Ph.D., director of the USDA's Human Nutrition Laboratories in Beltsville, Maryland. Dr. Mertz unknowingly first triggered the idea for this book several years ago during an interview by expressing his faith in the credibility of a trend toward expanding pharmacological investigations into foods and the legitimacy of much food folklore.

My warm gratitude also to three Bantam editors: Grace Bechtold for her long-time friendship and support of this and my other Bantam books; Michelle Rapkin for her enthusiastic and superb editing of the manuscript; and Donna Ruvituso who makes the production process as efficient and painless as possible.

As always, this book would not have been such a pleasure without the support and comfort, as well as judgment, of my agent, Raphael Sagalyn, and my friend Thea Flaum.

CONTENTS

Introduction   xi

PART ONE   **1**
THE NEW FOOD FRONTIER
Garlic and Other Medicinal Wonders   3

PART TWO
HOW FOODS FIGHT DISEASE   **21**
Twelve Tales of Scientific Investigation   23
    1. Enough to Make Your Blood Run Thin: The Case of
        the Chinese Mushroom   24
    2. Onions for the Heart   30
    3. Barley, Oats, and the Vegetarian Secret   35
    4. Chili Peppers' Yin-Yang Therapy   43
    5. The Great Fish Discoveries   49
    6. The Cabbage–Cancer Connection   56
    7. The Nuts and Seeds Defense   64
    8. The Search for the Mysterious Carrot Factor   71
    9. The Cranberry's Strange Antibiotic   79
    10. Wine, Tea, and the Marvelous Phenols   84
    11. More Fantastic Yogurt Tales   91
    12. Milk and Eggs: A Curious Look at the Future   100

PART THREE
THE FOODS: A MODERN PHARMACOPOEIA   **109**
    Apple   114
    Apricot   118
    Artichoke   120

CONTENTS

Banana and Plantain	122
Barley	126
Beans	132
Beer	139
Blueberry	143
Broccoli	146
Brussels Sprouts	148
Cabbage	150
Carrot	156
Cauliflower	160
Cherry	162
Chili pepper	164
Coffee	169
Corn	178
Cranberry	180
Currant	184
Eggplant	186
Fig	188
Fish	190
Garlic	198
Ginger	207
Grape	211
Grapefruit	213
Honey	216
Kale	220
Lemon and Lime	222
Melon	224
Milk	226
Mushroom	234
Nuts	237
Oats	239
Olive Oil	242
Onion	246
Orange	251
Pea	253
Potato	256
Prune	258
Rice	261
Seaweed, or Kelp	264
Shellfish	269

CONTENTS

Soybean 273
Spinach 278
Squash 280
Strawberry 282
Sugar 284
Tea 289
Tomato 297
Turnip 299
Wheat Bran 301
Wine 305
Yam 310
Yogurt 314

PART FOUR
DISEASE AND FOOD 319

A Capsule Guide to Cures and Prevention 321

References 328

Index 351

INTRODUCTION

For thousands of years, food has been regarded as potent medicine. But in the last century, pharmaceutical drugs have taken over as magic bullets, making us forget much of our rich heritage in the medical uses of foods. The ancient idea that foods have distinct pharmacological properties that can be used to promote health often seems like folklore, decidedly deficient in the rigorous scientific proof required in the twentieth century. That is, until you start looking.

To my amazement, I found that scientists worldwide are routinely discovering remarkable medicines in our food. That such food chemicals can alleviate and prevent disease was confirmed by about three hundred leading scientists and physicians, as well as more than 5000 scientific papers and abstracts, that I consulted for this book. As a medical and nutrition writer, I have long been fascinated by the connections between food and disease. In 1985 I undertook an investigation to find out where modern science stood on that question and to examine what evidence had been collected on the pharmacology of foods—not herbs and esoteric plant substances used as drugs—but everyday foods in everybody's diet.

Here's what I found:
- Foods are full of pharmacological agents.
- Foods do act as drugs in the body.
- Which foods you eat can make a health difference at the cellular level.

- Food folklore is full of wisdom that is now scientifically confirmable.
- Taking clues from food folklore, prestigious scientists are investigating food-disease connections and finding amazing powers in the food pharmacy.
- Some physicians and scientists are "prescribing" foods on the basis of new understandings of disease mechanisms.
- You can direct your own health by taking advantage of the new scientific information about the therapeutic powers of food.
- By making small changes in your diet—by deliberately eating more of foods known to have positive health effects (instead of always worrying about what is bad for you), you may prevent and alleviate both acute and chronic maladies such as infections, heart disease, high blood pressure, cancer, constipation and other gastrointestinal diseases, ulcers, arthritis, skin disorders, headaches, low energy, and insomnia.
- In short, an exciting revolution in the way the world's scientists look at food and its medicinal powers has begun. And these new scientific findings about the food pharmacy are destined to dramatically change our eating habits and ideas about how we can use food to ward off disease.

Never before in history have scientists around the world united in such an exciting investigation into the chemical basis for food's remarkable impact on human health. What was once regarded as quackery, folklore, and medical heresy is being explored with intense seriousness: the theory that food is indeed our largest, most complex pharmacy—a monumental drugstore stocked with an elaborate display of nonprescription drugs of nature's mysterious design.

We are talking about a food pharmacy of unimaginable versatility and complexity, made up of natural laxatives, tranquilizers, beta blockers, antibiotics, anticoagulants, antidepressants, painkillers, cholesterol reducers, anti-inflammatory agents, hypotensives, analgesics, decongestants, digestives, expectorants, anti-motion sickness agents, cancer inhibitors, antioxidants, contraceptives, vasodilators and vasoconstrictors, anticavity agents, antiulcerative agents, insulin regulators, to name a few.

The research comes from all corners of the world, showing that foods and their individual constituents perform in similar fashion to modern drugs—and sometimes as well or better—without the dreaded side effects. For example: when antibiotics fail to heal a wound, sugar almost always works. Yogurt boosts immune functioning better than a drug designed for that purpose, cures diarrhea more quickly than a standard antidiarrheal drug, and contains agents that are stronger antibiotics than penicillin. Onions raise beneficial HDL-cholesterol levels in the blood more effectively than most prescription heart medicine including the latest wonder drug. Garlic compounds match aspirin in preventing blood clots that may lead to heart attacks and strokes. Fish (notably mackerel) equals most diuretics in depressing mild high blood pressure. Ginger surpasses Dramamine in suppressing motion sickness. A couple of tablespoons of sugar at bedtime are as effective as a sleeping pill. Red wine knocks off bacteria about as well as penicillin.

This global inquiry into the therapeutic powers of food is not a trivial pursuit. It is heady and heavy scientific stuff, commanding the attention and energy of some of the world's leading scientists and physicians. It is already producing a remarkable new understanding of the power of common foods to cure and prevent numerous diseases. It is also leading to the extraction and synthesis of natural active agents in foods that can be used in concentrated form for therapeutic purposes.

The important point is that much of this knowledge is ready for use now, as you will discover in *The Food Pharmacy*—the result of my two-year investigation. This book is different from every other food or nutrition book, I believe, in reporting on radical new knowledge about food's potential health impact apart from its traditional nutrient benefits. In *The Food Pharmacy* you will be able to tune in on those scientific conversations going on all over the world about one of humanity's most fascinating commonalities—food and its impact on your health.

It is the intention of this book to:
- alert you to the explosive new explorations of food's pharmacological effects
- chronicle some of the most dramatic discoveries
- give you an understanding of some possible mechanisms by which foods can exert therapeutic power
- give you the most comprehensive information about the pharmacology of those foods about which there is scientifically sound evidence, and their possible therapeutic uses

In other words, this book provides vital new information about making choices from the food pharmacy that can help you stay healthier, feel better, and live longer.

Important: No single food, or foods of one type, should be eaten at the exclusion of others for the purpose of preventing or treating a specific disease or maintaining health, except on the advice of your own physician, whom you should consult before starting any medical treatment or diet. The information in this book is not medical advice and is not given as medical advice. Various types of food provide known and unknown substances vital to health; thus, varying your diet is an essential part of maintaining and achieving better health.

PART ONE

THE NEW FOOD FRONTIER

GARLIC AND OTHER MEDICINAL WONDERS

Let food be your medicine
and medicine be your food.
—Hippocrates

The smell of garlic in Georgetown University Hospital was almost more than Dr. Garagusi could bear. And, after all, it had been his idea. There was garlic in the petri dishes, the hulls of crushed cloves in the wastebaskets, and an odor so strong it was enough to make your eyes water as it drifted through the clinical labs, where blood and urine are analyzed for signs of disease, and into the patients' waiting room.

Who could blame the nurses for wondering if the noted doctor, an expert on antibiotics, had taken leave of his senses. What does garlic have to do with the Hippocratic oath? Garlic is the stuff that keeps vampires away. Garlic is the stuff that gives you bad breath, and it was giving this hospital bad breath.

"Whew!" said Dr. Vincent F. Garagusi, director of infectious diseases at the hospital and a professor at Georgetown University's School of Medicine, as he recalled the incident. "It was pretty bad, wasn't it, Ed?" Ed—Edward C. Delaha, chief microbiologist at the hospital—is the fellow who had to go to the supermarket, buy all that garlic, grind it up, and offer it to the bacteria which found it so offensive, they promptly died.

Yes, Ed agrees, but it *was* the smelly part of the garlic that killed them. Touched by the garlic extract, they disappeared, just kind of dissolved right there in the petri dishes. It was amazing—even to two men who knew a lot about the demise of bacteria. So, mused Dr. Garagusi, the Chinese were right.

3

It began for Dr. Garagusi as it has begun for many other scientists worldwide. Because of some intellectual puzzle, strange observation, or association with ideas of a different culture, they become fascinated with the mystery surrounding the curative and preventive powers of foods. Nearly all have been trained in the modern Western tradition to trust the magic of the pharmacopoeia of synthetic drugs. Now, for one reason or another, they are attracted to probing the secrets of that inadvertent pharmacy—our diet—which may in the end yield information that makes the erratic hits of modern drugs on the body seem mild in comparison.

In perspective, it seems like hubris not to have done it before. Just think of the enormous possibilities. The brains of human chemists in less than fifty years have come up with marvelous life-giving pharmaceutical drugs by stringing together molecules in new arrangements. What their creations can do to our physiology is awesome. Why should it seem so strange to take a closer look at the creations of an ancient cosmic brain that has strung chemicals together for hundreds of thousands of years in mysterious configurations and incorporated them into plants and other foods that we take into our bodies every day?

These are not just bits of pharmaceutical herbs we are talking about, but the great gobs of chemicals in vegetables, fruits, grains, nuts, seeds, fish, and animals and their eggs and secretions that determine our biological makeups every minute of the day.

Eating turns out to be the world's greatest pharmacological experiment.

GARLIC ON THE BRAIN

One day Dr. Garagusi had noticed an article in the *Chinese Medical Journal.* Chinese doctors in the province of Changsha, lacking the money and resources to obtain amphotericin, an antibiotic, resorted to an ancient practice of administering garlic. They fed and injected garlic into patients with a serious infection called cryptococcal meningitis. Of sixteen who got the garlic, eleven survived, for a cure rate of sixty-eight percent. Not bad. Really darn good considering that this infection gets in the spinal cord and into the brain, and even some powerful antibiotics can't cross the blood-brain barrier to attack the bacteria. That meant garlic, or at least some chemicals in garlic, probably did travel from the bloodstream or spinal fluid and into the brain, where it destroyed the bacteria. And it caused no serious side effects, unlike prescription antibiotics.

Dr. Garagusi, intrigued, looked up the medical literature and found that garlic was once extensively used to treat tuberculosis which, like cryptococcal meningitis, is a fungal infection. In fact, in the days before manmade antibiotics, garlic was the "drug of choice" against TB. At the turn of the century the head of a large tuberculosis ward in Dublin reported remarkable cure rates from eating, inhaling, and smearing garlic on the chest as an ointment. Around the same time in New York City a physician compared the effectiveness of fifty-five tuberculosis treatments and found garlic the best.

Dr. Garagusi, a student of medical history, also knew that garlic has had a long reputation as a magical cure-all. The ancient Egyptians worshipped it. Pliny the Elder, a Roman administrator and naturalist living in the first century A.D., recommended garlic for no fewer than sixty-one ailments. And what better company could one want: Even Louis Pasteur in 1858 put a dollop of garlic in a petri dish and recorded that the bacteria died.

Through the years numerous researchers have looked at the effect of garlic on the blood, showing that it lowers blood pressure and combats clotting. Indeed, Dr. Garagusi knew that researchers across town at George Washington University had confirmed the presence of chemicals in garlic that thinned the blood. There have been lots of reports in the medical literature on the antibiotic powers of garlic, attributed mainly to allicin, the chemical that produces the smell. A recent upsurge of interest has stirred researchers into trying to figure out just how garlic does it. Some hope to turn the active ingredients into pharmaceutical drugs.

Still, the Georgetown garlic experiment was different. Dr. Garagusi has a special interest in a type of fungal bacteria called mycobacteria. This particular class of bacteria had not been adequately subjected to garlic in the lab. Who knows? They might react differently to garlic's death threats. Just because garlic harms one family of bacteria, that does not mean it has the same effect on others.

Garagusi and Delaha also knew that the human destruction from these fungus microbes is growing more worrisome. Tuberculosis is on the upswing in the United States, often infecting those with acquired immune deficiency syndrome, AIDS. Another of the opportunistic infections that fells AIDS victims is caused by a fungal bug called M. avium, previously seen only in birds. Fungal infections in the United States have doubled or tripled in the last five years. Why this is so nobody knows, but Garagusi and Delaha were seeing more blood samples infected by these strains of fungus bacteria. If garlic were as effective against fungi as the Chinese medical report said, it surely was worth further investigation. Dr. Garagusi was eager to find out how these deadly fungi would react to intimate contact with garlic in the laboratory.

That's how it happened that the chief of Washington, D.C.'s prestigious Georgetown University Hospital lab went shopping for garlic.

The punch line of the story you know. The garlic's killer instinct was on target. Delaha peeled and ground up ten bulbs of garlic in a Waring blender. He extracted the active ingredient, allicin, from the garlic pulp, and after many chemical shenanigans ended up with a frozen extract of garlic. He put thirty strains of seventeen species of mycobacteria in sterile petri dishes and then introduced the garlic compound in various concentrations. (There were also comparable numbers of petri dishes with bacteria that received no garlic.)

The researchers sat back to watch the bacteria grow or not grow. Those in the nongarlic dishes thrived. And, of course, those face-to-face with the garlic extract withered, died, and failed to reproduce. The garlic did grave damage to every single one of the fungal bacterial strains to varying degrees, including those that cause tuberculosis. In fact, it was extra potent against the TB bacteria. (It was less effective against avium bacteria.)

Chalk up one for folk medicine and all those early doctors who used garlic against tuberculosis.

But that's not enough for modern science. That foods have biological impact is not in question to scientists like Dr. Garagusi. The problem is: how on earth do they work? How potent are they?

Exactly how did the garlic go about its lethal task? Precisely what happened to the cells of bacteria that made them cease growing? How did the allicin, that smelly chemical released when garlic is cut, effect its assassination—the same kind of act it performed against the bacterial cells in the bodies and brains of the Chinese suffering from meningitis?

Ah! To Dr. Garagusi, that is the interesting question.

Perhaps, like standard antibiotics, garlic rips apart the mycobacteria's cell walls or interferes with their enzymes so they starve to death.

"I wish we knew," says Dr. Garagusi. "It is the most major question, something we must find out."

Dr. Garagusi is not unlike countless other scientists and physicians throughout the world who are asking the same questions about the inherent curative and preventive powers in foods, and for essentially the same reasons. In fact, the main reason to tell you about his work in this area is not because it is so unusual, but precisely because it is not.

In his case, the research on garlic occupies a small fraction of his time, wedged in between the daily chores of running a large-scale clinical diagnostic laboratory. It's generally what's called "bootleg" research, unpaid for out of any particular budget and done in a scientist's spare time. A lot of this is going on in academic institutions. At the same time, the massive machinery of governments in the United States as well as in other countries is stimulating the search for disease antidotes in the diet in a big way.

It is a thunderous event.

The pursuit of knowledge about the food pharmacy is not an inconsequential event. It is engaging some of the best scientific minds in the world.

BACK TO THE FUTURE

Historically, it makes sense. The new scientific thrust simply restores food to its prominent place in medicine after a brief interval of therapeutic monopoly by pharmaceutical drugs. The medical profession's romance with food is ancient. Prescriptions on stone and papyrus dating back to 4000 B.C. list foods as cures for common diseases. The father of modern medicine, Hippocrates, proclaimed food and medicine inseparable. The great Jewish physician-philosopher Maimonides of the twelfth century in his treatise on asthma included recipes for chicken soup as remedies (some of which are scientifically valid today). For forty centuries Oriental cultures have regarded food and medicine as indistinguishable. In fact, it is instructive and humbling to remember that the modern tendency to draw a firm line between food and drugs is of amazingly short duration. As Irwin Ziment, M.D., a professor of medicine at the University of California at Los Angeles (UCLA) College of Medicine, notes: "The use of food as a drug had always been important until the modern drug industry arose in the nineteenth century." Dr. Ziment, who views foods as potent drugs, now sees a return to the concept of foods as medicines.

The new scientific fascination with the food pharmacy is emerging, especially in the United States and other strongholds of Western medicine, for at least three reasons: an infusion of scientific ideas from other cultures, notably the Far East; a revival of fascination with things natural (holistic medicine, health foods, and so forth), and stunning scientific advancements in the understanding of the diet's impact on disease.

Western scientists are finding out that the ancient cultures contain numerous verities. In the last ten to fifteen years, the heritages of other countries, like China, have had time to rub off on Western scientists. Consequently, there is a resurgence of respect for traditional medicine. Undeniably, scientists, especially in China, Japan, Thailand, India, even Russia and Middle European countries, are more apt to recognize medicine's debt to herbal and plant medicines, and are not one whit embarrassed to assign therapeutic powers to foods or wax rhapsodic about the curative values of a food like plain old tea.

A CASE OF THE GREEN TEA FACTOR

Many high-caliber scientists take it for granted that folklore mixes well with modern science. For example, in 1985, several prominent scientists from Japan's National Institute of Genetics published a paper with a fanciful title, "A Case of the Green Tea Factor." It was a rave review for a factor isolated from Japanese green tea leaves called "epigallocatechin-gallate," which in lab culture tests is an antagonist to cancer-producing chemicals. Nestled in the paper was a paragraph calling attention to the fact that "in China, green tea has been considered as a crude medicine for 4000 years." The investigators did not quarrel with reports that green tea could protect blood vessels, suppress cancer, and prolong the life span.

The point is not whether tea *does* all these things—although there is strong evidence that it is potent therapeutically—but that top-notch scientists are no longer reluctant to entertain the thought that it *could*.

Much of the new scientific interest in the food pharmacy is linked with ancient and current folklore.

THE OYSTER'S SEXUAL SIGNATURE

Sometimes the ancient wisdom examined in terms of modern scientific knowledge can draw you up short. There's a very old concept called the Doctrine of Signatures. According to medical historian Benjamin Lee Gordon, M.D., in the book *Medicine Throughout Antiquity* (1949), "This doctrine was probably the earliest therapeutic system in the history of medicine." Translations of medical texts from the seventh century B.C. show that physician-priests depended on it to choose remedies in ancient Assyro-Babylonia.

Its simplicity is appealing. The idea is that for every part of the human body there is a corresponding part in the world of nature. That concept flows from the ancient belief that man's "little world," or microcosm, is a direct reflection of the "larger world," or macrocosm. Thus, in nature you will find a counterpart for every bit of human anatomy.

Man's challenge in dealing with illness is to be smart enough to find that counterpart with which to heal himself. "To make the search easier," writes Dr. Gordon, "the Creator stamped all objects medically beneficial to mankind" to resemble the diseased part in shape, color, structure, or some other symbolic way. That means if you had jaundice, you might be treated with a mixture based on eviscerated yellow frog. Red skin blotches might call for animal blood or red fruit juice. Liverwort plant, with leaves shaped like a liver, would be proper treatment for liver ailments. In traditional Oriental medicine ginseng root became known as a "whole-body tonic," a source of vitality and long life, because it is said to often resemble a whole human form with a head, trunk, and arms and legs. Of all the herbs of China, ginseng root, since antiquity, has been the most highly prized as an "elixir vitae."

Now consider oysters. Actually, it was Dr. Harold Sandstead at the University of Texas who triggered the idea. Oysters have been heralded for centuries as an aphrodisiac—as a key to potency and fertility. How could that possibly be? Why would oysters be a sexual food? Dr. Sandstead, a leading expert on zinc, said he had never thought much about it, but the most logical reason popped into his head: "Probably because they look like human testes."

That would end the story, except that oysters are nature's most concentrated packages of zinc. They are richer in zinc than any other food by far. Three ounces of raw oysters have sixty-three milligrams of zinc compared with only three milligrams in the same amount of beef liver, another concentrated source. Experts say it's tough to get enough zinc unless you eat oysters.

And what happens to males who don't eat enough zinc? They don't mature sexually; their gonads shrink up. Also, normal males with zinc deficiencies fail to produce enough male hormone testosterone and sperm, and can become infertile or impotent. Dr. Ananda A. Prasad, a researcher at Wayne State University in Detroit, and a leading zinc authority, finds that even a mild zinc deficiency can induce dramatic declines in testosterone and sperm counts, producing infertility. In other research, a group of impotent men given more zinc almost immediately pepped up sexually. Aphrodisiac? Doctrine of Signatures? Coincidence?

Although the concept may strike modern Western sensibilities as ludicrously primitive, it is undeniable that men for thousands of years who followed the Doctrine of Signatures would have gobbled up zinc, boosting their chances of sexual and reproductive success.

Yet, folklore remains just that—superstition, silliness, worthless—in modern eyes until someone finds a plausible explanation for why it could work. It is not enough for Dr. Garagusi to have a hunch, or even agree with some of the greatest physicians of history, that garlic fights infections. Without an understanding of how food works on the body at the very basic cell level, the effects will forever seem nebulous and just a little bit like magic. It is the formulation of theories and a collection of supporting facts that raises the deliberations out of the realm of folk medicine and quackery.

What distinguishes current food knowledge from folklore is an understanding of the mechanism by which foods control the human physiology.

PLANT BONANZA

One eight-million-dollar-a-year industry has successfully forged that link between folklore and hard biological science: the pharmaceutical industry. The discovery and synthesis of profitable new drugs based on plants confirm that folk medicine is hardly hokum.

Many of our most widely used drugs come from plants. A field of study called pharmacognosy in schools of pharmacy is devoted to natural product research. Scientists investigate current and historic folk use of plants usually in places like China, Africa, and South America. If it looks as if there is something to it, they try to identify and isolate active chemicals producing the effect. Sometimes they then copy the molecular structure and turn out an artificial version of the pure compound. It's sold in concentrated doses as a pharmaceutical drug.

Dr. Norman Farnsworth can tell you anything you want to know about this subject. It's his life's work. He's director of the program for collaborative research in pharmaceutical sciences, College of Pharmacy, Health Sciences Center, University of Illinois at Chicago. He has set up a computer data base called Napralert, with about 50,000 scientific references on foods and their active chemicals.

Sure, folk medicine is right a lot of the time, he says. That's proven by the fact that about twenty-five percent of all prescription drugs used in the world are derived from natural plant substances, he says. He did a study of these 140 pure drugs derived from ninety species of plants and found an excellent correlation with folk remedies. In seventy-four percent of the cases the purified active chemical is used to treat the same disease as the plant was reputed to cure in folk medicine.

Our debt to plants is formidable. Science first forced a plant to yield up a chemical, benzoic acid, in the sixteenth century. In 1804 the opium poppy gave us morphine. After that, plant pharmacology went into high gear. Today Western medicine counts on stolen plant blueprints to turn out such common drugs as acetyldigoxin, allantoin, bromelain, codeine, digitoxin, L-Dopa, leurocristine, papain, physostigmine, pseudoephedrine, quinine, reserpine, scopolamine, strychnine, theophylline, and xanthotoxin. That doesn't include lesser plant drugs such as camphor, menthol, and capsaicin or over-the-counter drugs based on food extracts such as prunes sold as laxatives.

Still only a scant number (five to ten percent) of the 250,000 plant species on the face of the earth have ever been examined, says Dr. Farnsworth. "And common sense tells you that if we got so many good drugs out of only ninety species, there is a rich mine of pharmaceutical agents out there going unexplored."

There's no question that plants, including those in the diet, are pharmacologically active as proved by the fact that we make their essences into drugs.

THE COMPLICATED PEA

A funny thing often happens, though, when you squeeze a pure chemical out of nature's pharmacy. It doesn't have the same pharmacological powers as the original plant extract. An extract is merely a ground-up part of a particular plant with its entire chemical complex intact. Let's say you suspect peas are a male contraceptive. (There's evidence for that.) You isolate a presumed sperm-suppressing chemical in peas. But in tests, the single compound doesn't sterilize nearly as well as feeding whole peas to animals. Or, says Dr. Farnsworth: "Let's assume you make an extract from a plant that people use to cure insomnia. The crude extract puts the experimental animals to sleep. You isolate ten compounds; five of them could put an animal or human to sleep; five of them could keep them awake. It all depends on how much of each was in the plant as to whether it would put you to sleep or keep you awake, and how they worked together."

Dr. Walter Mertz says the same thing about vitamins and minerals. You can mix up a batch of nutrients to simulate a food, but it just doesn't work. "We know how much zinc is in human milk on which a baby grows beautifully. Now we put that same amount of zinc in an infant formula that we make, and we find that the infant will not grow. It's identical, for the main criterion for baby foods is to make them as close to human milk as possible. And they are close, but the zinc won't do it. There is something else in human milk that renders that zinc more effective. We don't know what it is."

Citrus fruits, too, cannot be defined by their vitamins alone. In 1985, Canadian researchers reported a meticulous study of patients with stomach cancer. They found that vitamin C doses (1000 milligrams a day) did help prevent stomach cancer, but little more than three fluid ounces of orange juice daily (containing only thirty-seven milligrams of vitamin C) was *twice* as likely to depress the chances of developing stomach cancer!

And fiber. You can extract pectin from apples and feed it to animals to lower their blood cholesterol. But it doesn't work nearly as well as the fruit pulp itself. And beans. You can eat either the beans or the gummy fiber from beans and get two different metabolic reactions in the intestinal tract. Even the form of the food matters. Coarse bran affects the body differently from fine bran. And the nearly identical nutrients made into pasta and bread have wildly different effects on blood sugar and insulin. Researchers find it amazing and inexplicable.

The chemical mixture of man's nourishment is something marvelously more complex and inscrutable than a collection of known nutrients or compounds. Most of Dr. Mertz's daily concern is advancing the study of individual nutrients at USDA labs. Yet it is very petty, and dangerous, indeed, he believes, to put faith in a faddish focus on individual nutrients at the expense of whole foods. People who think they can remedy their poor diets by taking vitamins and minerals do not realize that this is an insult to the complexity of the universe. Each food is a vast chemical factory of perhaps 10,000 or more elements.

For about the first half of the century scientists shunned whole foods for the study of their individual nutrients. Now that trend is reversing: food itself, not nutrients, is becoming the major concern.

"Exclusive concern with individual nutrients is not only unscientific but also potentially dangerous," says Dr. Mertz. "Foods are more than the sources of the now known nutrients. We are beginning to realize that foods which may be nearly identical in their nutrient composition can have very different health effects."

He also appreciates the emerging scientific wisdom behind some ancient tales. Writing in the July 1984 issue of the *Journal of the American Dietetic Association,* he noted: "The age-old belief that garlic and onions are good for the circulatory system is supported by modern experiments showing hypocholesterolemic (cholesterol-reducing) and anticoagulating (blood-clot preventing) effects of extracts from those sources. The unproven association between consumption of yogurt and longevity is beginning to sound plausible on the basis of recent animal experiments demonstrating increased resistance against infections in yogurt-fed animals."

So we should definitely pay attention to food folklore?

"Yes. I think we learned to recognize the good and bad health aspects of foods by very ancient experiences passed on by tradition. That knowledge is precious and serious. What Grandmother used to tell us is much more than a fairy tale passed on by an old lady. It is a distillation of centuries-old wisdom handed down through generations. We are only now beginning to understand it scientifically."

Dr. Mertz agrees that dissecting foods into individual nutrients to study their metabolism, health effects, and requirements is necessary to this scientific pursuit. But he warns: "This approach presents the risk of substituting incomplete scientific knowledge of individual nutrients for the lessons learned from our historical experience with foods." He is throwing his lot in with the latter.

Scientists, who once saw foods as mere collections of individual nutrients, are now vigorously beginning to explore their larger pharmacological complexities.

BEYOND VITAMINS AND MINERALS

It is no longer enough to know how much protein, fat, carbohydrate, vitamins, and minerals are in foods. Now there are "food factors, X factors, food compounds, co-travelers, desmutagens, antimutagens, anticarcinogens, and minor dietary constituents." In the chemist's hands, the complexities of plant and animal life are unraveling just as surely as the secrets of life unraveled in the laboratories of Watson and Crick. The quest for the composition of food is yielding new secrets of life and health. It is perhaps not as romantic as the unraveling of DNA, but it could be equally important in promoting health and longevity.

These newly discovered food compounds are distinct from nutrients; most have no nutritional value at all; rarely, as with beta carotene, they possess separate nutritional and drug effects. They are usually present in infinitesimal amounts. Although physiologically potent, the minor food constituents are probably not essential for life; you won't instantly perish without them. Nobody ever died from an allicin deficiency due to not eating garlic. But these mysterious dietary compounds can subtly and radically influence physiological mechanisms that are the keys to longer life and optimal health. Some may actually cure disease, but mainly they are thought to prevent the long and persistent erosion of bodily tissues that eventually end up as chronic diseases such as cancer, heart disease, arthritis, diabetes, and intestinal and neurological disorders—our greatest and least treatable medical threats. Unlike single-purpose modern drugs, the drugs in foods are more likely to act as lifelong antidotes to that accumulated cellular damage known as disease.

At any moment in your body there is monumental chemical-biological warfare going on in your cells. Disease is essentially a collection of cell disturbances, a conglomeration of cellular events that add up to a whole body event. Although you do not perceive disease until you see the symptoms, these symptoms appear only because enough cells have lost the battle to evil forces. Whether your health is promoted, sustained, or defeated depends on the perpetual struggle for possession of single cells.

Pharmacologically active food chemicals can guard individual cells by cutting the enemy off at any number of biological passes. Whether you are fighting off infections, arthritis, cancer, heart disease, diabetes, ulcers, or even depression or fatigue, you are carrying on that battle in unseen places by fending off tiny assaults against individual cells. How well you do that depends upon unfathomable biological activity.

Scientists are beginning to understand how food and food chemicals can exert influence against disease at a cellular level.

NEW THEORIES OF FOOD POWER

What makes this new perspective on food possible is the technological ability to detect potent chemicals in foods in infinitesimal amounts and test their biological activity, as well as the new understanding of the basic mechanisms by which these chemicals can affect disease. Science cannot see beyond its technological capabilities. Many of the new discoveries about food's potential could have come only in the last few years. One piece of chromatography equipment is so accurate, it has been described by its inventor this way: "If you threw a sugar cube into a reservoir, I could tell you from analyzing a few drops of the water exactly what chemicals were in the cube and how much." This means that virtually every compound in food can be measured in minute quantities. Scientists can also track the flow of chemicals throughout the body, analyze the basic mechanisms of life, such as the activity of enzymes. There are much quicker screening tests for the antibiotic and anticarcinogenic activity of chemicals.

At the same time, advances in understanding the underlying mechanisms of disease reveal the grand possibilities for controlling destructive cellular activity. Scientists probing those theoretical depths run into Jules Verne-like astonishments. It is like entering the world of Dr. Seuss or the fantasy world of Epcot Center's Journey of the Imagination, where unfamiliar creatures pop up at every turn. In the uninhibited land of medical hypothesis, theories fly, collide, unite, stick to each other to form strange appendages, then drift on, all in an effort to explain the causes, connections, and possible remedies for human ills.

Both drug research and the burgeoning field of food pharmacology strive to keep up with and adapt to these kaleidoscopic views of the human system's continuous battle with disease. For example, it is now known that much cell activity is governed by the presence of receptors on the surface of the cells. You can imagine these as perfectly crafted docking sites, where other molecules and cells land and insinuate themselves into a perfect geometric fit—like a Rubik's Cube coming together or a spaceship attaching to a space station. These receptors accommodate only those biological entities with a matching mooring shape. How precise the fit determines how tightly they lock together and thus how well they carry out their intended mission, which is a biochemical interaction.

Myriad molecular and cellular reactions depend on the existence, availability, and efficiency of receptor sites, thus determining the state of your health. Nature created these receptors not for the convenience of microbes, but so hormones, enzymes, and other vital substances could interact with cells. But clever bacteria and viruses through eons of evolution developed mooring apparatuses so they, too, can use receptor sites to attach to the cells. Without such attachment bacteria may not break down cell walls and viruses cannot penetrate and capture healthy cells in a destruction-replication ritual.

Enzymes, those catalysts without which chemical reactions do not occur, also need to alight and lock into receptors to initiate proper physiological actions. If your liver cells have too few or poorly functioning receptors for sucking "bad-type" LDL cholesterol out of the blood, excessive numbers of cholesterol globules circulate aimlessly, eventually ending up on artery walls, and promoting heart disease. Defining the importance of receptors in metabolizing blood cholesterol won a Nobel prize for Drs. Michael S. Brown and Joseph L. Goldstein of the University of Texas in 1985.

Anything that interferes or promotes the mooring with receptors obviously has an impact on biological processes. Suppose, for example, you could institute a "receptor blockade," placing something between the receptor site and the mooring configuration to prevent the two from fitting together. That's a concept being extensively pursued by pharmaceutical companies in attempts to create more effective drugs, especially agents against those intractable 200 or more common cold viruses. Finding a substance to plug up the receptor site would prevent microbes from attaching to and destroying healthy cells. Or you could send decoys into the system. Some compounds, including some in food, have receptor sites so similar to those of the human cells that they fool microbes into attaching to them instead of to vulnerable cells. Then they carry the organism harmlessly out of the body.

Scientists increasingly discover how and why the blood flows; they are defining the intricate mechanisms of clotting, which entails the actions of disclike cells called platelets that live but five to ten days and the blood-clot-dissolving mechanism (the fibrinolytic system) that operates constantly. Affecting the clotting tendency of blood at any of numerous stages can have profound effects on susceptibility to heart disease and stroke. Researchers have learned that some of the viruses and carcinogens that we are all exposed to must be activated or enlivened in the human body before they can do damage. Interfering with this activation through food compounds has exciting possibilities for thwarting both acute and chronic disease. Enzymes can be squelched or encouraged by compounds, including many in foods, thereby helping manipulate biological processes of all kinds.

Within the last few years medicine has leapt forward with the recognition of the immense power of body hormones called prostaglandins that are often the behind-the-scenes manipulators of a dazzling array of biochemical processes. These prostaglandins can cause pain, inflammation, skin disorders, sluggish blood, and infertility, among other things. Other groups of prostaglandins can protect the stomach from noxious chemicals and other intestinal damage. Anything that regulates the activity of these prostaglandins, as some foods can, is bound to have far-reaching effects on your state of health. Additionally, thrilling breakthroughs have shown that food chemicals get into the brain and fool around with neurotransmitters, thus affecting the state of your mind and mood.

Some of the most amazing theories floating in that subchamber of medical phantasia find common roots in disparate diseases, suggesting that the same foods could help fight varying ailments. There appears to be a strange interconnectedness and perhaps a common basis among diseases that seem wildly different. Researchers at the New York University Medical Center find evidence that heart disease may be another form of cancer, or at least the two may coexist in arteries. NYU's Dr. Arthur Penn and researchers elsewhere have found cancer activity in the plaques removed from the arteries of patients during coronary bypass surgery. Tumor activity in the arteries may predispose to the accumulation of cholesterol on the walls and clogged, hardened, inflexible arteries characteristic of atherosclerosis. Another hypothesis: Perhaps the high circulating levels of insulin in the blood of diabetics may damage artery walls, helping explain why they are so prone to cardiovascular problems. Then there's the idea that a particularly active group of enzymes in the body called proteases may form a common mechanism, turning on both cancer and infectious agents of various sorts. Inhibitors in foods may switch proteases off.

Viruses may be an underlying link to a plethora of maladies with entirely different symptoms. Although we think of viruses as the villains in acute infectious diseases such as colds, flu, and smallpox, actually they have been implicated in any number of chronic diseases, including cancer, atherosclerosis, arthritis, and as promoters of autoimmune diseases such as insulin-dependent diabetes, systemic lupus erythematosus, multiple sclerosis, and myasthenia gravis. It's been suggested that viruses may help throw the immune system out of whack or "turn on" disease factors that would otherwise remain dormant. Certain food constituents can boost immunity.

There is a prominent theory that the body ages, falling prey to cancer, cardiovascular disease, and numerous chronic diseases partly because of the release of charged particles that rip apart cells and DNA, the genetic matter in cells. These free radicals race around the body, as medical writer Larry Thompson described in *The Washington Post*, "like participants in a molecular demolition derby. They randomly bounce around inside cells, causing damage to the first molecule they touch. Radicals can inactivate enzymes, hormones, and other proteins and the fats in cell membranes." These free radicals perpetually assault the body, causing lifelong damage to cells and organs, creating bodily disintegration that we call aging.

However, these havoc-wreaking free radicals are retarded by antioxidants, chemical scavengers that also roam the body scarfing up the attackers. The body can produce antioxidants internally, and many foods also contain antioxidants that protect cells from destruction and aberrant changes leading to cancer.

Fantastic discoveries in both the underlying mechanisms of disease and the drug activity of foods are merging to inject new validity and vitality into the food pharmacy.

LUCKY VEGETARIANS

Partly because of such science, the emphasis on the health aspects of food is undergoing a subtle, soon-to-be-dramatic shift from negative to positive. Scientists fresh from their laboratory successes are witnesses to the fact that food, if it can bring terrible disease (such as high-fat-induced heart attacks) can also mitigate and prevent it. If there are villains in the food supply, there are also saviors. Deliberately enlisting the powers of the latter is becoming an accepted way to combat the anticipated ill effects of the former. We are no longer at the mercy of the bad guys. We are learning to better orchestrate those inner cellular battles, liberating us somewhat from the tyranny of chronic disease.

Many experts are convinced that certain foods can cancel out the damaging effects of other foods and alien compounds and act as partial antidotes to our dangerous environment and lifestyle. For example, it's known that many foods contain mutagens that may cause genetic cell damage leading to cancer. But recently, extensive tests, especially by Japanese scientists, have shown that foods are also full of powerful antimutagens that can neutralize the cancer threat. Japanese screenings found broccoli, green pepper, pineapple, shallot, apple, ginger, cabbage, and eggplant all "remarkably effective" in blocking cancer-promoting cell mutations. Cauliflower, grapes, sweet potato, and radish were "moderately effective." Just by luck some people are already beneficiaries of "pharmacological serendipity."

Nowhere is this better illustrated than by vegetarians. They have lower rates of cancer, heart disease, stroke, and a number of other chronic diseases than meat eaters. At first one explanation was that they eat less saturated fat. That evolved into the theory that maybe the higher-fiber foods they eat counteract some of the effects of the fat. Then it began to dawn that maybe vegetables, fruits, legumes, nuts, and other plant foods containing pharmacologically protective agents—the "minor dietary constituents," as Dr. Lee Wattenberg of the University of Minnesota labels them—are plenty potent in counteracting cellular assaults that foster disease.

This is becoming such a credible notion that some scientists foresee a not-too-distant future in which foods will be individually prescribed and designed to dramatically improve health. Dr. David Jenkins, a professor at the University of Toronto and a leading expert on diet and blood sugar, sees foods as inadvertent packages of drugs. He notes that "in pharmacology, people often talk in terms of combination therapy. Yet we have not realized that that is exactly what some foods are doing already—providing a combination therapy of their own." It's just, he says, that we do not yet use foods specifically and scientifically. But, he says, that will come with advanced knowledge.

Sounds pretty revolutionary—prescribing foods.

"Either revolutionary or evolutionary. But, actually, all we are doing is taking the sort of thinking understood by pharmacists for centuries and applying it to food. I mean food is a drug we take every day. We should find out its pharmacological effects and direct them to our individual needs and benefits, just as we do drugs."

Many commercial interests see a bright future for the food pharmacy. Some companies are analyzing and testing their food products for their specific health-promoting potential. Others are fortifying certain foods pharmacologically. For example, the Miller Brewing Company is taking the residues of barley left over from beer brewing and making it into cholesterol-lowering flour to put in cereals and bread. Academic scientists talk of extracting anticancer chemicals from foods like soybeans and adding them to milk. Dr. James Tillotson, head of research at Ocean Spray, where cranberry juice research is of high priority, believes that one day the government may insist on labeling not only nutrients in foods but also a food's total health effect based on solid studies of its pharmacological powers.

All of us are now using trial and error in the food pharmacy with virtually no knowledge of the outcome. In the future we will no doubt learn to assess biochemical responses so precisely that applied food pharmacology will be as routine as drug pharmacology. That is a long way off, but many experts see it as the exciting end point of the pioneering investigations into the food pharmacy.

Much wisdom contained in folk medicine now comes full circle, verified and vindicated by vigorous new investigations into food's biochemical activities. As a result, we can all take the food pharmacy more seriously than at any time in history and use that knowledge to promote our own health.

There is a revolution going on in the way we think about food. And what a wonderful revolution it is! Like Hippocrates, we, too, are beginning to realize that food is potent medicine.

PART TWO

HOW FOODS FIGHT DISEASE

TWELVE TALES OF SCIENTIFIC INVESTIGATION

What proof is there that food can actually intervene at basic levels to preserve health? The evidence is tumbling forth, usually as much by accident as by design. But once food's secret mechanisms are revealed, its unlimited potential is undeniable. Here are a dozen cases of how pioneering scientists have uncovered precise ways in which food can fight disease—from combatting viruses to curbing cancer.

These cases of scientific investigation do not explore all of food's possible pharmacological mechanisms by any means; but they dramatically illustrate numerous ways foods can conceivably affect cellular processes to ward off disease. The scientists' adventures chronicle the food pharmacy's variegated possibilities of performance as anticoagulants, blood-clot dissolvers, cholesterol reducers, expectorants, prostaglandin-inhibitors (like aspirin), cancer blockers, antioxidants, antibiotics, antiviral agents, immune-system boosters and antibody manipulators. Thus, old food folktales are being transformed into new scientific facts. They are destined to forge new connections in the way we think about food and its ultimate impact on our lives.

1.

ENOUGH TO MAKE YOUR BLOOD RUN THIN: THE CASE OF THE CHINESE MUSHROOM

For Dr. Dale Hammerschmidt it was the opposite of a blood-curdling experience. It, in fact, started off as routine. You see, Dr. Hammerschmidt, when he is not attending to his duties as a hematologist and associate professor at the University of Minnesota Medical School, has been known to cook up a wicked batch of mapo doufu, a Szechuan dish also called Pock-Marked Ma's Bean Curd. It's salty, hot, sweet, and pungent. Enough to make your throat burn, your eyes tear, and, as Dr. Hammerschmidt discovered, your blood do strange things. It took him several days to figure it out.

Dr. Hammerschmidt had done the experiment several times without incident. Using blood from patients with chronic myelogenous leukemia, he was trying to find out how certain cancer cells, called basophils, interacted with ordinary healthy blood platelets. (Platelets are disc-shaped cell fragments involved in blood-clotting.) It would give clues about how the cancer actually destroyed the body.

That day, as he sometimes does, Dr. Hammerschmidt used his own blood platelets as "targets," sure that they were healthy and untainted by antiplatelet drugs such as aspirin. But he quickly noticed that something was drastically wrong. His platelets did not interact as expected with the leukemia cells; in fact, his blood platelets were not normal, according to several tests. They were in a grave state of dysfunction. For an instant the dread thought passed through his mind that it might be leukemia. But another look showed that the *number* of

24

platelets—an indication of leukemia—was fine; only the way they functioned was messed up. Within two days his blood platelets were normal again.

In trying to solve the mystery, he recalled that he had had a nosebleed that morning and bled unusually long after nicking himself with a razor. Ordinarily, when you cut yourself, emergency squads of platelets rush to the site and stick together, or aggregate, forming plugs to patch up the breach. His easier, longer bleeding meant that something had blocked the normal aggregation of the platelets, and thus their tendency to promote clots. But what? Since it could not be drugs, perhaps food. He remembered that the night before he had eaten, perhaps overindulged in, one of his favorite Chinese Szechuan dishes called mapo doufu. Could that have anything to do with thinning his blood?

In typical scientific fashion, he invited several of his colleagues to an unusual dinner party and a controlled experiment. Some of them—the control group—got sweet and sour pork and the others, including himself, got mapo doufu made from the same recipe as previously. A few hours later they all gave blood. As expected, the sweet-and-sour-pork eaters had normal platelet function. And all four of the mapo doufu eaters had platelets with little inclination to aggregate. The cells were definitely not releasing the usual substances, such as serotonin and adenosine diphosphate (ADP), that cause other platelets in the vicinity to rush together in a heap of gluey camaraderie.

Determined to find the specific cause, Dr. Hammerschmidt and his curious colleagues systematically subjected bits of each mapo doufu ingredient to the test. They added extracts of ginger, bean curd, tree ears (the mo-er mushroom or black tree fungus), and sar quort (also known as jicama, a radishlike vegetable Dr. Hammerschmidt had substituted for water chestnut) to normal platelets to see what happened in the test tube. Two foods were incriminated as anticlotting agents: the tree ear mushroom and the sar quort.

The next step: proof by eating. (What scientists don't have to go through!) Dr. Hammerschmidt and others ate 400 grams, fully fourteen ounces, of sar quort. Result: upset stomach but no platelet dysfunction. The plot thins. After a decent interval they downed seventy grams (about two and a half ounces) of the mo-er mushroom. Within three hours their blood again went through analysis, and the tracing that ordinarily records a sharp increase if blood platelet function is normal lay flat and lifeless.

The platelets were in little condition to aggregate; they released no measurable serotonin, the stuff that signals the urge to stickiness. The black fungus used in many Szechuan and Mandarin dishes and called mok yhee in Cantonese had asserted its godgiven powers and been found out. Good heavens, these platelets behaved a lot like those exposed to aspirin, a well-known blood-thinning drug. *The black mushroom was an anticoagulant!*

To be sure, Dr. Hammerschmidt tested seven other samples of the tree ears bought at different Chinese food markets; all suppressed, to varying degrees, the platelets' desires to aggregate in a test tube. When an ordinary American button mushroom, the type you commonly pick up in the supermarket, was tested, it had zero effect on platelet clumping. Only the exotic Chinese mushroom worked.

Intrigued, Dr. Hammerschmidt discovered that the big black mushroom has a formidable reputation and long history in traditional Chinese folk medicine, and, lo and behold, its therapeutic uses correspond with the laboratory effects he had observed. Some Chinese from Taiwan and Hong Kong living in Minneapolis said simply that mo-er was "good for you," or "makes you live longer." Others reported specific uses, namely to cure headaches or to prevent postpartum thrombophlebitis. Said one woman, "It thins the blood."

Inquiring further, Dr. Hammerschmidt found that mo-er is reputed to be a longevity tonic, according to Florence Lin's *Chinese Vegetarian Cookbook*. In Minneapolis the white tree fungus, pei-mo-er, is promoted by some Chinese herbalists as a prophylactic after a heart attack. And *A Barefoot Doctor's Manual* recommends mo-er for dysmenorrhea, difficulties menstruating.

Dr. Hammerschmidt had a good time writing up his case for the *New England Journal of Medicine*. He raised the tantalizing possibility that low rates of coronary artery disease in parts of China might be tied to the habitual consumption of foods that interfere with platelet stickiness, not only the black fungus but also scallions and garlic (other known anticoagulants)—all conspiring to help keep the blood flowing and free of dangerous clots. Its blood-thinning capability probably also explains, he says, why the fungus is revered as a longevity tonic. But he did not even guess what the potent chemical in the Oriental "tree ears" was.

When you publish in the *New England Journal of Medicine*, a journal of worldwide repute, you can count on lots of other top researchers seeing your work. The Hammerschmidt adventure was of particular interest to a couple of prominent investigators at George Washington University who had isolated active anti-platelet clumping substances in garlic and onions. They jumped on the black mushroom case. They soon isolated an active anticoagulant chemical in the black mo-er called adenosine—the same blood-thinning compound they had found in onions and garlic. "No question," says Dr. John Martyn Bailey, professor of biochemistry at GWU, "we find that adenosine in these foods acts just like an anticoagulant; it's very similar to aspirin."

No question either that the black tree ear very subtly affects the blood of those who eat it in small amounts; it changes the character of cellular reactions that can have a *profound effect on the disease process over a lifetime.* Increasing evidence finds that hyperactive platelets can clump together too readily and create thick, sluggish blood, clots, and, along with cholesterol, layers of cardiovascular garbage known as plaque on the walls of arteries and cerebral vessels. Such food-borne anticoagulants thus may help *prevent* narrowed arteries, thick, sluggish blood, and obstructive clots—the stuff that strokes and heart attacks are made of. Yet, the effect of the mo-er is so secretive and benign that its powers would not have been discovered had it not messed with the blood of someone smart enough to notice.

Although such a discovery is a fluke, the presence of anticoagulants such as adenosine in food is not. Tests show that even the adenosine in the mo-er accounts for only sixty percent of its anticoagulant activity, says Dr. Hammerschmidt, meaning that the fungus contains other unidentified blood-thinning drugs. Thus, if we started actively looking, we unquestionably would find countless other foods that dispense unseen and undetected anticoagulants into our circulatory systems, commanding platelets to refrain from obscene accumulations that hasten our deterioration and demise. Such foods could help save us from heart attacks and strokes just as effectively as aspirin or anticoagulant prescription drugs—and with many fewer side effects.

Dr. Hammerschmidt still makes his mapo doufu, and it thins his blood just as centuries of Oriental physicians said it would—long before anyone ever heard of a chemical called adenosine or blood fragments called platelets.

DR. HAMMERSCHMIDT'S BLOOD-THINNING MAPO DOUFU*

¼ cup dried tree ears (mo-er or black tree fungus)
1 cup boiling water
3-inch piece fresh ginger
5 scallions, chopped (Set aside one chopped scallion, to be used separately.)
½ pound ground pork or beef
2 tablespoons soy sauce
1 teaspoon sesame oil
1 tablespoon Chinese rice wine or cooking sherry
8 or more cloves of garlic
6 fresh water chestnuts (optional)
2 teaspoons cornstarch
¼ cup cold water
6 squares fresh bean curd
1 tablespoon cornstarch
6 tablespoons peanut oil
1½ teaspoons hot pepper flakes
1 tablespoon hot pepper paste
1 teaspoon granulated sugar
3 tablespoons soy sauce
½ cup water
1½ teaspoons ground, roasted Szechuan peppercorns
1 teaspoon sesame oil
1 teaspoon salt, or to taste

Put the tree ears in a small bowl and pour the boiling water over them. Let them soak for about 15 minutes, until they become soft and gelatinous.

Peel the ginger, then chop it into tiny pieces, about the size of a match head.

Add one tablespoon of the chopped ginger and one chopped scallion to the ground pork along with the soy sauce, sesame oil, and wine. Mix thoroughly, then set aside for about 30 minutes.

Peel the garlic, then chop coarsely. Combine it with the rest of the chopped ginger and mince them both together until they reach the consistency of a thick paste. (This may take several minutes, but Mrs.

*From: E. Schrecker, J. Schrecker, and J-F. Chiang, *Mrs. Chiang's Szechwan Cookbook* (New York: Harper & Row, 1976 revised 1987), pp. 220-224.

Chiang insists that the finer you chop the garlic and ginger, the more interesting the finished dish will be.)

Cut the dark skin off the outside of the water chestnuts, then chop them into pieces about the size of a match head.

Combine the cornstarch and water in a small bowl and set aside.

Cut the bean curd into ½-inch cubes.

Drain the tree ears, then rinse them and pick them over carefully to remove the tiny impurities, like little pieces of wood, that might still be imbedded in them. Then mince into little pieces the size of a match head.

Just before you are ready to begin cooking, add the cornstarch mixture to the meat mixture and blend thoroughly.

Heat your wok or pan over a moderately high flame for about 15 seconds, then add the peanut oil. It should be hot enough to cook with when the first small bubbles begin to form and a few small wisps of smoke appear.

When the oil is ready, quickly throw in the garlic and ginger and vigorously stir-fry them over a medium flame for about 30 seconds, using your cooking shovel or spoon to scoop the ingredients from the sides of the pan and then stir them around in the middle, so they won't burn or stick.

Continue to stir-fry while you add the hot pepper flakes, the hot pepper paste, the water chestnuts, and the tree ears. Then stir-fry for another 30 seconds.

Add the meat mixture and keep stirring it as it cooks, taking special care to break up any large chunks of meat that may stick together.

After the meat has cooked for about one minute and has lost its pinkish color, throw in the bean curd and the chopped scallions and stir-fry everything together for about 45 seconds. Then add the sugar and stir-fry for another 30 seconds.

Pour in the soy sauce and the water and wait for the liquid to boil, then let the contents of the pan cook over a moderate flame for two more minutes.

Add the Szechuan peppercorns and stir thoroughly.

At this point, determine how much sauce is in the pan. If the dish seems watery, you should get ready to add the cornstarch and water mixture you have already prepared. But if there does not seem to be much liquid, you won't need the cornstarch.

Make sure that you stir up the cornstarch mixture before you pour it into the pan, then stir-fry everything over a medium flame until the sauce becomes clear and slightly thickened.

Add the sesame oil and stir it in thoroughly; then, just before serving, taste the dish for salt. It should taste sharp and clear, with just a hint of sweetness. Stir the salt in and serve.

2.

ONIONS FOR THE HEART

Never mind that onions have been used for 5000 years to cure virtually everything under the sun. Never mind that neither the Food and Drug Administration nor the American Medical Association lists onions as cardiovascular drugs. Never mind that the subject is not a hot topic at heart meetings. If you had been cardiologist Victor Gurewich, you, too, might have accepted inspiration from an Egyptian papyrus.

Dr. Gurewich, a professor of medicine at Tufts University, was discouraged over the blood profiles of his patients who had suffered heart attacks. Most came in with extremely low levels of HDL (high-density lipoprotein) blood cholesterol; that's the good type that acts as a scavenger in the blood, scarfing up and carrying cholesterol to the liver, where it is destroyed. People with high HDL cholesterol levels enjoy a protection from the ordinary ravages of blood cholesterol and heart attack. Some experts call HDLs the most critical indicator of heart disease risk. Low levels of HDLs promote coronaries.

But raising HDLs in heart-disease patients is tough. Dr. Gurewich and his staff were not having much luck. "That's when a fellow in my lab, from Poland, where natural remedies have more of a heritage, said, 'Let's try onions,' " says Dr. Gurewich. "He had run across material in the folklore literature saying it might work. Specifically, it was recommended in an ancient Egyptian papyrus, and it seemed to me if it had survived for two thousand years, it might have some validity. So we said to our patients, 'We are going to feed you onions.' "

Prescribing onions for heart patients is hardly routine among the nation's leading cardiologists. But Dr. Gurewich has impeccable medical credentials. He is also director of the vascular laboratory at St. Elizabeth's Hospital in Boston, and he knew that onions had other beneficial effects on the blood. Moreover, onions lack the risk of serious side effects common in therapeutic drugs. If they worked, it would be better than anything they had tried; if not, nothing lost.

So the patients started out eating a medium-size raw onion every day. Later, some preferred to take onion juice in capsules.

Usually blood cholesterol responds rapidly to drugs and changes in diet. But a month dragged on, and another month. Some of the patients were losing heart, so to speak. But then, whammo, the first results came in from the lab showing a perceptible rise in HDLs. Then more. "We got striking results," says Dr. Gurewich. In the original group of twenty onion-therapy patients, all of them had sagging HDLs of less than twenty percent; normal is at least twenty-five percent. With the onion therapy, their HDL levels went up an average of thirty percent, sending most of them into the normal range. Onions did not always lower the *total* blood cholesterol, but they triggered shifts in the ratio of good-to-bad cholesterol, replacing a substantial amount of the destructive LDL (bad-type cholesterol) with heart-protective HDL cholesterol. In other words, something in onions flicked a biological switch that said produce more HDL.

It was clear from the start that the HDL boost in some—about one in four—was dramatic, but in others it was virtually nonexistent, for unknown reasons. One fellow in the group whose HDLs did not go up suffered a heart attack. But in others onions produced remarkable improvements in their blood profiles, doubling, even tripling their HDL levels. One man then in his thirties with a history of heart disease in his family had extremely low HDL levels of fifteen percent. When he took the onions, his HDL cholesterol level shot up to thirty percent, where it stayed for a year. Then he went off to Mexico on a business trip for three months and gave up eating onions. When he returned to the lab for his blood test, his HDLs had skidded again to sublevels of fifteen percent, the same as in pre-onion days. Naturally, when he resumed the onion therapy, the HDLs soared again and remained there as long as his blood was regularly supplied with onion chemicals.

To Dr. Gurewich, his onion experiment is an enormous success. Onions have become routine therapy for his heart patients; seventy to seventy-five percent of them, he says, see a rise in their HDLs. And he now finds that only half a medium raw onion a day (fifty grams, or a couple of ounces) is fully as potent as a whole onion.

How this wonder bulb triggers the body to make more HDL cholesterol, thus accomplishing what the best brains in the pharmaceutical labs
have generally failed to do, is still a total mystery. "We simply don't
know enough about the synthesis of HDL and what regulates it even to
guess what the mechanism of action in the body might be," says Dr.
Gurewich. As to the identity of the natural chemical producing this blood
miracle, Dr. Gurewich has attacked that problem in his vascular laboratory.
He and his lab technicians have identified about 150 compounds in onions,
but says Dr. Gurewich: "We still don't know which one raises the HDLs."

They do know a few of its characteristics, though. Heat can kill the
chemical's activity. The HDL boost is greatest from raw onions, and
lessens with cooking. Onions cooked to limp and tasteless have virtually
no effect on HDL cholesterol. Also, the active agent is one that gives
onion its strong taste. The major effect comes from the hotter white and
yellow onions; mild red onions don't work nearly as well. The stronger
the onion taste, the sharper the elevation of HDLs.

But that is not the end of the onion tale. Dr. Gurewich says the
onion possesses a lively concoction of chemicals that perform complex
chemotherapy on the cardiovascular system. Onions, he says, contain a
compound known to lower blood pressure. The onion, like the black
Chinese mo-er mushroom, also contains adenosine and maybe other
chemicals that keep platelets from sticking together. Equally important,
the onion works on another function of the blood; it revs up the body's
fibrinolytic, or blood-clot-dissolving, system. Just as some onion
chemicals keep platelets from getting together, others actively work to
dissolve clots as they form. This clot-dissolving chemical in onions, says
Dr. Gurewich, is not destroyed by heat; thus, onions—both cooked and
raw—contain chemicals that promote clot breakup.

Such anticlotting activity is more critical than previously recognized. New evidence from the famous Framingham Heart Study in
Massachusetts shows that men with high blood levels of fibrinogen—
the basic substance from which clots form—are more likely to suffer
strokes and coronary artery disease. Thus, researchers say, too much
fibrinogen in your blood may be as hazardous as high blood pressure.
Onions combat fibrinogen.

More exciting, foods that activate the fibrinolytic system—helping
destroy the dangerous fibrinogen—can offset some of the ill effects of
artery-damaging fatty foods.

It may come as a surprise to learn that eating a high fat meal makes
your blood measurably more sluggish; the amount of clot-promoting
fibrinogen increases, the fibrinolytic activity slows, blood takes less

time to clot, and cholesterol levels go up. In 1966, Indian investigator Dr. N. N. Gupta at K. G. Medical College in Lucknow first drew scientific attention to the fact that onion could *counteract* some of the expected detrimental changes in blood brought on by high fat meals. He took blood samples from a group of men before and several hours after they ate a meal with ninety percent fat—butter, cream, and eggs. Then he added about two ounces of fried onions to the same high fat meal, again drawing blood samples before and after. The onion proved a powerful antidote. Not only did blood cholesterol levels sink when onion was added, but the onions also prevented the high fat from promoting the detrimental steps leading to blood clots: platelet clumping and formation of fibrinogen, the clotting substance. Onions were particularly potent at revving up the body's fibrinolytic (clot-destroying) mechanism.

A string of subsequent studies showed that boiled, raw, and dried as well as fried onions also partially cleared blood of the ill effects of dietary fat. That's why it makes good sense to top your hamburger with a slab of raw onion or stir up a few onions with your steak.

Naturally, scientists have been searching for the active ingredients in the onion (and its close cousin, garlic) that cause these profound alterations in the blood. Several have been identified. In 1975 a British team of heart specialists and biochemists at the University of Newcastle upon Tyne isolated several onion chemicals that promoted clot dissolution. They fed low doses of one, an odorless cycloalliin, to humans and found it did stimulate the fibrinolytic activity.

At the same time, scientists have been tracking the fascinating route by which the onion—mainly its blood-thinning chemical agents— accomplishes its pharmaceutical activity. That brings us back to the research team at George Washington University who tagged adenosine as the blood-thinning agent in Dr. Hammerschmidt's black fungus, tree ears.

First, you have to know that George Washington University's School of Medicine is a major center for the study of the most exciting class of biological agents to come along in years. Prostaglandins, as they are called, defined only in 1964, now dominate the medical bio-chemical scene. They are hormones with diverse powers, so named because they were first found in the prostate gland in 1930. Because they are present in tissue in such minute quantities, nearly thirty years passed before chemical techniques became advanced and sensitive enough to separate out and measure them.

These multifaceted chemicals have a dazzling array of effects on a number of bodily functions. If you were opening boxes within boxes in search of the ultimate precipitating cause of biochemical reactions in the body, one of the smaller boxes would be labeled "prostaglandins." These chemicals direct complex interactions that control the lives of cells. The prostaglandins are inter- and intracell messengers, always whispering instructions, commanding the release or shutoff of one or another arcane chemical substance. Shutting off these chemical messengers can have monumental effects on the body. For example, after centuries of ignorance, scientists, with the advent of prostaglandin research, discovered how aspirin works. It suppresses the secretion from the cells of certain prostaglandins that turn on processes causing inflammation, pain, and platelet aggregation. In fact, aspirin blocks cells' production of a prostaglandin A called thromboxane that orders cells to start sticking together. That is the rationale for suggestions that aspirin, by thinning the blood, may help prevent strokes and heart attacks. Compounds in onions do precisely the same thing.

That's what GWU's crack team of prostaglandin experts and biochemists, Drs. Jack Y. Vanderhoek, Amar N. Makheja, and John Martyn Bailey discovered. Dr. Bailey explains how they happened to be looking: "We had come across reports that onion and garlic prevented blood clotting. Since we were primarily interested in the effect of prostaglandins on platelet aggregation, we said, 'We wonder if extracts of onion and garlic will block both the platelet aggregation and the synthesis of a particular prostaglandin in the platelets called thromboxane.' Indeed both onion and garlic did block both." That was pretty good proof that the platelets failed to stick together because they did not produce the thromboxane that would order them to.

The investigators, boring deeper into the chemical process, uncovered what the onion-garlic oils did to block the critical prostaglandin from being made; they suppressed the activity of enzymes needed to initiate production of the prostaglandin. And that, they say, explains one way onions can behave as an anticoagulant to protect the heart.

Small wonder that in France it was once common to feed horses onions and garlic to dissolve blood clots in their legs. It is a large wonder the practice is not more common among humans who die in unprecedented numbers from cardiovascular disease. Dr. Gurewich's unorthodox experiment—and the extensive research in other countries on onions and garlic—show that a food can succeed where standard pharmaceuticals fail. Only one anticholesterol drug (gemfibrozil) substantially boosts HDLs—and then by an average ten percent. As Dr. Gurewich asserts, onions are a potent multipurpose heart medicine, confirming ancient folklore that there is more to eating onions than culinary wisdom.

3.

BARLEY, OATS, AND THE VEGETARIAN SECRET

If there were vampires among the food pharmacy scientists, they would surely fly every night to the beds of vegetarians, drawing their blood to discover why they enjoy such a special place in the health universe. Undeniably, vegetarians have it all over meat eaters when it comes to escaping chronic diseases such as heart attacks, strokes, diabetes, high blood pressure, and certain cancers. In a heart study, for example, reported in the July 6, 1985, *British Medical Journal*, scientists tracked 11,000 vegetarians and carnivores for seven years; death rates were much lower among the vegetarians. If you take the experts' word for it that the major reason is diet and not laid-back lifestyle, you can chalk up credit to two possibilities: the omission of harmful meat and/or the addition of plants.

Do specific factors in vegetables build a body less vulnerable to disease? One way to find out is to look for physiological signs that distinguish vegetarians from others. To this aim, avowed vegetarians have had their arms bound and stuck, shedding their blood into countless vials for laboratory probes. Such tests show unquestionably one distinctive difference: vegetarians have markedly lower blood cholesterol, especially the detrimental LDL type; lower cholesterol cuts the risk of heart attacks. And dramatic new evidence confirms that reducing destructive LDL type and raising HDL good-type cholesterol can even help unclog damaged coronary arteries.

For years scientists have been searching for a unifying theory to

35

explain how vegetables help control blood cholesterol. They have come up with two compelling theories—one that grew out of investigations of barley, the other of oats.

Dr. Asaf Qureshi and a small enclave of scientists at the United States Department of Agriculture's Cereal Crops Research Unit in Madison, Wisconsin, are convinced they have found the answer to the vegetarian riddle in barley. Dr. Qureshi, formerly a senior researcher at the USDA lab and now a private consultant, says that's no surprise. Barley, after all, has a long history in Pakistan, his native country, as a heart protector. "My father was a physician, and he always insisted that his patients from the villages of Punjab who ate so much barley rarely had heart disease," says Dr. Qureshi, "and I now know why." Dr. Qureshi maintains that certain compounds widely dispersed in vegetables, including barley, act as powerful drugs to suppress the liver's internal production of cholesterol. "This is a major reason vegetarians have much less heart disease, we think: they are on a constant regimen of cholesterol-lowering compounds."

The theory is based on the rarely professed belief that if you can save people from the excesses of their own livers, you help save them from heart disease. It's largely unappreciated that *liver synthesis and not the consumption of high fat, high cholesterol foods* is the main source of cholesterol in the body. If you dampen the liver's manufacture of cholesterol, blood levels of the bad fatty stuff usually drop, along with your risk of heart disease. As the liver pours less cholesterol into the bloodstream, cells needing LDL cholesterol are fooled into behaving as if there is a shortage. Consequently, they suck more LDL cholesterol out of the bloodstream.

That's the way one of the hottest new heart-disease drugs on the market works—Merck's Mevacor (lovastatin); it blocks an enzyme in the liver that stimulates LDL cholesterol output. Wouldn't it be great if nature were thoughtful enough to provide chemical regulators in the diet also—like the drug—to stifle the liver's ability to churn out destructive cholesterol? That's what the scientists in Wisconsin thought too.

The exciting quest began in 1977, when Dr. Qureshi decided to test the cholesterol of chickens being fed oats, corn, wheat, rye, and barley to see how fast they grew. It was not part of the experiment, but he blesses the day that he demanded that memorable blood sacrifice. As Dr. Qureshi scanned the cholesterol counts of corn-fed chickens, he found nothing unusual. Wheat and rye depressed cholesterol slightly. Oats even more so, but wow! Barley pushed cholesterol way down to 76 milligrams per 100 milliliters—nearly half that of corn-fed chickens. The barley-fed birds could be poster starlets for an aviary heart association. Something in barley packed a cholesterol-lowering wallop.

At first the scientists thought the magic ingredient was fiber. Numerous studies show that food fiber, namely of the soluble gummy type, depresses blood cholesterol. But when they took all the fiber out of the barley kernel and fed it to the chickens, their cholesterol still fell dramatically. Fiber, heck. The scientists knew they were onto something brand new in the food pharmacy, a potent new cholesterol-fighting compound.

The secret, they were sure, lay in the liver's failure to synthesize more cholesterol, which could be traced to lazy enzymes. It was as if the factory had shut down because the workers went on strike. The enzymes failed to assemble the molecular chains forming a substance called mevalonic acid that turns into cholesterol. It takes sequential reactions of about twenty chemicals to ultimately produce cholesterol in the liver. A key compound in the early stages of the metabolism of cholesterol is mevalonic acid. As Dr. Warren C. Burger, once a core member of the research team, notes: "If you knock out or partially impair the HMG-CoA reductase enzyme, it doesn't produce the mevalonic acid that in turn produces cholesterol."

The synthesis of cholesterol in the liver decreases?

"That's right."

The scientists did a slew of studies to make sure their results were no fluke. They fed more chickens the corn, wheat, rye, oats, and barley and got the same results. They stretched their budget to test a couple of dozen pigs (that have a cardiovascular system quite like humans) and found that barley sent their blood cholesterol into an eighteen percent dive.

The inescapable conclusion: something, God knew what at that point, in these foods (and it was not fiber, they contend) was deactivating the enzyme needed to turn the liver into an energetic cholesterol factory. And most important, it turned down the urge to make the LDL type that destroys artery walls. HDL levels that help wash away dangerous cholesterol remained intact.

But what was causing it?

After many frustrating attempts to extract barley's pharmaceutical essence, in 1983—breakthrough. Dr. Qureshi isolated an active compound in barley (and wheat, oats, and rye) that indeed suppressed the liver's ability to synthesize cholesterol. It is called tocotrienol, or, in the Wisconsin team's lingo, "inhibitor 1." The Wisconsin Alumni Research Foundation (WARF) licensed the rights to the patent, hoping the chemical might evolve into a profitable anticholesterol drug. The Wisconsin researchers went on to discover "inhibitor 2," a triglyceride, and "inhibitor 3"—in the grains. All are present throughout the kernels of barley, rye, and oats. But by far the greatest amounts are found in the oils of the coarse outer layers of the grains—what we call fiber. A coincidence? Is fiber simply an inert carrier of compounds with formidable anticholesterol action? Is that why so-called high fiber grains and vegetables lower blood cholesterol? Not because fiber has great physiological activity of its own, but because it wraps itself around cholesterol-reducing chemicals? Dr. Qureshi thinks so. But others maintain that certain types of fiber also perform as potent cholesterol-lowering drugs helping explain the vegetarian secret.

Meet James Anderson, M.D., a famous name at the University of Kentucky College of Medicine. "Dr. Fiber" himself has spent a decade trying to penetrate the pharmacological essence of high fiber foods. He heartily recommends them to diabetics to lower blood sugar and to everybody else to combat the cardiovascular disease epidemic. Dr. Anderson contends that food fiber has plenty of pharmacological power on its own—independent of its chemical co-travelers—and that certain types of fiber, too, can turn down the liver's synthesis of cholesterol. To him, it is mainly fiber, which is found exclusively in plants, that gives vegetarians the health edge.

Actually, Dr. Anderson's is a moderate American franchise of an idea that has been percolating in England since the early 1970s among a group of physicians, including Denis Burkitt. The hypothesis is that fiber deficiency is a prime cause of modern ills and that fiber can cure or prevent almost anything that ails you, including diabetes, coronary artery disease, high blood pressure, obesity, hemorrhoids, varicose veins, diverticular disease, hiatus hernia, gallstones, constipation, irritable bowel syndrome, appendicitis, and cancer, especially of the colon.

It's not the first time humankind has heard this.

Vegetarianism—encompassing fiber, although it was not called that then—dates back to the classical Greeks. In nineteenth-century America, a vegetarian preacher, Sylvester Graham, whose legacy is the graham cracker, praised fiber as the primary reason vegetables, fruits, legumes, and grains are healthful. He drew on scientific investigations into fiber by the respected physiologist William Beaumont, who in 1833 praised "bulk as perhaps, nearly as necessary to the articles of diet as the nutrient principle." At the time the charismatic Graham's bread recipes were the fiber talk of the day.

The fiber talk of today is Jim Anderson's oat bran muffins.

Dr. Anderson stumbled onto oats because he noticed a funny thing when diabetics ate high fiber foods; not only did their blood sugar and insulin improve, their blood cholesterol and blood pressure fell. But their triglycerides—another type of fat—went up, which was worrisome. Around the same time, something remarkable dawned on him. He had assumed that the precipitous drops in blood cholesterol and pressure happened because eating more carbohydrates by necessity squeezed fat out of diets; a person can eat only so many calories, so if more go into carbohydrates, fewer go into fat. Since cutting down on fat, notably saturated animal fat, is known to depress blood cholesterol, Anderson had not thought much about it, even though the blood cholesterol counts were dropping far more than expected from fat deprivation. Then it struck him—of course! Maybe the added fiber was the main factor pushing down blood cholesterol—not the omission of fat. Maybe the fiber, therefore, could be manipulated to better achieve the reductions, and even wash away triglycerides and artery-destroying LDL cholesterol while boosting the good HDL type.

It was a hunch that led him to the Quaker Oats Company and a product they were putting into pet food. Dr. Anderson had tried wheat bran without luck. (As it turns out, wheat bran does not lower blood cholesterol.) Then he remembered the Dutch oat millers. Reports were coming out of Holland that they often eat prodigious amounts of oatmeal—six or seven bowls a day. And they are blessed with exceptionally low blood cholesterol. Dr. Anderson knew that oats have a gelatinous fiber quite different from that of wheat. "You know when you cook oatmeal, the stuff that sticks to the pan is gummy fiber," explains Dr. Anderson. (Oats are extra high in soluble fiber, wheat in insoluble fiber.) But that was a heap of oatmeal to eat. Dr. Anderson suspected he could get a greater effect from oat bran, the concentrated fiber left after the oat flour is shaved off. He contacted Quaker Oats and asked for bran. After a little searching they located some in their pet food processing plant. They shipped a one-hundred-pound drum of oat bran to the University of Kentucky's Medical College in 1976.

After Dr. Anderson figured out what to do with it, it was precisely enough for 533 servings. In a few weeks he ate thirty-five of them himself. Like many scientists, his professional interest was also a personal one. His blood cholesterol had stretched as high as 300 and at the time was about 285. He began watching his diet a little more closely and eating a morning porridge made from three dry ounces of oat bran. (Later, he learned to make oat-bran muffins.)

His eyes sparkle when he tells it: "My blood cholesterol plummeted 110 points in five weeks, from 285 to 175. I was the first human as far as I know to eat oat bran to lower cholesterol. The fellow who did my blood chemistry at the university lab brought the analysis over personally—he was so stunned by the results. He wanted to know what the devil I was doing."

The type of cholesterol attacked by the oat bran was on target, as further tests showed. "With oat bran, in our first four people, we saw a fifty-eight percent reduction in the bad guys, the LDLs, and really, this is one of our true surprises, the HDLs almost doubled—went up by eighty-two percent. That's right, we saw a selective reduction in LDL and a rise in HDL. We said this is really exciting. This is what we need to fight heart disease."

In the next few years the doctor fed oat bran to hundreds, sometimes made into muffins; their cholesterol dropped an average twenty percent. Even when people did not cut back on eating fat, the oats still pushed their blood cholesterol down. Dr. Anderson also tried legumes, high in soluble fiber; they were spectacular too. Fiber was a cholesterol-lowering drug—or, more precisely, says Dr. Anderson, a very large class of drugs.

Scientists could spend their careers—and many, like Dr. Anderson, are—trying to figure out the machinations of that stuff we call fiber, or roughage.

Fiber seems unspeakably dull. But the physiological consequences of eating it are enormous. After escaping disintegration by stomach acids, particles of fiber arrive in the colon, where things get pretty exciting. Fiber's fate there determines your fate—from such immediate matters as bowel movements to long-term prospects of colon cancer. For one thing, the fiber along with other undigested compounds ends up strewn throughout the lower intestine, where it is bare to attack from multitudes of bacteria. These microbes literally devour the material, breaking it down into simpler chemical substances, a process called fermentation. From this microbial feast emanate all kinds of metabolic by-products with physiological properties, including gases and a slew of metabolically active volatile short-chain fatty acids.

Scientists are intensely curious about these short-chain fatty acids, which can be absorbed from the colon into the rest of the body. Some shoot directly to the liver. It is believed they have awesome potential in regulating functions related to blood cholesterol and cancer. One such, called propionate, has been tested by Dr. Anderson in rats. The rodents that drank water with added propionate had less cholesterol in their blood and liver. Dr. Anderson theorizes that the fiber, after some chemical shenanigans, metabolizes into the propionate, turning down the liver's production of cholesterol (just as Dr. Qureshi's barley chemicals do). Dr. Anderson believes this is the way beans reduce cholesterol. But oats, containing similar amounts of soluble fiber, do not work that way at all. Oats evidently lower cholesterol by washing away bile acids in the intestinal tract that otherwise would be converted to cholesterol, much the same way the drug cholestyramine does.

Fiber, of course, also produces bulkier stools and speeds their passage through the intestinal tract. That is a primary reason fiber is believed to prevent colon cancer. Carcinogens in the larger stool are more diffuse and have less exposure to the colon wall. Some scientists also theorize that plant fiber per se or its metabolites act as anticancer drugs, for example, by helping regulate estrogen levels, which are related to breast cancer.

Even the type of fiber that produces a bulkier, moister stool is debatable. Fiber in the colon absorbs water. For years doctors assumed the bulkiest stools came from plant fibers that held the most water. Commercial bulk laxatives were tested for effectiveness by their ability to mop up water. But extensive work by Dr. John H. Cummings of the Dunn Clinical Nutrition Centre, Cambridge, England, one of the world's leading fiber authorities, finds otherwise. He demonstrated that if you smash up foods, extract their cell walls, and expose those to water, their ability to soak up water varies about tenfold. For example, a gram of cell-wall substance from potato, banana, or bran holds only three grams of water. One gram of cucumber, carrot, and lettuce fiber soaks up twenty to twenty-four grams of water. That should make lettuce a terrific laxative and bran not much good at all. But bran, although unable to absorb much water in a test tube, by far produces the greatest increase in stool bulk, and is the best stool-bulking dietary preventive of constipation, and accompanying ills, known.

Dr. Cummings discovered fiber's activity may also hinge on an inexplicable drug effect from a chemical called pentose. He found that people who ate fibers with the most pentose, a sugar in cell walls, had bulkier stools. No surprise: wheat bran, nature's best laxative, is rich in pentose.

Thus, many roads lead to the reasons that vegetarians are freer of all kinds of chronic diseases. It seems sure that complex compounds in plants as well as fiber function like the latest sophisticated drugs to turn down the liver's production of cholesterol, leaving the blood less cholesterol polluted. Dr. Qureshi thinks his barley discoveries are not the end, merely the beginning. He says nature spread her favors widely, creating a plant kingdom, and thus a food supply full of cholesterol dampeners that exert a tremendous cumulative benefit on the cardiovascular system. Chemicals that clamp down on the liver's manufacture of cholesterol have been reported in garlic, orange peel, ginseng, anise, lemon grass oil, alfalfa, olive oil, beer (from the hops), grapes, wine, milk, and yogurt—as well as, of course, barley, rye, oats, and beans. And science has only begun to look.

The moral is not only that vegetarians enjoy good health, but that by eating plants, including grains, you infuse your body with a perpetual dose of pharmacologically active compounds that act as natural drugs to keep your heart and vascular system functioning better, your blood freer of dangerous cholesterol, your digestive processes working better, and your system less prey to certain cancers.

DR. ANDERSON'S CHOLESTEROL-LOWERING OAT-BRAN RAISIN MUFFINS

2½ cups oat-bran cereal
2 teaspoons brown sugar substitute
½ cup raisins
1 tablespoon baking powder
½ teaspoon salt
1 cup skim milk
4 ounces egg substitute
1 tablespoon vegetable oil

Preheat oven to 425 degrees F. Grease bottoms only of 10 medium-size muffin cups or line with paper baking cups. Combine dry ingredients and raisins. Add skim milk, egg substitute, and oil and mix just until dry ingredients are moistened. Fill prepared muffin cups ¾ full. Bake at 425 degrees for 17 minutes or until golden brown. Makes 10 muffins.

4.

CHILI PEPPERS' YIN-YANG THERAPY

If you have a cold, build a fire in your stomach. The crazy notion that this will work stems from an ancient medical concept of balancing opposites. In ancient Greco-Roman medicine, every physician worth his salt knew that if you had phlegm characterizing a "cold disorder," the treatment of choice was something "hot." The traditional Oriental yin-yang theory of therapeutics calls for hot pungent "yang" spices to treat "cold yin" respiratory diseases. That there could be validity to such a seemingly unscientific idea intrigued one modern medical theorist and pharmaceutical expert, leading him to some fascinating investigations of chili peppers.

Irwin Ziment, M.D., comes from Great Britain where the diet is usually bland, just the kind of thing the English don't need, he says, because they also have a damp climate—two factors he thinks conspire with others, such as smoking, to make chronic bronchitis among the Brits rampant. Bronchitis, he says, for many years was so common in Britain, it was called "the English disease."

But Dr. Ziment now lives in California where the diet is far from bland—punctuated with lots of hot Mexican sauces, Japanese wasabi (that pungent, green horseradish-mustard served with sushi and sashimi), Szechuan chili peppers, spicy Indian curries, and Thai foods that make your eyes water. He approves. It's all good for your lungs, he says. In parts of the world where the cuisine is hot, pulmonary disease rates are low, he adds. According to his surveys, Mexican populations

43

around Los Angeles have less respiratory trouble, despite their smoking, and when they do develop chronic bronchitis, they require less
therapy. Why? Because they eat hot foods. In fact, if they don't
already, Dr. Ziment advises his patients with pulmonary problems such
as emphysema and chronic bronchitis to eat a hot spicy meal at least
once a day, or down a glass of water sprinkled with ten or twenty
drops of Tabasco sauce, or chew on chili peppers. And if you have a
cold or sore throat, Dr. Ziment tells you to grind up a teaspoon of
horseradish, add a glass of warm water and a little honey, and drink it.
Or mix up some garlicky-rich chicken soup with a hefty dash of red or
black pepper. It's the standard, he avows, against which all other
therapeutic cold remedies should be judged. "It's probably the best
there is."

Take note that Dr. Ziment is professor of medicine at the University of California School of Medicine at Los Angeles—one of the
nation's most prestigious training grounds for physicians—and chief of
medicine and director of respiratory therapy at Olive View Medical
Center in L.A. He is also an authority on pulmonary drugs, and is the
author of several textbooks on the subject, including *Respiratory Pharmacology and Therapeutics*. If you ask such a noted authority if he
sees anything strange about recommending chili peppers, he points
out that their ancient use makes them a more credible drug than many
current drugstore remedies that have not a whit of proven therapeutic
benefit and may have side effects.

Indeed, much of his interest in chili pepper therapy grew out of an
intellectual odyssey resulting from the research for the textbooks. He
began tracing the medical history of the use of expectorants, a special
interest of his. Expectorants are those agents like Robitussin that help
you cough up phlegm or mucus out of your lungs. Stronger prescription
expectorants are critical therapeutic agents in chronic obstructive pulmonary disease.

When Dr. Ziment looked into it, he found "an international concur-
rence of thought on the way drugs are utilized as expectorants." And
to his surprise, the agreement stretches back in history. "What impressed me," he says, "was that most standard pharmacopoeias from
Europe and the Orient mention spices and garlic as expectorants.
These comments are so frequent that one has to consider their validity. And the second thing that became very obvious is that many of the
chemicals in these spices have a remarkable similarity to chemicals we
use today as orthodox expectorant drugs."

No question, says Dr. Ziment, hot foods have been used to treat pulmonary diseases since antiquity. He found that ancient Egyptian medical writings recommended mustard in respiratory therapy. Hippocrates prescribed vinegar and pepper as respiratory drugs. The great Roman physician, Galen, favored the use of garlic for chest pain. In the Middle Ages mustard was a potion used against asthma, coughs, and chest congestion. The well-known twelfth-century Jewish physician Maimonides, an expert on asthma, recommended spicy chicken soup for that condition and "the stirring up and ejection of pulmonary phlegm." In 1802 the distinguished English physician Herberden recommended garlic and mustard seed, among other agents, to treat asthma. Oriental medicine uses capsicum peppers, black pepper, mustard, garlic, turmeric, and other spices to treat colds, sinusitis, bronchitis, and asthma. Russians use horseradish to cure colds.

Dr. Ziment discovered that such folk remedies, just like modern drugs, have a common action: they invariably affect the viscosity and consequent movement of mucus in the lungs—not something most people dwell on unless they have problems. Normally, the journey of mucus in the lungs is so subtle and unobtrusive, you are not conscious of the routine clearance that pushes mucus up out of the lungs and to the back of the throat, where you swallow it. Rhythmically propelling the mucus along through breathing passages are cilia, tiny hairlike projections on cells. Like the synchronous oars from millions of tiny rowers, the cilia stiffen and rapidly sweep upward, then flex back, hoisting the mucus up and out of the bronchial tree. All goes well if the mucus is thin enough for the cilia to move.

In chronic bronchitis—often due to smoking—the mucus becomes thick, sticky, and profuse, clogging breathing tubes. The cilia, also impaired by the disease, lose the power to waft the secretions against gravity. Mucus accumulates and stagnates in the small airways, irritating the lungs, producing coughing, and after a while, infection. Air passages become inflamed; breathing is difficult; unless the mucus is somehow coughed up or expectorated, the lungs, overwhelmed, eventually fail.

Thus, critical to lung function is the proper consistency and regular removal of secretions. The ancients discovered that certain pungent foods possessed so-called *mucokinetic* (moving mucus) agents that thin, regulate, or propel the mucus out of the lungs. Modern drugs that promote the removal of sputum from the respiratory tree are described as mucokinetic.

It's this mucokinetic effect that explains the pharmacological secrets of hot pungent spices. They literally thin down the lung's secretions so they can be coughed up or normally expelled. As do modern drugs, the spices may work by a dozen or so mechanisms; probably most common, says Dr. Ziment, is through an instant communication system from the stomach to the lungs. In his historical search, Dr. Ziment was struck by the fact that commonly prescribed respiratory remedies are also emetics—in large doses they make you vomit. Take ipecac, for example. In small doses it is an old-fashioned cough remedy, one of the early treatments for asthma. It increases the production of fluid in the lungs, and is typically used today in larger doses to produce reflex vomiting in case of poisoning.

Here's Dr. Ziment's theory of what happens: a spicy food hits a "receptor button" in the stomach, flashing a signal through the vagus nerve to the brain, back to the lungs, where it stimulates bronchial glands to release a flood of watery fluid. Since nerves can be signaled all along the ingestion route—from mouth to stomach—the same reflex turns on glands that also cause the nose and eyes to water. As Dr. Ziment says, that's why "horseradish, pepper, or a spicy meal cleans out your nose and sinuses in a jiffy." In the lungs, the sudden outpouring of fluids thins the mucus or causes the glands to produce less sticky mucus, so it flows more easily. The pungent, aromatic foods, especially members of the fiery hot pepper family—in contact with the stomach—trigger an internal flash flood of tears that cleanse the system, breaking up nose and lung congestion, flushing out sinuses, and washing away irritants. "I think spicy foods are good for any condition in which these secretions in airways are thicker than normal," says Dr. Ziment, "and that would be sinusitis, a cold that produces thick secretions, and, of course, chronic bronchitis."

It appears that hot spicy foods may act both as a preventive of and therapy for bronchitis. Dr. Ziment believes that many people develop serious bronchitis partly because they do not like hot spicy foods. When he urges patients to try them, he reports "sometimes profound effects." He advises them to "start out on ten drops or so of Tabasco sauce in a glass of water or tomato juice, and if they tolerate ten, I then suggest twenty. Many of them find they are then able to cough up the secretions much more easily."

The component in such hot sauce that probably triggers this lung-cleansing process is capsaicin, the mouth-burning stuff in hot red pepper. Dr. Ziment notes that capsaicin is derived from a compound that is the basis of the chemical structure of a drug called guaifenesin. The *Physicians' Desk Reference* lists guaifenesin as an expectorant and an active ingredient in about seventy-five over-the-counter and prescription cough syrups, cold tablets, and expectorants, including Robitussin, Vicks cough syrup, and Actifed.

But mustard, horseradish, curry, and garlic, he says, perform essentially the same way. All can act as emetics and trigger bronchial gland secretion.

One of Dr. Ziment's favorite chest medications is garlic, an intriguing natural drug to help cure colds, he believes. He points out that the major flavoring agent in garlic, alliin, is chemically a close cousin of a drug called S. carboxymethylcysteine, or Mucodyne, a well-accepted European drug prescribed for regulating the flow of mucus. Garlic may be an even more potent anticongestant when combined with vitamin C, he maintains, because vitamin C may help break down alliin into a compound that is chemically very similar to Mucodyne. This, he says, provides a rational pharmacologic basis for utilizing garlic (potentiated by vitamin C) as a natural mucokinetic agent. For greatest potency, he advises, use the garlic cloves whole or zap them into a microwave oven before adding them to soups. That prevents the breakdown of alliin into allicin, the odiferous chemical, which has other therapeutic traits. Crushing or cutting the garlic clove causes a rapid conversion to allicin. Mustard, a traditional expectorant, also contains allyl isothiocyanate, similar to garlic's alliin.

Hot spicy foods may also help the lungs in other ways. One study found that giving rats capsaicin before exposing them to cigarette smoke "abolished airway edema and bronchoconstriction induced by cigarette smoke and other irritants." Further, as Dr. Ziment notes, evidence mounts that lung damage, including emphysema, may be partly due to free radicals—those active oxygen molecules that literally rip cells apart—which might be mopped up by sulfhydryl agents derived from chemicals in foods like garlic. "If that theory is borne out," he says, "maybe it's true that garlic will help prevent emphysema or damage from bronchitis by performing as an antioxidant to mop up the free radicals." For that reason, an editorial in a prestigious medical journal recently suggested incorporating garlic in cigarettes.

Dr. Ziment's prescription: Eat hot pungent foods if you have a cold, sinus problems, lung congestion, asthma, bronchitis, or emphysema—or if you think you are vulnerable to any of the above. Or try the Ziments' special chicken soup, a modern remedy in the ancient tradition.

DR. ZIMENT'S PRESCRIPTION GARLIC CHICKEN SOUP FOR COLDS AND COUGHS

28 ounces chicken broth
1 bulb garlic (about 15 cloves)
5 sprigs parsley, minced
6 sprigs cilantro, minced
1 teaspoon lemon pepper
1 teaspoon minced mint leaves
1 teaspoon minced sweet basil leaves
1 teaspoon curry powder

Peel the garlic cloves, and place with the other ingredients in a pan without a lid. Boil, then simmer for about 30 minutes. The infusion can then be filtered free of solid constituents. Alternatively, the garlic and herbs can be ground up and left in the soup. It may be preferable to grind up all the herbs and add them to the chicken broth initially.

Instructions for use: The fumes of the boiling soup can be inhaled during its preparation. The soup and its constituents can be divided into 4-8 equal portions, each of which should be taken at the beginning of a meal, one to three times a day. Patients are encouraged to add additional ingredients (for example, carrots, bay leaves, chili pepper flakes) to taste. A more dilute preparation may be deemed preferable, both personally and socially, until adaptation to this therapy occurs.

A HOT BONUS FOR THE CALORIE CONSCIOUS

Hot spicy foods may give you an unexpected bonus—an increased metabolic rate that burns off calories faster. It's no secret that certain food constituents can speed up metabolism, the process that produces heat by burning calories. In a test with twelve volunteers, British researchers at Oxford Polytechnic found that adding three grams of hot chili sauce and three grams of ordinary yellow mustard (about three-fifths of a teaspoon of each) to a meal caused the subjects to increase their metabolic rate an average twenty-five percent, burning an average forty-five more calories in the following three hours. One person burned up ten percent more calories or 76 out of a 766-calorie breakfast after adding the hot stuff.

5.

THE GREAT FISH DISCOVERIES

Anyone with half an ear cocked to health matters has to know that fat is the enemy. We've been told that too much fat will clog and stiffen our arteries, bringing forth wrathful events that choke off blood to the brain and deaden the throbbing glob of muscle known as the heart. But the intricate ways fat in food is metabolized into a cascade of bodily messengers that carry instructions to every cell in an endless disease process are undergoing intense scrutiny and stimulating revisionist thinking. Whether your arteries are wrecked—and your body suffers considerable other long-term chaos—may depend on the chemical makeup of the fat and its consequent disposition by the body. Fats are different, and, in particular, fat from the sea is a thing unto itself.

Consider for a moment that the fat you eat has undreamed of consequences, in fact, may constitute a drug of pharmaceutical genius able to sweep away the ills of dozens of disparate diseases. This prospect is being seriously entertained by scientists all over the world and is supported by millions of dollars in research grants from the National Institutes of Health.

Never mind that the idea of a single remedy for a variety of diseases from arthritis to psoriasis is the epitome of quackery, the antithesis of the revered drug model, where specific chemicals shoot down specific symptoms. The discovery of prostaglandins, those amazing cellular communicators, has totally destroyed that narrow notion, leading to revolutionary concepts about the widespread powers of the food pharmacy and one food in particular.

49

To think that one thing, let alone common fish, could be linked to blocking so many seemingly unrelated disease processes, would, until recently, have invited charges of scientific lunacy. It is an astonishing discovery. The awesome fact is that our vital bodily functions are intimately connected with the physiological characteristics of marine creatures, once our comrades in the evolutionary trip, and now a source of food.

The sustenance offered up by the sea is different from that of the land. Ocean plants—seaweed and phytoplankton—that feed the fish that we then feed on differ chemically from the seeds and grains of the earth. When we eat the fish, we, too, are altered at the very inner workings of our bodies—the way our blood flows, our arteries constrict, our cells repair themselves, and our immune system functions. The fish oils actually flow into our cell membranes like atavistic invaders, changing the basic composition of our bodies.

As these oils are smashed by the enzymes of the body, the resulting chemical reactions create pharmaceutical-like activity that is almost identical to that of common drugs like aspirin, steroids, painkillers, diuretics, antihypertensives, and anticoagulants. These metabolic by-products released by fish oils may make or break health in subtle ways, and, in fact, control basic underlying mechanisms common to numerous diseases. The inescapable conclusion: Nourishment from the sea is an ancient, powerful, and long-neglected antagonist to disease in ways scientists are only beginning to discover.

It all started nearly forty years ago with some musings over a medical oddity among the Eskimos. As early as 1950, an embarrassing paradox was spotted: The Eskimos had virtually no heart disease and yet ate a high fat diet of blubber and seal meat; their blood cholesterol levels, especially among Alaskan Eskimos, were fairly high, only slightly lower than that of Americans, Danes, and others who were dropping dead from heart attacks. Clearly, these Eskimos could not pose as role models in a low fat, low cholesterol, heart disease prevention campaign—even though they rarely suffered heart disease.

Between 1950 and 1974, hospital records in Greenland showed that only three Eskimos in a population of 1800 died of heart attacks. From comparable numbers, you'd expect forty fatal heart attacks among Danes and one hundred among Americans. Records further revealed that Eskimos escape other diseases modern man is heir to: psoriasis, bronchial asthma, diabetes, peptic ulcer, kidney disease, multiple sclerosis, arthritis, and other immune-related diseases.

Unable to ignore the paradox any longer, a few curious souls began to wonder about a peculiarity of Eskimo blood noticed by physicians some 500 years ago. Eskimo blood is not as sticky and does not clot as readily. When cut, Eskimos bleed longer. The same phenomenon shows up among families in Japanese fishing villages who also are remarkably free of heart disease. This was a clue for some scientists that the amount of cholesterol in the blood—though a vital indicator of cardiovascular health—is not *everything*. Other blood factors may be equally or more critical in warding off heart attacks and strokes.

Thus, while the anticholesterol bandwagon rolled on through the fifties and sixties and into the eighties, certain researchers found solace in a parallel inquiry that went beyond cholesterol and into more arcane reasons why that awful debris called plaque defaces artery walls, why arteries suddenly clamp in a deadly spasm, and why cells hustle together in blood-flow-stopping clots. Coming to heart disease from another direction, they ran smack into a unifying theory of how marine fat actually protects Eskimos—and others serendipitously—from grungy arteries and maybe everything else.

It has to do with the fact that Eskimos stuff themselves with a unique oil found in seafood. They typically devour thirteen ounces of seafood every day, all of it heavily packed with molecular chains of fatty acids called omega-3's because of their chemical structure. (The last double bond is on the third carbon from the end of the chain; the end is symbolized by omega, the last letter of the Greek alphabet; thus the chain becomes omega minus three or omega-3.) In contrast, the fat or oil in land plants and meat from animals raised on such plants are dominated by "omega-6" fatty acids that are broken down differently in the body.

Now, as far as your cells are concerned, what you eat is what they are. If you eat a lot of fish, your cells are infused with omega-3's; if you eat a lot of land foods, your cells are awash in omega-6's. Critical is a delicate balance. If the omega-6's get the upper hand, as is common in Western land-locked diets, they incite the cells to frenetic activity, spewing out excesses of hyperactive prostaglandins and similar hormones that wreak havoc on the body.

Theory goes that an overzealous production of prostaglandins and similar hormonelike messengers called leukotrienes signal cells to perform a multitude of complicated biochemical reactions that show up as multiple diseases. Of course, prostaglandins and leukotrienes in proper balance are good guys, too, commanding reactions that promote health. But in excess, certain types can ravage the body, causing cells to run amok and build inappropriate blood clots, constrict and dilate blood vessels and bronchial passages on whim, create heart spasms, and send squads of antibodies to attack perfectly good tissue, setting up inflammation to ward off nonexistent threats. In other words, run-amok prostaglandins and similar cell messengers can be underlying creators of diverse disease processes.

And what is the origin of the dangerous hordes of prostaglandins? In a medical breakthrough, Swedish researchers discovered in 1965 that prostaglandins are made from a fatty acid called arachidonic acid. When you eat unsaturated fat in foods from land plants or animals reared on such plants the fat is modified in the body to a substance called arachidonic acid. Enzymes further change this arachidonic acid into extremely potent physiological agents, prostaglandins and leukotrienes.

Obviously, if you dampen arachidonic acid's enthusiastic conversion to disease-generating prostaglandins, presto, the disease process may be stopped dead in its tracks; symptoms disappear or don't appear. And how can you do that? By eating seafood, scientists believe, you inject more omega-3 marine fat into cells, where it checks the potential destruction from too much omega-6 land-type fat, whence springs arachidonic acid. When more omega-3's are available, they dilute the ability of land vegetable 6's to get out of control. Omega-3's climb inside cell membranes, displacing the overzealous vegetable 6's and sometimes sit on prostaglandin receptor sites, blocking their errant behavior. Thus, the omega-3's cool down the speed at which land-based 6-type fatty acids stimulate the mighty arachidonic machine to spew out too many potentially destructive prostaglandins. The omega-3's also can selectively clamp down on the overproduction of some of the bad-guy prostaglandins and rev up production of counteracting good guys.

Thus, modern theory has it that most Eskimos are in such great shape and protected from chronic diseases because their regular intake of the fabulous omega-3 type fat blocks arachidonic acid's metamorphosis into potent disease-promoting agents. Even though their sea-fatty diet does not promote extremely low blood cholesterol, it nevertheless creates a cellular situation that overpowers other fats' ability to trigger heart and other chronic diseases. In the Eskimos' case, not all fat is always bad for you.

Although a small cadre of scientists have long been on the trail of the fish story, it attracted little attention until lately. Inquiries aimed at basic mechanisms that would elucidate seafood power began in the 1970s with a rash of discoveries about the wiles and control of prostaglandins.

Think of it this way: omega-3 fish oils are a lot like aspirin (and other antiinflammatory agents, immune regulators, and anticoagulants). Although aspirin has been used since ancient Greece, it was not until 1971 that John Vane, who later won a Nobel prize, uncovered the healing mechanism. Aspirin blocks enzymes that produce prostaglandins that lead to aches and pain. Everybody paid attention.

Virtually nobody paid attention the following year when a young scientist from Michigan announced at a scientific conference in Vienna that certain components of fish oil do essentially the same thing. While scrutinizing various fatty acids, he found that the polyunsaturated fat known as omega-3 also suppressed arachidonic acid's ability to spin off prostaglandins. The profound implications seemed clear to the scientist William Lands, Ph.D., now professor of biological chemistry at the University of Illinois at Chicago, that eating omega-3's predominant in fish would curb prostaglandins too, creating untold biological ramifications. Dr. Lands's was the first substantial clue to how fish oil can manipulate human biology. But "it fell flat," he recalls. Few then grasped the commonality of fish oils and aspirin. It was an idea ahead of its time.

But with the discoveries in 1975 of thromboxane, a prostaglandin that tells blood cells to clump up into dangerous thrombi that plug up blood vessels, and in 1979 of leukotrienes, cell messengers that help control the immune and inflammation process, the research heated up.

Two Danish researchers, Jorn Dyerberg and Hans Olaf Bang, began in 1977 their now famous studies of Eskimos. They drew Eskimo blood, confirming that it ran thin, was lower in bad LDL-type and higher in good HDL-type cholesterol; they attributed it to the high fish diet. University of Oregon researchers fed a group of Americans about six and a half tablespoons of salmon oil daily and found it depressed blood cholesterol slightly, triglycerides mightily, and increased bleeding time from seven minutes to ten minutes.

Dr. Lands went to work feeding omega-3-rich mehaden fish oil to dogs, cats, and mice for about three weeks with spectacular results: fewer heart attacks and thrombotic incidents and less damage to arteries. For example, blood vessel blockage shuts off blood flow, causing inevitable damage. But the fish oil lessened the damage. In cats, fish oils lessened the brain damage from strokes. Dogs fed the omega-3 oils suffered a mere three percent damage in heart muscle, compared with twenty-five percent in those not fed omega-3's. One possible reason: fish oils make blood less viscous, so it flows more readily. A fascinating phenomenon: cell membranes full of omega-3's are more fluid and pliable; thus such deformable cells are better able to squeeze through constricted capillaries, keeping tissues supplied with oxygen. If your blood vessels are narrowed, as most are after a certain age, this can be a lifesaving maneuver.

Unquestionably, fish oils may protect against thrombosis—clots that block off blood, hence life-giving oxygen to tissues. As an early test, Dr. Lands found his own blood less inclined to aggregate into clumps that form the treacherous thrombi after he took a tablespoon of fish oil morning, noon, and night for a month. Many other studies, notably in Japan, show the same thing. Japanese who fish for a living, and eat their catches, have blood with less of a tendency to form clots than Japanese land-locked farmers.

Dr. Lands, an internationally recognized theorist in this subject, notes that prostaglandins and leukotrienes also seem to play a part in the buildup of arterial plaque, in angina, and in vascular spasm, an increasingly recognized cause of death. The prostaglandin thromboxane, for instance, has been known to constrict blood vessels, induce coronary vasospasms, and angina. And the intracellular communicators are thought to help direct cells to paste themselves against artery walls and then snag circulating cholesterol to make even bigger piles of occlusive debris. By interfering with all of these heart disease provoking processes, seafood may save multitudes of lives.

The evidence that fish, even in modest amounts, protects against cardiovascular disease is now so credible that it is given wide circulation in the world's leading medical journals. Report after report supports it. What gave the idea the medical stamp of respectability were three articles in the prestigious *New England Journal of Medicine* in May 1985. The blockbuster was a study by investigators from the Netherlands who found that over a twenty-year period deaths from coronary heart disease were more than fifty percent lower among a group of men in a small Dutch town, Zutphen, who ate at least thirty grams of fish (a little over an ounce) a day compared with those who ate no fish. That means, said the investigative team headed by Daan Kromhout, Ph.D., of the Institute of Social Medicine, University of Leiden, that eating as little as one or two fish dishes a week may help prevent heart disease!

Scientists all over the world have taken up the fish oil quest, particularly in Japan, West Germany, and Denmark. But omega-3's impact on cardiovascular disease is no longer the half of it, says pioneer Lands. He and others have begun to contemplate all the other things the run-amok descendants of arachidonic acid do. If fish oils, presumably the omega-3 component, could so powerfully interfere with the basic mechanics of heart disease, wouldn't it, by turning down the prostaglandin engine, simultaneously have repercussions for other disease processes?

Imaginations, attention!

Cancer, asthma, rheumatoid arthritis, lupus, psoriasis, allergies, immune inflammatory disorders, headaches, high blood pressure, and multiple sclerosis are all disorders related to overenthusiastic production of prostaglandins. The possibilities are thrilling: fish oils, by curbing prostaglandin formation, may control the underlying metabolic mechanisms that set off these diseases too. Recognizing the vast potential, the National Institutes of Health is funding research on the impact of fish oils against such diseases in which prostaglandins are implicated.

So far the omega-3's have achieved remarkable successes in both humans and animals in fighting numerous prostaglandin-regulated maladies. (For a rundown of these, see Fish, page 190)

Nothing has ever come on the nutrition-medical scene to match the fish oils. Are they a panacea? Unknown. But experts emphasize that it is critical to distinguish between potential *preventive and curative* effects. Once chronic disease is full blown or advanced, it is doubtful that fish or its omega-3 oils have the power to reverse it, although they may arrest it. In other words, foods from the sea may not act as potent drugs to *cure* the result of decades of cellular assaults on the body. But *prevent* disease? That's another matter, says Dr. Alfred D. Steinberg, an arthritis expert at the National Institutes of Health. "Preventing the onset of a disease and treating the disease once it has occurred are very different." As an analogy he points out that certain drugs not powerful enough to cure nevertheless easily *prevent* the same disease. Marine fat may fall into that category of a natural prophylactic pharmaceutical.

Dr. Lands agrees that focusing on fish as a cure-all misses the point. He sees fish's main potential as blocking the continual assault on cells from hyperactive prostaglandins that over the years build up into symptoms of chronic diseases. The future of dealing with chronic diseases is in prevention, not treatment. His belief: "Many of these chronic diseases are accumulated insults that your body has suffered over the years. If you prevent those cumulative nicks and bangs day after day—by curbing the continual onslaughts from prostaglandins, for example by infusing your tissues with counteracting omega-3 fish oils—it's likely that you can forestall a lot of chronic disease." That, he says, is the real message of the great fish discoveries.

6.

THE CABBAGE–CANCER CONNECTION

Honestly now, if you were fate perusing nature's drugstore in search of a new pharmaceutical to thrust into the limelight to fight one of the world's worst scourges, cancer, would you even pause over cabbage? or broccoli? or brussels sprouts? or cauliflower? Plus their other funky cousins, all members of a plant family officially named brassica, also called cruciferous because their four-petaled flowers reminded somebody in the Middle Ages of a cross, or crucifix?

Well, once upon a time most people viewed such a prospect as ridiculous.

A mere twenty-five years ago it was near scientific heresy and unthinkable cruelty to suggest that cancer could in any way be shut off by diet. Now scientists know that molecules of compounds in foods are potent players in the life-and-death cellular wars. Food compounds can perform a remarkable variety of anticancer activities: they can capture and snuff out roaming "free radical" oxygen molecules that promote cellular damage and cancer; they can neutralize agents that would activate carcinogens; they can stimulate enzymes to set up elaborate systems for flushing carcinogens from the body; they may interfere with messengers that would switch on oncogenes in the cell nucleus, starting and encouraging the cancer process.

Scientists now say that food compounds can fight cancer at virtually every stage—from the first "initiation" of the cell by a cancer agent to the growth rate of tumors decades later. In fact, certain foods, because of their unique collection of compounds, may be site specific, that is, like drugs, they may be best able to protect certain organs from cancerous assault. In that most somber of fields, cancer, scientists are now thinking big, even envisioning the day when anticancer diets and other preventive measures will be individually prescribed depending upon your genetically identified susceptibility to certain cancers.

Building a stronger biological fortress against cancer is the flip side of doom. It is human intelligence's bold response to a twentieth-century cancer plague inflicted by ignorance, carelessness, and, for some, just plain genetic ill fortune. Hidden, complex chemical manipulations by food substances promise some salvation, softening the consequences of littering the air, land, food, water, and our bodies with chemicals that change living cells into predictable lumps of malignancy. Since we are bombarded by carcinogens, why not infuse ourselves with anticarcinogens, creating a perpetual police force to meet, bully, corral, and force hazardous chemicals out of the body before they inflict irreparable damage on cells. If we use chemotherapy to kill cancer cells after the fact, why not *chemoprevention*—the deliberate and controlled use of substances, including those abundant in foods, to block the effects of carcinogenic poisons around us—before the fact—before cancer has usurped the body.

It is a thrilling idea. Credit it to Lee Wattenberg, M.D. Everybody else does. Dr. Wattenberg, a professor of pathology at the University of Minnesota Medical School, is the acknowledged pioneer of this concept to save us from cancer, much of it self-inflicted. Since the late 1960s, and until recently little recognized, he has carried on intricate and often tedious experiments, defining mechanisms by which chemicals in simple foods like cabbage and broccoli could reach into the living cells and stop cancer. Dr. Wattenberg is the intellectual center of an exploding universe of scientists searching for ways to erect internal shields against the human vulnerability to cancer.

It didn't start with cabbage. But it was cabbage that galvanized scientific imaginations and lent credibility to a once incredible notion.

Dr. Wattenberg's work quite by chance was boosted by the findings of a first-rate epidemiologist, Dr. Saxon Graham, chairman of social and preventive medicine at the State University of New York at Buffalo.

In the mid-1970s Dr. Graham and his associates interviewed 256 white male patients with colon cancer at the Roswell Park Memorial Institute, and 783 patients of identical ages who did not have cancer, selected at random. They asked them all how often each month they ate nineteen vegetables, including coleslaw, tomatoes, cabbage, lettuce, cucumbers, carrots, brussels sprouts, broccoli, turnips, and cauliflower.

The men who reported eating the most vegetables had the lowest risks of colon cancer. In fact, the chances went down steadily, the more vegetables eaten. A man who ate any of these vegetables more than a couple of times a day was only half as likely to have colon cancer as a man who never ate them or ate them less than twenty times a month. It was fascinating because the vegetables produced what is called a "dose response." The more taken, the greater the therapeutic effect. Scientists love this because it indicates, much like a drug, that this is a reliable finding and not just a fluke. Drugs, for example, when tested, are expected to give measurable dose responses, otherwise there is suspicion they are unreliable. So Dr. Graham and his colleagues were tickled pink to see their experiment so neatly follow a dose response.

Then they decided to take a look at the vegetables separately, and lo and behold, cabbage stood out and it, too, almost perfectly followed a "dose-response" pattern. The bottom line: If you ate cabbage more than once a week, you were only one third as likely to develop colon cancer as someone who never ate cabbage, at least if you were male and white. In other words, one serving of cabbage a week could cut your chances of colon cancer by sixty-six percent! Even if you ate cabbage once every two or three weeks, the risk dropped by forty percent. Sauerkraut and coleslaw, as well as broccoli and brussels sprouts, also showed a dose-response protection against colon cancer.

Dr. Graham did a wrap-up commentary on this work as the lead article in the January 1979 issue of the *American Journal of Epidemiology*. It was the same month as a national diet and cancer conference of scientists in New York City. Everyone was agog over Dr. Graham's finding. But its significance was cemented by the intellectual bridge linking it to Dr. Wattenberg's then recent revelations.

Dr. Wattenberg's work was the eureka, the brain click that made sense of Dr. Graham's findings. Dr. Wattenberg, since the early 1970s, had been feeding small amounts of cruciferous vegetables (cabbage, broccoli, brussels sprouts, cauliflower, and turnips) to rats and mice, injecting them with well-known carcinogens, and watching to see if they developed cancer or had metabolic changes in organs that would block the formation of cancer. Many did not develop cancer; they were oddly protected by the vegetables. "Interesting, but . . ." mused his colleagues.

Then in the May 1978 issue of *Cancer Research*, Dr. Wattenberg hammered home the implications. He had isolated chemicals called indoles from the cruciferous vegetables and given these to animals as a chemopreventive "hors d'oeuvre" before administering the cancer-causing chemicals. The pure cabbage compounds also proved potent antidotes to developing cancer.

The protection was impressive. Without indoles, of rats subjected to the chemical carcinogen, ninety-one percent got breast cancer; with the indoles the rate dropped as low as twenty-one percent. In another test with a lower dose given over a longer period to mice, one hundred percent without indoles succumbed to tumors, compared with only forty-four percent who were fed indoles.

Dr. Graham, as well as everybody else in the field, saw the striking parallel between his finding in humans and Dr. Wattenberg's in animals. Dr. Wattenberg offered a perfectly reasonable scientific explanation of how such funky vegetables as cabbage might exert such a potent physiological effect on the machinery of cancer. The message reverberated loud and clear in the community of scientists who study cancer. Cancer and diet research was off and running in a new direction, with cruciferous and chemoprevention—Dr. Wattenberg's term—the new watchwords. Today the National Cancer Institute spends millions investigating the cruciferous vegetables and invites scientists to submit grants on the subject.

Dr. Wattenberg went on to decipher the elegant tricks cabbage compounds employ to defeat cancer and to reveal like potential in other common foods. As he and others show, food chemicals have plenty of chances to intervene in the long, slow cancer process with its incubation period of twenty to forty years or more.

First, cells must be "initiated" to cancer—their DNA—genetic material—altered by "hits" from carcinogens such as ionizing radiation, cigarette smoke, pesticides, and unknown genetic factors. The mutated cells may then start to divide inappropriately, proliferate, and cluster into forerunners of cancer called precancerous lesions, exploding later into full-blown malignancies. Whether this aberrant cell division and progression happens and how quickly depends on encouragers or "promoters." Cigarette smoke, for example, is a classic promoter. The point is that cancer development is a multistage, longtime event, and interfering with it anywhere along the line can retard or halt its deadly march.

That's what food's "minor dietary constituents," as Dr. Wattenberg calls them, do with imagination and variety. Some can halt cancer at its cellular conception. If, when a carcinogen comes calling on a cell, a proper food chemical or offspring is present, it may save the virgin cell from rape and corruption of its DNA, thereby thwarting cancer at the earliest stage. Other food compounds acting as antioxidants may track down, entrap, and destroy the cancer promoters that are cheerleaders for enlarged and metastatic damage, leading to spreading of the cancer. Some foods produce both early blockers and late-stage suppressors in a marvelous "fail-safe" system. Thus, if the first brigade fails to fully disarm the carcinogenic invaders, other forces take over to slow the deadly progression.

In meticulous experiments, Dr. Wattenberg has mapped one of the wondrous ways food chemicals triumph over cancer. Many food anticancer agents, including cabbage and its cousins, deploy their forces through the body's exquisite detoxification system, he explains. It's this little-appreciated defense system for disposing of foreign noxious compounds that for eons has enabled us to eat plants and survive. It lets nutrients through while sloughing off the plants' other less agreeable substances. The system likewise blunts assaults from everyday modern carcinogens such as air pollutants, pesticides, occupational chemicals, and food contaminants. In fact, how well this detoxification system functions may strongly influence how well you resist cancer. Increased activity and complex metabolic processes of certain enzymes shoo dangerous chemicals right out of the body. In Dr. Wattenberg's words: "Enhancement of the activity of this system could increase the capacity of the organism to withstand the neoplastic effects resulting from exposure to chemical carcinogens."

Here's the bottom line: Foods like cabbage seem to push the vital detoxification system into high gear. Cabbage compounds, including indoles and chemicals with the jawbreaking name dithiolthiones, exert a mighty influence on enzymes that have their hands on the throttle of the detoxification system. Prodding the enzymes revs up the detoxification system, causing it to release a flood of molecules called glutathione—a natural body substance that can engage and destroy toxins, including carcinogens—as well as enzymes that glue the glutathione to the carcinogen molecule. Think of the scene as a crowded dance floor populated by both DNA and glutathione molecules. Along comes a nasty fully activated carcinogen. If it bumps into a DNA molecule, trouble. But if it encounters a glutathione molecule, the twosome are often terminated by a chemical reaction; the carcinogen is neutralized, detoxified. Obviously, the more glutathione molecules in tissue, the greater the statistical chances that they will meet and destroy a carcinogenic molecule, leaving vital DNA untouched. Thus, not keeping enough glutathione molecules available in the darkest interior of your being could be an event of potential doom.

Dr. Wattenberg and others have demonstrated many times over experimentally that if you feed animals cabbage and other cruciferous vegetables, their enzyme detoxification mechanism speeds up. Feed them the pure cabbage chemicals, same thing. In both cases, the animals are much less prone to develop cancer when later exposed to cancer-causing chemicals.

Dr. Thomas Kensler, associate professor of toxicology at Johns Hopkins University School of Hygiene and Public Health, feeds afla-toxin, a potent carcinogen, to animals. He gives others a dose of cabbage-type dithiolthiones before the aflatoxin. He examines the cells of the dithiolthione-fed animals and finds twice as much glutathione and ten times more of the enzymes that cement the glutathione to the carcinogens. Further, he finds that aflatoxin damage (binding) to DNA drops by ninety percent. Consequently, there are fewer cancerous changes in cells and in the end many fewer tumors. As Dr. Kensler says: "Dithiolthiones are as potent an anticancer agent as we have ever looked at. It's quite dramatic."

Dr. Wattenberg's experiments on animals show conclusively that both raw and cooked cruciferous vegetables as well as their pure chemicals increase enzyme detoxification activity. But, he notes, certain cabbage indoles protect only if they arrive in the body *before* a carcinogen. If the indole comes on the scene *after* the carcinogen has attacked cells, its powers appear limited. It cannot clean up the mess. But other cruciferous chemicals called isothiocyanates did suppress colon cancers in rats when given a week after a certain cancer-causing agent. Cells apparently need consistent low-level doses of the right food substances to maintain biological barriers to cancer development.

Also sure to buck up the case for cabbage and its cousins is an unusually fascinating and impressive Norwegian look at precancerous signs in the colons of people who do and do not eat cruciferous vegetables. Doctors believe full-blown colon cancer erupts from small colonic growths called polyps or, in more advanced stages, called adenomas. Not all such benign growths become cancerous, but most experts agree that since the growths are the foundation of colorectal cancer, if you can eliminate the appearance or expansion of polyps, you zap the possibility of colon cancer.

Norwegian scientists tracking down a diet-cancer connection in 1986 examined the colons of people with no symptoms of cancer for signs of polyps—those tiny colonic growths. First they screened 155 men and women aged fifty to fifty-nine by sigmoidoscopic examination (insertion of a lighted instrument into the colon) to spot polyps or adenomas, their size and extent of abnormality. Then, for the next five days, without telling the participants the test results, investigators asked them to meticulously record everything they ate.

Seventy-eight, or about half, had polyps. But, strikingly, the half *without* the precancerous signs of colon cancer ate *more of their calories in the cruciferous vegetables*—cabbage, broccoli, cauliflower, and brussels sprouts, and more fiber in general. The vegetables seemed to suppress both the growth of the ominous clumps of cells and their degree of abnormality. Those with the largest, most abnormal adenomas—over five millimeters in diameter—for example, ate the least cruciferous vegetables, says chief investigator Dr. Geir Hoff of the Medical Department of the Telemark Sentralsjukehus in Skein, Norway.

Cabbage, as are all of these vegetables of the cross, is taken seriously at the National Cancer Institute, notably to prevent primarily colon and possibly stomach cancer. An internal NCI analysis made in 1987 noted that fully six of seven major epidemiological studies similar to Dr. Graham's find that people eating more cruciferous vegetables have less chance of colon cancer. The studies came from Israel, Greece, Japan, and Norway, as well as the United States, and most frequently mention cabbage, along with kohlrabi, sauerkraut, brussels sprouts, and broccoli.

Other population surveys add cancers of the lung, esophagus, larynx, rectum, prostate, and bladder to the malignancies possibly prevented by the large cruciferous family.

Where will it all end? Dr. Wattenberg proposes that eventually some of the cruciferous chemicals be extracted, synthesized, and possibly given to people at high risk of cancer such as those occupationally exposed to cancer-causing chemicals.

In the meantime, it is foolhardy to ignore the persuasive messages from the labs and academia: people who eat more vegetables of the type chock-full of known anticancer chemicals are less apt to have cancer. The ancient Romans even more drastically followed their beliefs; on one occasion they ran their doctors out of town and for years reportedly maintained their good health by eating cabbages. Science once again is catching up with folklore.

THE ANTICANCER CRUCIFEROUS TWELVE

They all have flowers with four petals that to botanical historians resembled a crucifix or cross; thus cruciferous. They also share common chemicals that can counteract some of the destruction from carcinogens.

Broccoli
Brussels sprouts
Cabbage
Cauliflower
Cress
Horseradish

Kale
Kohlrabi
Mustard
Radish
Rutabaga
Turnip

7.

THE NUTS AND SEEDS DEFENSE

If you go to lunch with Dr. Walter Troll, he will steer you to the salad bar where you can load up on chick-peas—one of his favorites. He's not so wild about plain old boiled soybeans, although they have made him famous among his colleagues; to him they taste a little blah. His wife sometimes makes tofu cake, which he says tastes a little like pineapple upside down cake. On a trip to Japan, the Trolls picked up some advice on cooking with soybeans from Japanese cancer researchers. The Japanese, after all, are the world's biggest consumers of soybeans, virtually all of them grown in the United States. Ironically, says Dr. Troll, *our* soybeans are probably one reason the Japanese generally have cancer rates lower than ours. (The prime exception is stomach cancer, which he blames on the Japanese practice of eating too much salty food.)

Dr. Troll, professor of environmental medicine at New York University, has been pushing beans, rice, legumes, and nuts in the diet since 1969—the year he made a landmark discovery about a group of compounds called protease inhibitors abundant in seeds and nuts. He insists these compounds may help squelch cancer by interfering with the activity of body functionaries, including oncogenes, and enzymes called proteases that can promote cancer.

Here's what happens after dining on chick-peas—or on any other legume, rice, nuts, corn, or grain—according to Dr. Troll. The chick-peas go to the stomach and into the intestinal tract, where their outer coating is ripped off and they are smashed to bits by digestive juices. But inside the chick-peas are indestructible molecules, the protease inhibitors, that survive in the intestinal tract. Dr. Troll knows; he has made them radioactive and traced them in animals—and "they come out totally intact," he says.

Protease inhibitors were not made for your convenience or safety but to guarantee the perpetuation of plant species. The protease inhibitors, for example, make precious seeds anathema to insects, and undigestible and thus indestructible if eaten by birds; thus, the seed is excreted intact so it can sprout new plants. So far about eight different types of protease inhibitors have been isolated from "seed foods," and that includes tubers such as potatoes.

You want these protease inhibitors hanging around, says Dr. Troll, for a multitude of reasons: one, there's evidence they monitor and squelch the activity of proteases that have the nasty habit of turning on and turning up cancer processes. Proteases, protein-splitting enzymes, carry on normal biological functions such as digestion of proteins. But certain proteases are also the helpers and caretakers of cancer cells. Because cancer cells are unwelcome newcomers lacking bodily protection granted normal cells, they exploit proteases in order to thrive. For example, collagen, a protein, is a tough material holding cell walls and organs together. Cancer cells, to spread, must smash down those walls, possibly by enlisting proteases called collagenase to batter the collagen, and thereby gaining entrance. Naturally, if corresponding protease inhibitors are on the scene, they tend to block collagenase's procancer activity.

Additionally, Dr. Troll finds protease inhibitors to have kaleidoscopic anticancer activity, even to tampering with the switch controlling the restless and mighty oncogenes. Oncogenes, cancer researchers' newly discovered intellectual playthings, are thought to be one of the elemental keys to cancer. Oncogenes reside in every normal cell—generally quietly. But if they undergo a specific mutation, they turn into cancer genes and incite the cell to proliferate wildly into a tumor. "If the oncogene is not activated, it does us no harm," says Dr. Troll. There are now about one hundred different known oncogenes. According to Dr. Troll, they take part in both the cell's baptism to cancer and the long, slow progression.

Since protease inhibitors also function as antioxidants they can counteract destructive, wide-ranging, super-charged oxygen molecules called "free radicals" that damage cells. Thus, protease inhibitors, says Dr. Troll, offer "umbrellas of protection," fending off the cancer process almost every step of the way—from blocking or reversing DNA damage to starving or destroying full-blown cancer cells.

But Dr. Troll's enthusiasm over protease inhibitors centers on their powers to intercept cancer at that time most critical for humans— after cells are initiated to cancer (their DNA is damaged) and are vulnerable to prods toward aberrant growth. "If we can prevent promotion, we will be all right," figures Dr. Troll. He believes it's too late to forestall initiation. "One has the feeling that all of us are probably initiated because of exposure to widespread carcinogens in the environment," he says. He's counting on our chances to keep that initiated cell from abnormally dividing and proliferating into a malignant mass, thereby blocking the long-time march of the cancer process after cells suffer initial damage but before the tumor gets out of control.

That's where oncogenes come in. Dr. Troll believes activated oncogenes can both change DNA and switch on cell proliferation, ending in cancer. In one experiment, Dr. Troll and NYU colleague Seymour Garte took a ras oncogene from the DNA of human bladder cancer cells and inserted it into normal cells, which then "divided into a neoplastic thing." But when the scientists added four different types of protease inhibitors, the cancerous changes did not take place.

So in effect you find that protease inhibitors stopped the oncogene from being activated and switching on cancer?

"Yes. The ras oncogene may be necessary for all cell growth and tumor growth. So if you inhibit it—turn off the switch in some fashion at exactly the right time—the tumor won't grow." Theoretically, this may be how protease inhibitors interrupt a broad range of cancers at various stages.

Dr. Troll is even convinced that protease inhibitors can slow down the very late stages of cancer progression in somewhat the same way chemotherapy does, but in a much more targeted, less toxic fashion. He speculates that infusing your cells with protease inhibitors by eating foods rich in these agents may help block cancer progression up until the time the malignancy spreads from the original site, or metastasizes. "Dietary interference is probably too late by the time of metastasis," he thinks. "Before that, it may work."

In a remarkable finding, another prominent researcher on protease inhibitors, Dr. Ann Kennedy at the Harvard School of Public Health, even found that protease inhibitors in tissue cultures can *reverse* the initial cancer-causing damage to cells—something scientists have previously considered impossible. Scientific consensus is that once a cell's DNA—its master genetic tape—has been altered by a cancer-causing agent, the destructive message can never be erased; it's indelibly inscribed, waiting for other events—such as cancer-promoting agents—to amplify it into malignancy. But Dr. Kennedy discovered in test tube experiments that applying protease inhibitors to cells with carcinogen-induced DNA damage actually made the cells return to normal; they behaved as if their DNA had never been assaulted. The protease inhibitors actually healed the genetic damage. And even after departure of the protease inhibitor, the cells remained normal, did not revert to their precancerous condition, and could not be stimulated to abnormally proliferate, launching the cancer process.

Some other evidence of why scientists are so enthusiastic about these food chemicals' anticancer powers:

Protease inhibitors, in lab experiments, have been shown to retard the growth of human breast and colon cancer cells. Feeding the soybean compounds to animals blocks breast, skin, and colon cancer. Injecting protease inhibitors saves mice from otherwise lethal irradiation. Soybeans, which contain protease inhibitors, block spontaneous liver cancers in mice. Painting mice skin with cancer promoters doesn't produce cancer if you also add protease inhibitors. This was Dr. Troll's big exciting discovery in 1969 that gave him a day "I will never forget," and launched numerous scientific probes of protease inhibitors.

In a later classic experiment, Dr. Troll and his colleagues proved the powers of soybean compounds against breast cancer in animals. Soon after birth, groups of rats were fed different diets. One group ate soybeans. Then at two months of age all were exposed to three hundred rads of total body X irradiation. Forty-four percent of the soybean-eating rats developed breast cancer compared with seventy percent on regular rat chow.

Dr. Kennedy showed that these food agents strongly suppressed oral cancer in hamsters. Dr. Kennedy and her team also added extract of soybeans to the diet of mice and found that legumes blocked colorectal cancer. She thinks that protease inhibitors are likely to combat all types of cancer except stomach cancer.

And there's backup human evidence that eating seed foods may help save you from cancer. An impressive look at the food patterns and cancer rates of forty-one countries was done by Pelayo Correa at the Louisiana State University Medical Center in New Orleans. He found a striking upsurge in per capita consumption of rice, corn (maize), and beans in countries with the lower rates of colon, breast, and prostate cancer. The more ardent bean, rice, and corn eaters also had less coronary heart disease. Dr. Troll says there is good theoretical evidence showing that protease inhibitors help control blood clotting, possibly cutting down on cardiovascular troubles. Other researchers who found less breast, uterine, and ovarian cancers in women eating more cereal and beans suggested the seed foods might partially counteract the ill effects of high fat diets suspected of promoting these hormone-regulated cancers.

Foods containing protease inhibitors may also mount a mighty defense against viruses. Here's why: Some viruses have to be activated before they can attach to human cells and become infectious. Cooperating in this venture, the pancreas produces proteases that are washed through a duct and into the gastrointestinal tract, where they live in large numbers. Although these protease enzymes regulate numerous life-sustaining metabolic activities, they also have a thing with viruses. A virus can sit dormant in the gastrointestinal tract, in the respiratory tract, or even on a Kleenex for long periods of time, but once it meets a protease under the right conditions, it's like Sleeping Beauty or the third phase of Ms. Pac-Man; they hug and kiss and the virus springs to life and starts replicating.

It seems logical to try to knock out the activating charm of some of these protease enzymes, leaving viruses in a stupor and nondangerous. Thus, the virus doesn't get activated, doesn't stick to cells, but is left to be swept along the intestinal tract and into somebody's sewer.

That's, of course, what a protease inhibitor does; it squelches the protease enzyme's ability to arouse viruses. According to one provocative image, the inhibitor may prevent a virus particle from taking off its outer protein coat, and it cannot invade a cell and inject its genetic material while wearing its coat. If a virus can't get this far, it can't gain access to the cell's genetic machinery and can't replicate itself. So the cell is safe. A virus, unlike bacteria, cannot reproduce on its own. To spread infection a virus penetrates a healthy cell, taking over its genetic machinery, which it uses to replicate itself, spewing out more viruses.

There's no question that protease inhibitors of the type found in foods—especially those in soybeans—can turn off viruses. Researchers at the Johns Hopkins University School of Medicine mixed human rotaviruses that cause diarrhea and general gastrointestinal illness with several protease inhibitors and let them incubate in human cells. All of the substances kept the viruses subdued. High concentrations of the soybean compounds obliterated nearly one hundred percent of viral activity. There were no sweet dances between the protease enzymes and the viruses, empowering them to invade human cells.

When the investigators gave the soybean constituents to mice infected with a virus, far fewer of the mice got sick and generally were less contagious. Interestingly, a single low dose of soybean substance worked only when given *before* inoculation with the virus—as kind of an antiviral hors d'oeuvre. But when administered in high doses several times after injection with the virus, it also squelched infections in the animals to a good degree.

Because numerous viruses need to be activated by proteases in order to be dangerous, the soybean inhibitors, by interfering with that basic mechanism, pack potential as very broad antiviral agents. Some examples of viruses that can't perform without the activation ritual are: myxoviruses, a large group of viruses that can cause influenza and mumps; retroviruses, associated with leukemia; coronaviruses that cause respiratory infections, and poxviruses that cause smallpox.

Natural protease inhibitors that disarm viruses are much safer than currently available antiviral drugs. Few pharmaceutical virus-fighters have ever been developed, and those that have direct their attack by interacting with the nucleic acids in the heart of the cell's genetic machinery. At the same time, there are fears they may mess up the nucleic acid synthesis in normal cells, leading to long-term damage, possibly cancer. On the other hand, researchers say the enzyme blockers in foods interfere with the splitting of proteins that allow the virus to break through cell walls instead of working within the cell nucleus. Thus, nature's therapeutic mechanism is gentler and safer.

Some say protease inhibitors themselves may be dangerous, but proponents say the fears are groundless. It's been asserted that heavy doses of protease inhibitors, especially in domestic animals, retard growth. There is also evidence that the compounds can promote pancreatic cancer in rats. But according to Dr. Troll, when protease inhibitors were fed to monkeys, which are biologically most similar to humans, there were absolutely no signs of harm. Also, the agents did not cause any type cancer in mice, pigs, or monkeys, he says.

The protease inhibitors are far-flung throughout the vegetable kingdom; that they are powerful drugs is undeniable. That they get into the gastrointestinal tract is also certain. At least in animals, they exert anticancer properties in several regions of the body. In experiments they turn off cancer-generating oncogenes and viruses. It doesn't take much imagination to suggest that heavy doses of these protease inhibitors may be another formidable reason why eating vegetables promotes health.

WHERE YOU FIND DR. TROLL'S ANTICANCER AGENTS

Look for protease inhibitors first in legumes. Soybeans and chick peas (garbanzo beans) have the highest concentrations. Other rich sources are broad beans, lima beans, tofu, black-eyed peas, kidney beans, fava beans, peas, lentils, and mung beans. All of the "seed foods" have protease inhibitors in varying concentrations: all kinds of nuts (peanuts, walnuts, pecans, etc.); tubers—white potatoes, sweet potatoes (yams), taro, banana; cereal grains—barley, wheat, oats, rye, rice, maize (sweet corn), sorghum grain.

Although the inhibitors are most concentrated in the seed foods, they are also found in high amounts in eggplant and in moderate amounts in spinach, broccoli, brussels sprouts, radish, cucumber, and pineapple. And recently, a prominent researcher in Washington state discovered that fifty percent of the protein in an unripe tomato was in the form of protease inhibitors! The compounds diminished as the tomato ripened. The truth is, because too few foods have been analyzed for protease inhibitor content, scientists are not sure which foods may turn out to be unexpected rich sources of the compounds.

Many types of protease inhibitors survive cooking and processing; for example, high levels have been detected in cooked soybeans and tofu, and even in baked bread, notably whole grain bread. Dr. Troll, however, says cooking significantly destroys protease inhibitors in potatoes. *Raw* potatoes are a much better source.

8.

THE SEARCH FOR THE MYSTERIOUS CARROT FACTOR

It seems almost too daffy an idea to be true—that infinitesimal amounts of druglike compounds in carrots and similar vegetables could arouse damaged cells to resist assaults that otherwise end up as deadly lumps of malignancy. Yet, in the last few years millions of cancer research dollars and vast brainpower have been devoted to answering an almost laughable question: How could one little C, as in carrots, possibly combat such a horrendous modern pestilence as the Big C? Neither the findings nor the consequences are silly. Astonishing as it seems, the cancer epidemic from the human foolishness of cigarette smoking and other environmental pollution may be partly offset by the simple ritual of putting in your mouth, chewing, and digesting modest amounts of orange or dark green plants every day.

While testing other plant compounds invariably takes place in animals and test tubes, the essence of carrot is already being widely tested *in humans* as a potential antidote to cancer. Although every food is a grab bag of chemicals that may attack cancer broadly, the carrot factor, it appears, interferes with the cancer process at later stages—during the promotion phase. And its orangeness may perform best against cancers peculiarly related to smoking. Nor is the "carrot factor" confined to carrots. Although the chemical family called carotene, or carotenoids, derives its name from carrots, it is the primary pigment of all deep-orange and deep-green vegetables. (Green chlorophyll covers up the orange or red hue.)

It is a synthetic carotenoid, beta carotene—naturally abundant in carrots—that scientists funded by the National Cancer Institute have handed out in capsules to select groups in the hope of blocking cancer. How did that happen? Because originally somebody noticed that people who eat carrots and other foods rich in carotenoids have less cancer. It is science's attempt to convert the observed powers of the food pharmacy into a pharmaceutical reality.

Trying to clarify the carrot factor has been a rocky intellectual ride with lots of twists and surprises, and it is far from over.

Actually, it all began not with carrots, but with liver—at least the type of vitamin A in liver. Crucial to the mystery is the fact that vitamin A comes in two forms: preformed retinol from animal foods such as liver and milk, and plant carotene which is converted in the body to usable retinol. In 1967 National Cancer Institute scientists discovered that retinol animal-derived vitamin A squelched respiratory cancer in hamsters. Very quickly scientists were sure they were hot on the trail of a potential cancer antidote.

Dramatically buttressing the case was a growing mountain of evidence from surveys linking higher cancer rates to diets low in vitamin A. During the 1970s fifteen studies from Israel, Norway, Japan, China, France, Iran, and the United States all suggested that people who ate more "vitamin A foods" had less chance of cancer, particularly of the stomach, lung, esophagus, colon, rectum, and bladder. A crucial clue—misjudged at the time—was the fascinating fact that consistently topping the lists of antidotal cancer foods were dark-orange and dark-green vegetables. Considered mere vitamin A factories with no other talents, these vegetables were simply lumped in with meat-type vitamin A foods.

Nobody worried. The theory made superb scientific sense. Vitamin A controls cell differentiation, which is what gets out of whack in cancer. Also, vitamin A protects the epithelial cells of the body's inner and outer linings, the skin, lungs, and throat—precisely the areas vitamin A foods seemed to guard from cancer.

But then scientists came up against major snags; animal studies were equivocal. Low blood levels of vitamin A were not consistently tied to higher risks of cancer. Shot through with conflicting data, the vitamin A–cancer theory began to fall apart.

Still, surveys pinpointing dark-green and dark-orange vegetables and fruits as weapons against cancer did not go away; they proliferated. Scientists scratched their heads in confusion—until Richard Peto and his colleagues at the Imperial Cancer Research Fund, Cancer

Studies Unit, in Oxford, England, rode to the rescue with a provocative paper in *Nature* in 1981. Peto solved the dilemma by suggesting
that it was beta carotene—the substance that *converts* to vitamin
A–and not the preformed vitamin A in animal foods—that lifted vegetables and fruits to their status as prime depressors of cancer rates.

Of course! His argument produced a scientific sigh of relief.
Vegetables and fruits are chock-full of a family of about 500 compounds
called carotenoids, of which about ten percent, including beta carotene,
are converted in the body to usable vitamin A. Of these vitamin
A–activity carotenoids, beta carotene is the superstar. And it's concentrated in carrots, sweet potatoes, winter squash, spinach, and kale.
Most of the world (the United States excepted) gets some ninety
percent of its vitamin A from such plant foods—green leafy vegetables
being the biggest source in Asia.

With a clearer picture of the carrot factor, new investigations
came up with some splashy stuff. A blockbuster: a study in *The Lancet*
in 1981 by noted epidemiologist Richard Shekelle, Ph.D., et al., now at
the University of Texas. The research clearly identified beta carotene,
not vitamin A, as dramatic protection against lung cancer. The researchers since 1957 had tracked 2000 men, how much they ate of 195
specific foods, and who got lung cancer. The conclusion: "A diet
relatively high in beta carotene may reduce the risk of lung cancer *even
among persons who have smoked cigarettes for many years.*" Specifically,
men eating the least carotene-containing foods were *seven times* more
likely to get lung cancer than men with the diet richest in carotene.
Dr. Shekelle made no bones about recommending "a half cup of carrots a
day" to help prevent lung cancer.

Because beta carotene is an old substance, long used as a drug in
dermatology, virtually nontoxic, and readily available from Hoffmann-
LaRoche, testing it on animals is a snap. The suspected anticancer
agent was bestowed on laboratory animals with sensational results. For
example, Eli Seifter, Ph.D., professor of biochemistry at the Albert
Einstein College of Medicine in New York, and his colleagues exposed
rats to carcinogens and then fed them high doses of beta carotene from
two to nine weeks later. Dr. Seifter describes beta carotene as a kind
of "morning-after" pill. The substance blocked tumors from appearing
and growing. Generally, the earlier given, the greater the potency, but
there was a grace period of about five to six weeks in which beta
carotene either worked in discouraging the "late stages of tumor
development and/or the early stages of tumor growth." In fact, beta
carotene when combined with therapeutic radiation even caused full-

size tumors to virtually disappear. This jibes with epidemiological evidence suggesting that beta carotene foods can somehow check damage after continual onslaughts from carcinogens like cigarette smoke.

Striking studies by both Micheline Mathews-Roth of Harvard Medical School and Andrija Kornhauser, Ph.D., at the Food and Drug Administration show that laboratory animals subjected to ultraviolet light simply do not develop skin cancers—if they are fed high doses of beta carotene.

Swayed by mounting evidence that beta carotene might intercept the human tragedy known as cancer, the National Cancer Institute in 1982 started extensive human experiments. The best-known test is headed by Dr. Charles Hennekens of the Harvard School of Public Health, in which about 22,000 physicians are taking either a capsule of beta carotene or a placebo (inert substance) for five years to find out whether beta carotene prevents cancers of all types. Additionally, there are beta carotene intervention tests for specific cancers—six studies on lung cancer, including a large one in Finland and one in China, two on colon, two on esophagus (including a large study in China), and three on skin. The results of the studies are expected between 1990 and 1992.

Meanwhile, both good news and new mysteries about beta carotene's cancer-fighting powers pile up. One problem plaguing scientists was that vitamin A levels in blood didn't consistently link up with cancer rates. But low blood levels of beta carotene do! It appears that the less beta carotene flowing through your veins, the greater your susceptibility to lung cancer. A 1987 landmark study by the late Marilyn Menkes, Ph.D., of the Johns Hopkins University School of Hygiene and Public Health, published in the *New England Journal of Medicine*, laid out a grim connection between low beta carotene in the blood and the appearance of lung cancer nine years later.

She and her co-investigator used samples of blood collected and analyzed for beta carotene in 1974; then in 1983 they located the blood donors and found ninety-nine with lung cancer. They compared the blood levels of beta carotene from lung cancer victims with those of similar donors who did not get cancer. To be sure, low beta carotene in the blood predicted lung cancer. Those with the lowest beta carotene were 2.2 times more likely to get lung cancer than those with the highest levels. More striking, low beta carotene in the blood was dramatically linked to squamous cell carcinoma—a sort of skin cancer of the lung lining—the most common killer from cigarette smoking.

Individuals with the least beta carotene in their blood had *four times* the risk of developing this smoker's cancer than those with the most beta carotene. How much beta carotene you eat is readily reflected in the blood.

Dr. Menkes calculated that upping intakes of beta carotene foods might prevent from 15,000 to 20,000 lung cancer deaths a year.

And how much more every day would people have to eat to accomplish that?

Roughly the amount found in one carrot, according to one analysis.

One carrot?

That's right.

As the potency of the carrot factor emerges, it seems most firmly committed to blocking epithelial cancers, notably of the lung. Scientists have united with astonishing unanimity in endorsing natural carotene against lung cancer. Ten out of eleven epidemiological studies worldwide find that *something*—investigators usually single out beta carotene—in deep-green leafy and deep-orange vegetables and fruits substantially slashes the risk of lung cancer. The average chances of lung cancer for those who skimp on high carotene foods doubles or triples. Carotene fare appears to protect nonsmokers, in particular ex-smokers, and, to a very slight extent, even current smokers, from future catastrophe. However, researchers shout to the rafters at every scientific meeting that any benefit from beta carotene is infinitesimal compared with the overwhelming power of cigarettes to push cells toward cancer. Diet is a futile screen against the carcinogenic disaster of filling the lungs with smoke.

Eating high carotene foods may also help prevent another typical smoker's cancer—of the larynx in that critical period after quitting smoking. Says Dorothy Mackerras of the University of Texas School of Public Health in Houston of her study among chemical plant workers: "Once you stop smoking, it would seem that carotene can help the larynx heal, so you're less likely to get laryngeal cancer." She found that of those who quit smoking two to ten years ago, the low carotene eaters had five and a half times the risk of developing laryngeal cancer as those with high carotene intake. But the beta carotene guarded only *former* smokers; it was not tough enough to overcome the cancer-causing powers of constant smoke bombardment to the larynx cells. Interestingly, she found no protection from taking vitamin A pills—which are made of retinol.

What is the source or nature of the power of these carotenoids, especially beta carotene? How do they work? How precisely can they fight cancer within cells? New discoveries bring surprises here, too, as well as promises of previously undreamed of health benefits. Originally, it was assumed that beta carotene's conversion to vitamin A was what made it a cancer antagonist. But it is more complex and exciting than that. Beta carotene, it turns out, unlike ordinary vitamin A, is an antioxidant. That makes it like a Mack truck in tracking down and snuffing out carcinogens. Beta carotene can quench dangerous molecules of supercharged oxygen that race around the body causing destruction. In other words, beta carotene's antioxidant drug effect in protecting cells is independent of its chameleonlike transformation into vitamin A.

That finding opens the floodgates to ever new and vast possibilities. The fact that beta carotene is an antioxidant stretches its potential pharmacological talents even beyond cancer protection to encompass all the physiological possibilities associated with antioxidants. Exciting new evidence suggests that beta carotene indeed has, according to Dr. Norman Krinsky, a noted authority on antioxidants and professor of biochemistry and pharmacology at the Tufts University School of Medicine, "widespread immunological effects." Researchers find that it stimulates production of T-helper cells, vital functionaries that guard against all infections. Japanese scientists note that beta carotene helps prevent both viral and chemical cancer by "augmenting the immuno-surveillance system," making tissue more immune to cancer damage. As an antioxidant, beta carotene foods predictably would guard the cardiovascular system, act as antiinflammatory agents, and even retard aging.

Moreover, this means that beta carotene can no longer be held up as the single, or perhaps even most potent, anticancer agent in high-carotene foods like carrots, spinach, kale, and sweet potatoes. For if vitamin A activity is not the main marker of cancer-fighting ability, all the other hundreds of carotenoid pigments in these foods may also find a place in the sun. Indeed, it appears that nearly all carotenoids in foods are antioxidants of various strengths. Dr. Krinsky, for example, tested canthaxanthin, a vegetable carotenoid that has no vitamin A activity at all. It, too, in test tubes prevented cells from becoming cancerous and in animals blocked tumors just as beta carotene did. Dr. Krinsky credits the carotenoid's antioxidant effects on unknown chemical powers unrelated to vitamin A. That means that beta carotene has no corner on anticancer activity.

In fact, some experts strongly suspect that other carotenoids, and not beta carotene, are the main cancer antagonists in certain foods.

According to Dr. Frederick Khachik, of the United States Department of Agriculture, analyses of the foods most uniformly linked to lower cancer risks in epidemiological studies—broccoli, brussels sprouts, cabbage, kale, and spinach—reveal that they have much higher concentrations of other carotenoids than of beta carotene. Only nineteen percent of spinach's and kale's total carotenoids are beta and similar vitamin A–type carotene. The figure is a mere ten percent for broccoli and brussels sprouts and eight percent for cabbage. However, all of these anticancer vegetables possess exceptionally high levels of another carotenoid called lutein. Dr. Khachik thinks lutein, not beta carotene, may be the main carotenoid that makes such foods champion cancer fighters.

And that really makes for a strange and exciting kettle of carrots. That suggests that protection by high carotenoid foods like carrots and spinach may not issue from a single beta carotene bullet but from a collusion of hundreds of untested, antioxidant carotenoids plus other unknowns. It's what British Columbia cancer expert Dr. Hans Stich calls "a cocktail effect," which he considers insufficiently explored. Nature does not fashion itself after Eli Lilly or Hoffmann-LaRoche or Searle. More likely, he philosophizes, foods release a shower of chemoprevention unmatched by a single drug. By mixing beta carotene, and other antioxidants, he expects a cumulative effect—greater and less toxic than from one food chemical alone. This cocktail effect, he says, "is what the diet probably already does." And he reminds us: at this point we do not know that beta carotene or any other specific carrot factor prevents cancer. All we do know is that eating fruits and vegetables seems to.

Thus, the elusive "carrot factor," despite current infatuation with one carrot essence—beta carotene—is quite likely the *whole carrot itself—and the whole broccoli floret, brussels sprout, and spinach and kale leaf.*

BEST SOURCES OF ANTICANCER CAROTENOIDS*

Apricots, especially dried (high in beta carotene)
Broccoli
Brussels sprouts
Cabbage, green
Carrots (high in beta carotene)
Kale (highest in all carotenoids)
Lettuce
Spinach
Squash (high in beta carotene)
Sweet potatoes (high in beta carotene)
Tomatoes

*Rule: The darker green the leafy vegetable and the deeper orange the fruit or vegetable, the richer it is in carotenoids.

9.

THE CRANBERRY'S STRANGE ANTIBIOTIC

Dr. Anthony Sobota, a microbiology professor at Youngstown State University in Ohio, was not seeking to make a name for himself as discoverer of the "cranberry antibiotic." He was looking for better treatments for urinary tract infections. He was running drugs through sensitive tests to see if they worked in a new way—not by killing bacteria but by preventing their adherence to the surface cells of the urinary tract.

The traditional way to curb infections is to kill the bacteria outright or disrupt their life processes, stopping them from reproducing. Thus, antibiotics like penicillin typically attack the bacteria's cell wall or interfere with the microbe's production of enzymes or nucleic acids that allow it to spread and establish strongholds within the body.

However, in the last decade, scientists have become extremely interested in combating bacteria another way: by stopping them from sticking to healthy cells in the first place. If the bugs can't stick to the cells, so the theory goes, they can't cause infections. Scientists in Sweden had found that bacteria causing urinary tract infections are particularly apt at working their damage by adherence; only those bacteria that managed to gain a foothold on urinary tract cells induced disease. So, Dr. Sobota reasoned, thwarting the bacteria's ability to stick would combat the disease process at the moment of inception, even before symptoms developed.

It was fairly simple to determine. He obtained bladder surface cells from the urine of women, then he mixed them with bacteria, and stained the bacteria red. By looking under a microscope he could count how many of the red-tinged bacteria were sticking to the cells. It was the same situation bacteria would face in the urinary tract. If they stuck, they would spread and cause infection.

Dr. Sobota had disappointing results with low or sublethal doses (not enough to kill bacteria) of antibiotics such as ampicillin, a synthetic relative of penicillin, that are traditionally used to treat urinary tract infections. When he looked under the microscope, the bacteria were still there, clinging happily to the cell surfaces. Then a student suggested he try cranberry juice, which a local hospital was using successfully to treat paraplegics, who are uncommonly susceptible to urinary tract infections.

Dr. Sobota knew it wasn't crazy. References in the medical literature on cranberries dated back to 1860. In 1923 two American physicians fed cranberries to humans and noticed increased hippuric acid, a reputed antibacterial substance, in their urine. Later researchers pinpointed quinic acid in cranberries as the agent generating the hippuric acid. A Wisconsin physician in 1962 reported great success by giving six ounces of cranberry juice twice a day to prevent and cure urinary tract problems; one patient, a sixty-six-year-old woman with a longstanding kidney inflammation (chronic pyelonephritis), was free of disease within eight weeks, and even after two and a half years refused to give up the cranberry juice, vowing it was the only medicine that helped her. In another experiment, about seventy percent of a group of women and men with acute urinary tract infections improved after drinking sixteen ounces of commercial cranberry juice for twenty-one days.

All of these decades of probing concluded that if cranberries worked, it was because they raise the acid levels of the urine. And as every medical student knows, acidified urine is like a mild antibiotic; it kills off or disables bacteria that hang around the urinary tract causing trouble. It's this commonsense theory that even now gives cranberry folk medicine credibility among physicians. "Sure, urologists tell people to use cranberry juice to prevent urinary tract infections and kidney stones. I think it's something all of us do. What the cranberries do is acidify urine," says Dr. Price Stuart, Jr., president of the American Urological Association.

But does this easily verified biochemical reaction state the total truth? Nature might be more subtle, still making doctors right, but for the wrong reason. More complex hidden chemistry might account for the legendary reputation of the cranberry. Dr. Sobota wondered. Maybe . . .

He went out, bought some cranberry juice cocktail at a supermarket, and also squeezed some juice out of whole cranberries. He then did the same thing with the cranberries he had done with the drugs he was testing. When he looked under the microscope, he could see the bacteria had slipped and slid off the cells like raindrops off a roof. They could not seem to get a grip.

"Here I was adding antibiotics, trying to knock the bugs off to prevent them from adhering, and the drugs were working only poorly. I tried the juice and it cleaned everything; it knocked everything off. I was just astounded. I could not believe it."

How much better did the cranberry juice do than the low doses of drugs?

"Dramatically, by a factor of ten."

The juice was ten times more effective?

"That's right."

The stronger the concentration of juice, the greater the effect. However, cranberry juice cocktail—from twenty-five to thirty-three percent pure berry juice—taken right off store shelves proved plenty potent. The bacteria were even rendered helpless when the juice was diluted to one part juice per hundred parts water, so powerful is the agent.

Here's what probably happened, says Dr. Sobota: The bacteria attach themselves to cells through thousands of hollow rodlike structures called pili. These pili are the docking tentacles that hook into cell surfaces. To effect a perfect connection, both the pili and the cells have receptors that fit perfectly, like a key in a lock. Somehow, an agent or agents in the cranberries plugged up those receptors, just like jamming gum into a keyhole, so the attachment could not take place. Dr. Sobota is not sure whether the cranberry factor envelops the bacteria or the cells or both, but the effect is the same—a "receptor blockade." Without stickum capabilities, bacteria are flushed harmlessly out of the body in a river of urine.

It was exactly what Dr. Sobota had been searching for—an agent to control bacteria in a new, ingenious way; only it didn't come from a pharmaceutical factory—it came from a food store.

But what if the cranberry agent is destroyed or inactivated in the digestive tract, and thus does not perform in the human body as it does in a petri dish? To be sure the cranberry factor was biologically active, Dr. Sobota tested both plain cranberry juice, and, more important, the urine from animals and humans *after* they had drunk cranberry juice. The active agent was still there and potent; the urine generally contained high levels of "the cranberry factor," and showed potent activity in keeping harmful bugs from sticking to cells. In one group of people, about seventy percent of those who drank fifteen ounces of cranberry juice cocktail had significant amounts of the antibacterial chemical in their urine. The factor showed up in the urine within one to three hours after the juice was drunk and there's some evidence it remained potent for twelve to fifteen hours.

That the cranberry factor survived in the urine is the essence of the breakthrough, according to Dr. James Tillotson, vice-president of technical research and development at Ocean Spray, a maker of cranberry juice. "That's what makes Sobota's work so new and exciting and proves cranberries have something unique," he says. In short, the active agent peculiar to cranberries gets in the urine, and subsequently into the bladder and kidneys, where it sits a while, and, in fact, moves through the entire urinary tract, washing against cells and bacteria, preventing their sticking together and thus, presumably, aborting an infection. It is like a chemical therapeutic soup that is flushed along the entire urinary tract.

At this writing, the precise "cranberry factor" has not been isolated and identified. Dr. Sobota is searching for it among thousands of chemicals in the urine of people who have drunk cranberry juice. So are workers in the Ocean Spray labs. And pharmaceutical companies have expressed interest in turning it into a drug when it is identified.

Unusual? Yes, in the fact that a scientist has at long last discovered a surprising new way that nature fights pathogens—by gently wrapping their prey in a Teflon-like coating so they can't attach to healthy cells—which is a mechanism only recently explored in pharmaceutical companies in attempts to develop new synthetic infection-fighters. But there is nothing unique about the *presence* of antibiotics in foods.

Penicillin itself was isolated from bread mold. Human populations on remote islands sometimes show a mysterious resistance to modern-day antibiotics, suggesting they have been subjected to large naturally occurring antibiotic doses in foods. And what about those discoveries that found tetracycline—yes, tetracycline—in the skeletons of Sudanese Nubians who lived on the flood plains of the Nile in A.D. 350? Anthropologists note that infections were remarkably low among these peoples, probably due to the periodic ingestion of natural antibiotics in grains and beer. Rates of infectious disease were also reportedly low among the laborers who built Cheops's pyramid—one anthropologist speculates this was due to their "radish-onions-garlic diet."

Many spices and herbs commonly used in traditional medicine are known to contain antibiotic properties. One analysis listed sixty different chemicals with antibacterial activity that occur naturally in foods and plants. Among common foodstuffs from which known antibacterial agents have been isolated are apples, buckwheat, chili peppers, water chestnuts, eggs, garlic, ginger, honey, hops, milk, onions, radishes, tea, and yogurt.

The cranberry is not the only formidable antibiotic surprise to pop out of nature's pharmacopoeia. It's just one of the most remarkable.

10.

WINE, TEA, AND THE MARVELOUS PHENOLS

Imagine a class of natural drugs so monumental, so extensive in the food supply, so biologically active that their potential in protecting health is absolutely dazzling. Scientists throughout the world are overwhelmed by their abilities to knock out viruses and bacteria, block the cancer process, and perform a multitude of functions that strengthen the cardiovascular system. These compounds are little publicized, yet they are one of the National Cancer Institute's top priorities for investigation as a natural anticancer compound. They are the mighty polyphenols that include astringent-tasting compounds called tannins, and their reputation is growing as a source of scientific fascination. They may be a secret weapon against a variety of diseases and if eaten judiciously could add immeasurably to health.

The battle between viruses and fruit-rich polyphenols produced some memorable research from Canada. In the 1970s two government virologists noticed that a virus touched by strawberry extract became paralyzed and unable to carry on its usual routine, that is, it could not penetrate a healthy cell membrane, inserting its DNA into the cell nucleus and directing the cell's vital genetic machinery to produce a flood of new viruses to ravage the organism. Thinking this had great implications for controlling viral infections with certain foods, Dr. Jack Konowalchuk, now retired, and Joan I. Speirs, at Canada's Bureau of Microbial Hazards, Food Directorate, set about testing several fruit extracts against common infection-producing viruses.

They grew a bunch of viruses in plastic dishes and then drew up a fruit salad shopping list for feeding the viruses: one pint of blueberries, 1½ pounds of blue Ribier grapes, one pomegranate, three quarts of fresh strawberries, two twenty-ounce packages of unsweetened frozen strawberries of different brands, and one half to one pound each of peaches, plums, crabapples, wild cranberries, and raspberries.

After some chemical purifications, the Canadian scientists ended up with several containers of the multicolored liquid fruit extracts, which they then added in various amounts to test tubes of waiting viruses in cell-tissue cultures.

After twenty-four hours they went with high hopes to inspect the fruit-virus mixture; they were stunned and excited by the desolation. It was clearly a virus Waterloo. Only a few survived. Dr. Konowalchuk theorizes that the fruit chemicals erected some sort of biochemical barrier around the viruses that prevented their breaking through the membranes of cells in the tissue cultures. Impotent to invade cells to get to their source of life, the viruses simply perished in large numbers.

Remarkably, every single fruit extract defeated the viruses. Although higher concentrations of fruit extracts were most virulent, even low doses were potent. Virtually none of the polioviruses survived (less than one percent) after being face-to-face for twenty-four hours in a test tube with extract of blueberry, crabapple, cranberry, grape, plum, pomegranate, raspberry, or strawberry. Even when the extract was diluted ten to one, practically all the viruses were crippled. Peaches were least effective: still, when diluted, peaches neutralized about eighty percent of the poliovirus.

The researchers concluded that "the antiviral components of various fruits and plants may act both on viruses and host cells to prevent infections."

Heartened by their unexpected results, they went on to test apples, grapes, wine, and nineteen commercial juices and beverages taken right off supermarket shelves. Freshly squeezed apple juice, commercial grape juice, as well as wine and tea proved extraordinarily potent against viruses.

Throughout the investigation, the researchers had been trying to identify the active antiviral agents in the fruits. In both apples and grapes, for example, they were sure the active compounds resided in the skin and pulp. They tested pure compounds of ascorbic acid, chlorogenic acid, gallic acid, vanillin, and tannic acid or tannin (the stuff that gives tea and wine its astringent taste)—all phenols. Tannic acid was an especially potent enemy of viruses. "There is no question that tannins will coat virus particles and neutralize them," explains Dr. Konowalchuk. "Somehow the tannin comes between the virus and the cell surface so the virus can't penetrate the cell. So the viruses kind of die off."

The Canadian researchers were sure the main virus antagonist in grape juice was the polyphenols, including tannin, and suspected it was also the case for apple juice and tea. In fact, they had tested pure grape tannin sent from France's Bordeaux region and found that it was antiviral against several viruses. Bordeaux. That smacks of wine. Exactly. Red wines are full of tannins. Although white wines also proved somewhat antiviral, red wines were much more potent. Later Dr. Konowalchuk screened some wines for tannin content and found that Italian red wines were richer than Canadian or French wines in tannins. He analyzed grapes used to make wines in Italy. He even discovered that red wine was, alas, even more antiviral than grape juice itself. "Something in the wine made it better; I never found out what."

By that time the research was an internal hot potato.

It is one thing to talk about drinking apple juice and tea for your health; those are like mother's milk, but wine! Is it really good public policy to search for the antiinfectious attributes of an alcoholic beverage? And what was all this about trying it out on the herpes virus? The newspapers had a good time with it.

Dr. Konowalchuk had also become particularly intrigued by tannin's ability to control the herpes simplex virus, the one that causes cold sores. "I said, hey, look at that; the herpes virus is extra sensitive." So one day when he had a cold sore, he dabbed on a little freeze-dried red wine concentrate used in the research (he says the sticky residue left after a little wine evaporates also contains concentrated tannins). "The pain disappeared instantly. The lesion shriveled up; no scab appeared. And that was the end of it." Dr. Konowalchuk believes the wine extract was able to penetrate the broken skin of the sore, reaching the virus and disabling it, just as occurred in test tubes. Other people in the lab started coming back and asking for wine extract to treat their cold sores. And one thing led to another.

Since, Dr. Konowalchuk says, viruses in the same family often react similarly, he wanted to test it on the herpes type 2 virus, the one associated with genital disease. He had even arranged with a gynecologist to do a small study of volunteers with herpes to see if the concentrated tannins worked as a topical application. But it never happened. The grape studies rotted on the vine. The controversy was too much for the government. Dr. Konowalchuk says the money was cut off. He retired, although he still uses freeze-dried red wine to heal his cold sores and ponders occasionally whether Italians who regularly drink red wine have fewer viral infections. He thinks it seems likely.

It also seems likely that many of the phenolics turn off cancer and generally protect body tissues from all kinds of harm. Phenolics are also formidable antioxidants—scavengers that round up those highly reactive oxygen-free radicals hell-bent on cell destruction. Thus, polyphenols, like other antioxidants, are general benefactors, guardians to ward off the everyday cellular attacks that cause the body to deteriorate and develop numerous symptoms of disease. Ingesting polyphenols is like giving yourself an internal shower with jet sprays of health-promoting chemicals.

Scientists are especially excited about the phenols' cancer-fighting properties because they provide a triple threat. They potentially defeat cancer by at least three mechanisms: they can shut off the formation of carcinogens, turn up the body's natural detoxification defenses, and suppress cancer promotion.

There's no doubt that certain phenolics widely present in common food—especially ones called caffeic acid, ellagic acid, ferulic acid, and gallotannic acid—block mutations or overt cancer in tissue cultures and animals. Dr. Lee Wattenberg, discoverer of the anticancer cabbage chemicals, has also extensively tested the plant phenols and their antioxidant capabilities in blocking cancer. For example, he found that giving mice caffeic or ferulic acid before exposing them to cancer-causing agents reduced the incidence of stomach cancers by forty percent. Japanese scientists in 1985 proclaimed a type of gallotannic acid in green tea the most potent natural antimutagen they had so far tested. In exquisite experiments, Michael J. Wargovich at the University of Texas and Harold Newmark, now at Rutgers, observed much less nucleic and DNA destruction in the colon cells of mice that were fed caffeic, ferulic, and ellagic acid prior to exposure to the cancer-producing agents. Thus the theory that plant phenolics may prevent cancer by pumping blocking agents into cells to shield DNA from harm and prevent them from actually being inoculated with carcinogens.

Food phenols can also act in their antioxidant capacity to thwart formation of one of the most powerful family of carcinogens, called nitrosamines. Nitrosamines can form when sodium nitrite or nitrate, in cured meats, chemically reacts with ubiquitous compounds called amines. In the 1970s there was a wide search, spurred by government fears of the cancer-causing nitrosamines in bacon and other cured meats, for a way of blocking that dangerous conversion of nitrites and amines to nitrosamines. Several scientists, including Newmark, then at Hoffmann-LaRoche, discovered that vitamins C and E, antioxidants, did just that, resulting in the routine use of vitamin C in processing cured meats. However, at the same time, just by accident, Newmark's group also discovered that two plant phenols, caffeic and ferulic acid, also "were superb in blocking nitrosamines—in fact, far better than anything else, even vitamins C and E."

Following up on that, Dr. Hans Stich, at the University of British Columbia, discovered that not only pure caffeic and ferulic acids, but also the *ordinary beverages tea and coffee,* rich in the polyphenols, inhibited the conversion to the carcinogenic nitrosamines in the intestinal tract of both animals and *humans.* Furthermore, Dr. Stich tested instant coffee, instant decaffeinated coffee, roasted coffee, one Japanese tea, one black Indian tea, and one Chinese tea—and found that all of them blocked the mutagenicity process preceding cancer in test tubes—*and in doses at which they are ordinarily consumed.*

Dr. Stich is convinced that "the importance of phenols are underestimated as anticarcinogenic agents." He points out that although beta carotene (on which he is also a prominent researcher) has stolen the limelight in the search for natural cancer antidotes; in fact, vegetables and fruits contain more polyphenols than they do beta carotene, and fruits particularly have little beta carotene, but are rich in phenols of various types. He notes that apples have large amounts of phenolics; yet they have never really been tested properly for anticancer activity. "And wine, tea, and coffee are loaded with phenolics."

So wine could be anticancer?

"It could be, especially red wine. And beer has a relatively large amount of phenolics from the hops."

A particularly intriguing type of tannin or phenol concentrated in tea, especially green tea, is called catechin. Dr. Stich thinks this tea catechin may be just as powerful as beta carotene in helping suppress the appearance of oral cancers among snuff users and tobacco chewers, a major problem in certain parts of the world. He has extracted catechin from green tea and put it in capsules for testing as a prophylactic in people at high risk for oral cancer.

In many worldwide studies, the polyphenols, especially tea catechins, have been building a formidable reputation as protectors of the cardiovascular system. For example, experiments show that ellagic acid can lower blood pressure in animals and control hemorrhage in animals and humans, apparently by activating blood coagulation. This is not surprising because tea catechins have been hailed in literally hundreds of experiments in Russia and India as strengthening capillary walls and slowing down atherosclerosis. Green tea catechins are therapeutically used in the Soviet Union to treat diseases resulting from "capillary failure." Tested in humans by Soviet scientists, a mixture of tea polyphenols and half the daily recommended allowance of vitamin C were found to increase capillary strength up to five times that of controls deprived of polyphenols and vitamin C. In fact, according to a recent Russian report, "It has been shown that tea catechins are superior to every known capillary-strengthening drug."

Tea infusions are also reported to have an antiinflammatory action. Green tea was much more potent than black Indian teas. Green tea polyphenols also, according to Russian studies, increase resistance to infections in animal tests, and have been used extensively in Japan to combat dysentery.

In a recent review of tea-health research, Mikhail A. Bokuchava of the Bakh Institute of Biochemistry, Academy of Sciences, U.S.S.R., summed up the findings of extensive studies of tea by two Russian scientists, attributing the therapeutic effects mainly to the properties of tea catechins: "It was ascertained that consumption of green tea brew had a therapeutic effect on infectious diseases, particularly dysentery. An application of green tea brew for treatment of hypertension decreased blood pressure, alleviated headaches, and improved the general health state of patients. Green tea brew beneficially influenced the cardiovascular system, fluid-electrolyte balance, hematopoiesis and renal function . . . with no cases of local blood congestion due to thrombosis, in spite of the fact that no anticoagulants were used. . . . An incorporation of green tea brew into the combined antirheumatic therapy at an active stage of rheumatism revealed its favorable effect on the general condition and subjective feelings of patients, as well as on their capillary resistance . . . and inflammatory processes. They also used green tea brew as a therapeutic method for chronic hepatitis, mainly of viral origin, and reported its beneficial effects. . . . The researchers concluded that tea liquor should be used as a prophylactic drug to prevent such common diseases as hypertension and atherosclerosis." No wonder Dr. Bokuchava commented, "tea beverage is often called an elixir of life."

As Dr. Stich notes: "Phenols have not had nearly the attention they merit."

WHERE TO FIND THE PROTECTIVE POLYPHENOLS

Because there are so many different phenols (around 200), and each may have different physiological effects, it is difficult to pinpoint which foods may be most therapeutic, and no thorough analysis of the polyphenol content of foods has ever been made. However, spot checks have found apples, dry tea shoots, potatoes, and brewed coffee to be extraordinarily rich in chlorogenic acid, confirmed to have anticancer properties. Grapes, certain nuts, and strawberries have high concentrations of ellagic acid, a powerful inhibitor of mutagenesis. Wine, especially red wine, is astoundingly high in gallic acid. (Red wine also contains chemicals that may promote cell mutations in test tubes.) Wheat bran and barley seed are high in ferulic acid, another laboratory-proven anticancer compound. Plums, cherries, apples, pears, and grapes are high in cinnamic acid, another phenol shown to be biologically active.

Tea is a formidable package of the phenols known as catechin, with green tea more than twice as potent as black tea. Green tea contains eighty to 170 milligrams of catechin per gram of dry tea compared with thirty to seventy milligrams in black tea. The longer the tea is brewed, the greater the infusion of catechin. Instant tea is also rich in catechin, green about three times as concentrated, according to one analysis.

11.

MORE FANTASTIC
YOGURT TALES

Dr. Elias Metchnikoff, Russian by birth, was a rather famous late nineteenth-century scientist, a close friend of the great bacteriologist Louis Pasteur, and subdirector of the prestigious Pasteur Institute in Paris. He discovered phagocytes, cells that help defend the body by ingesting microorganisms and foreign particles, and won a Nobel prize in 1908 for his work in immunology. In 1916, when Dr. Metchnikoff died, *Nature* magazine hailed him as "one of the most remarkable figures in the scientific world."

It's safe to say that few today can recite his vast scientific accomplishments, but virtually everyone has been left, whether they know it or not, with a legacy of his fertile brain—all because in the early 1900s he wrote two popular books, *The Nature of Man* and *The Prolongation of Life*. In them he propounded his theory that much disease is caused by microbial putrefaction in the intestines. The process, he believed, literally poisoned the body by releasing toxins that destroyed artery walls and caused senility and early death.

However, he was convinced that the destructive intestinal microbes could be counteracted—prevented from proliferating and secreting their poisons—by other microbes in fermented or "sour" milk, better known to us as yogurt. In *The Prolongation of Life*, he wrote: "From time immemorial human beings have absorbed quantities of lactic microbes by consuming in the uncooked condition substances such as soured milk, kephir, sauerkraut, or salted cucumbers which have undergone lactic fermentation. By these means they have unknowingly lessened the evil consequences of intestinal putrefaction."

He and his colleagues at the Pasteur Institute set out to test their theory on mice using a sour milk called yahourth from Bulgaria. In the course of the research, they isolated from the yahourth a lactic-acid-producing microbe, which they dubbed *Bulgarian bacillus.* As part of the yahourth experiment, they gave groups of mice lactic acid, a variety of microbes, and the new Bulgarian yahourth microbe. Sure enough, the mice eating the Bulgarian bacilli from yahourth thrived the best, had the most offspring, and exhibited the least intestinal putrefaction, a sign to Dr. Metchnikoff that he was indeed right. He began drinking a pint or so of the special "sour milk" every day. In 1900, sure he had found one of the secrets to long life, he arranged for the commercial marketing of a "sour milk" but scrupulously refused to share in any profits.

To his great delight, stories corroborating his faith in yogurt's life-stretching powers poured in—tales of people in Africa, France, Eastern Europe, even America, who ate curdled milk and had extraordinary longevity. He reports: "M. Nogueira has written to me to say how much he was astonished on revisiting after a long period of absence the district of Massamedes, to find the natives so well preserved and displaying so few traces of senility. (They use sour milk copiously.) . . . And M. Grigoroff, a Bulgarian student at Geneva, has been surprised by the number of centenarians to be found in Bulgaria, a region in which yahourth, a soured milk, is the staple food."

Yes, it is the late, great Nobel prize-winning immunologist, Dr. Metchnikoff, whom we must thank for those haunting, indelible images of old, wrinkled centenarians tromping through the Balkans, fit as twenty-year-olds and destined to outlive us all because of their prodigious consumption of yogurt. Yogurt's ties to longevity did not rise from the nebulous haze of folk medicine, after all, but from the scientific genius of one Dr. Metchnikoff, the first to assert that yogurt's bacterial activity was the key to the food's legendary health powers.

To some of his peers, it was not his finest contribution: In his obituary, *Nature* lamented that "this small though valuable adventure of his in dietetics has been unfortunately, but perhaps inevitably, the one and only feature . . . which has impressed itself on the somewhat erratic intelligence of the man on the street."

Alas, the author of the *Nature* obituary and Dr. Metchnikoff might be amused to learn that three quarters of a century later, scientific minds renewed their quest for yogurt's ancient secrets, and rodents throughout the world are still busily lapping up yogurt, yahourt, kefir, yakult, koumiss, dahi—as it is variously called, in the service of science. Yogurt is proving to be one of nature's most pharmacologically potent foods. Even in ways Dr. Metchnikoff did not touch on. The yogurt tales are growing.

That is not to say that Dr. Metchnikoff had all his facts straight. To be clear, nobody has studied yogurt eaters for a lifetime and documented an abnormally long life span. In fact, because birth and death records among Balkan peasants are in such disarray, there's no proof that, as Dr. Metchnikoff's sources claimed, they do live longer. Furthermore, though Dr. Metchnikoff insisted that lactic acid was the main therapeutic agent in yogurt, he suspected that other mysterious, unknown antibacterial products were also present. True. Recent scientific investigations find that yogurt contains plenty of knock-'em-dead antibiotics as well as other health properties—a fact that would undoubtedly please Dr. Metchnikoff immensely.

Not surprisingly, much current research tries to explain yogurt's reputed infection-fighting properties, and there is no question the evidence is compelling. For example, for nearly a decade, until 1985, United States Department of Agriculture scientists at Beltsville, Maryland, carried on an intensive study of the longevity and infection rates of rats made to dine on yogurt. (And you thought those fellows at Agriculture were dull!) In one recent test, civil servants at Agriculture fed rats yogurt or milk, then injected them with massive doses of salmonella bacteria—the same bugs that can infect humans. The rats who ate yogurt did not get as sick as those on the milk diet. And fewer of the yogurt eaters died. Decidedly, a yogurt factor made them more resistant to infection and kept them alive longer.

Romanian scientists at the Institute of Virology in Bucharest recently reported essentially the same thing in mice injected with lethal doses of influenza bugs. Mice given a yogurt substance with the viruses survived the flu infection much longer and had much lower mortality rates than mice deprived of yogurt. In one facet of the experiment, one hundred percent of the mice exposed only to the virus died, and one hundred percent of the infected mice fed yogurt lived.

There's evidence, too, that yogurt battles bacteria in humans. At the Medical Research Institute of Michael Reese Hospital in Chicago, two gastroenterologists fought off a citywide epidemic of diarrhea in the early 1960s with a preparation of lactobacillus acidophilus, one of the common bacteria types used to make fermented milk. Where conventional antibiotics had often failed, the concentrated lactobacillus acidophilus capsules worked remarkably well. Of fifty-nine patients with severe diarrhea, all but two got better almost instantly. Included were some whose diarrhea was associated with antibiotic use and serious bowel diseases such as diverticulitis and ulcerative colitis, as well as those who had had colostomies.

In some tests yogurt has surpassed routine drugs. Physicians at New York City's Jewish Memorial Hospital in 1963 fed forty-five infants who had been hospitalized with severe diarrhea one hundred milliliters (a little over three fluid ounces—or between a third and a half cup) of skim milk yogurt three times a day. In contrast, a control group of infected infants got appropriate doses of the drug Neomycin kaopectate. The average recovery time for those fed yogurt was 2.7 days compared with 4.8 days for those given the kaopectate. Yogurt, containing lactobacillus bulgaricus and streptococci thermophilus, was nearly twice as effective as the drug in speeding up recovery time.

A string of experiments done in the 1970s confirm that yogurt can be potent against organisms in the gastrointestinal tract. Several studies in Poland, Yugoslavia, and Japan—where fermented milk has been intensively studied—found that milk containing lactobacillus acidophilus alleviated dysentery. Treated with such milk, half of a group of Polish children with salmonella dysentery and two thirds of those with shigella dysentery were quickly cured. Furthermore, as long as they continued to drink the milk, none came down with the infection.

For six months in 1975 a group of 500 Japanese servicemen daily drank about a cup of yakult, a popular liquid fermented-milk drink. Not a single one had dysentery; fifty-five, or ten percent of another group of 500 servicemen who did not drink yakult came down with dysentery.

Since the days of Dr. Metchnikoff, scientists have credited yogurt's most potent antimicrobial activity to lactic acid, a by-product formed by adding bacterial cultures to milk. But scientists now know the process is more complex; the fermentation process spawns unique antibiotics, just as moldy bread yielded penicillin.

Dr. Khem Shahani, professor of food science at the University of Nebraska, has spent most of his professional life probing yogurt's health secrets, much of it searching for explanations about why the ancient food is a centuries-old remedy for infant diarrhea in countries along the Mediterranean Sea and was commonly drunk in watered-down form by shepherds in the Middle East to prevent intestinal diseases. In that pursuit, he and others have plucked from yogurt and other fermented milks, and tested in the lab, agents that act as antibiotics.

In 1963 Dr. Shahani isolated an antibiotic he dubbed acidophilin because it was formed in fermented milk by the L. acidophilus culture. He remembers it well. He was immediately besieged by drug companies hoping to make it the new penicillin. He hooked up with the pharmaceutical firm the Merck Company, which he says spent a lot of money on the project. He patented the antibiotic, but after five years it had not become the magic bullet. He subsequently found another antibiotic from yogurt, which he named Bulgarican because it came from the L. bulgaricus bacterial strain.

To date, investigators, including Dr. Shahani, have located at least seven distinct natural antibiotics in yogurt capable of killing a variety of intestinal-disease-causing microorganisms. Additionally, the yogurt lactobacilli spew off other microbe killers such as lactic acid, acetic acid, benzoic acid, and hydrogen peroxide.

How potent are they?

Dr. Shahani: "The antibiotic quality of acidophilin has been compared with the killing power of streptomycin, penicillin, Terramycin, and others."

Does it compare well?

"Oh, yes, extremely so."

Is it as potent as the drugs?

"More potent."

Dr. Shahani's most exciting moment came when he purified the acidophilin; he was the first person to extract the pure antibiotic substance from the fermented milk cultures. Until that is done, there is no hope of its being made into a drug. That the antibiotics never rivaled penicillin in the marketplace does not disturb Dr. Shahani now. The bloom is off the period when everything had to be distilled into a drug. It is far better, he says, to eat the pure yogurt—because, after all, the antibiotics are not everything. Yogurt promises far more.

THE IMMUNITY FACTOR

As a start, recent studies in Japan, Italy, and Switzerland, as well as in Dr. Shahani's labs, suggest that yogurt may fend off infections, not only through antibiotic action—by killing microbes outright (the Rambo approach to bacteriology)—but also by boosting the immune system's response to disease threats. The recognition that agents, including drugs, can make the body a better fortress against disease is a new frontier. In cancer therapy, such new agents are called biological modifiers; they are also termed immunostimulants (to spur the immune system to action) or immunopotentiators (to boost current immune functioning). Numerous drugs designed to buck up faltering immune systems have come on the market in the last few years.

In fact, in Japan, certain lactobacilli found in yogurt are already used as immunopotentiating pharmaceuticals, according to a prominent Italian immunologist, Dr. Claudio DeSimone at the University of Rome. Dr. DeSimone, too, has new respect for the bacilli's effect on immune functioning. In sophisticated laboratory studies on both mice and human blood cells published in 1985, he discovered that yogurt dramatically revved up the immune system's production of antibodies and other infection-fighting agents. In particular, the lactobacillus bulgaricus in yogurt gave rise to great numbers of so-called natural killer cells that combat infections, and tripled the amount of interferon manufactured by cells. (Interferon, one of the body's natural infection-fighting agents, has been found effective against a wide range of infections. It has also been tested with much less success in fighting cancer.) The yogurt bacteria, said Dr. DeSimone, improved immune functioning in the cells just as effectively as did a synthetic drug, Levaelsole, a so-called immunopotentiator expressly designed to boost human immune functioning.

When yogurt was added to their normal diets, within fifteen days mice showed an improved immune functioning both locally and systemically—in the digestive tract and in the bloodstream. This double response indicates yogurt might influence not only intestinal infections but infections throughout the body.

Dr. DeSimone admits he was quite surprised when he first saw the effects of the yogurt on the T cells of mice, and even more so when he learned that animals fed yogurt, when challenged by infectious antigens, developed more antibodies than those fed only milk. "I admit I was a skeptic," he says. "At the beginning of the work, I was on the other side. I thought it really doesn't work."

Do you eat yogurt now?

"Yes."

Did you eat yogurt before your studies?

"No." (A broad smile followed by uproarious laughter. A scientist caught in a personal interpretation of his data.)

You must believe in your work?

"You are right. I did suggest to my wife she eat yogurt too."

If you raise the body's immunocompetence, could that theoretically fight all kinds of infections, from both bacteria and viruses?

"Yes, I think so. I think it could be effective. When you give yogurt, maybe you stimulate in some way the immune system—that the body's struggle against bacteria is potentiated."

And do you think yogurt could make you live longer?

"It may be that if you have a better response, a better defense, you can live longer, maybe because you have fewer infections." At least Dr. Simone's yogurt-eating mice lived longer.

The yogurt longevity factor may also be linked to the fact that yogurt compounds can fight cancer. One of the earliest reports, in 1962, came from Bulgaria and claimed that L. bulgaricus, a yogurt-making bacteria commonly used in that country, possessed potent antitumor activity. Supposedly of 258 mice implanted with sarcoma, 180 (fifty-nine percent) were cured by the L. bulgaricus. Yogurt as a cancer fighter! It thrilled Dr. Shahani. For more than five years, in collaboration with researchers at the Sloan Kettering Institute for Cancer Research in New York City, he tried to isolate anticancer compounds from yogurt. Strains of L. bulgaricus and L. acidophilus did show anticancer activity, but not enough to interest drug companies or cause a splash among medical experts. His later studies found that yogurt (with L. bulgaricus) and acidophilus milk did squelch the growth of cancer cells in mice by about thirty percent.

In 1986 French scientists at the National Institute of Health and Medical Research in Paris uncovered the possibility that yogurt might somehow help ward off human breast cancer. They compared the diets of two groups of women: 1010 women with breast cancer and a comparable group of women without breast cancer. An outstanding difference in diet: Those women who ate yogurt the most often had the lowest risk of breast cancer, and the risk decreased as yogurt consumption increased.

In the 1970s evidence began accumulating around another mystery. The Finns eat an unenviable diet—high in meat, fat, protein, and low in fiber—the exact fare some scientists blame for high rates of colon cancer. But not in this case. Just the opposite. The incidence of colon cancer is extraordinarily low in Finland. Their diet also is full of dairy products, especially yogurt. And they reportedly harbor large numbers of lactobacilli in their intestines. Could there be a connection? Perhaps.

Quite frequently, carcinogens, like viruses, needing activation to be dangerous, have that rite performed by enzymes in the intestinal tract. Recent microbiological studies in animals and humans find that eating high levels of L. acidophilus can dampen certain enzymes' ability to convert otherwise harmless substances in the colon into potent cancer-causing agents. Further good news: rats exposed to heavy carcinogens and then fed yogurt were not so apt to develop cancer.

Crackerjack investigators who have spent more than a decade on this work are Dr. Barry R. Goldin and Dr. Sherwood L. Gorbach at the Infectious Disease Service, New England Medical Center, in Boston. Their latest study has fired the imaginations of cancer theorists. Under the two researchers' supervision, twenty-one healthy adults under age thirty-four with no intestinal disorders drank two glasses of plain milk a day for about a month. Then for the same period they switched to two glasses of acidophilus milk a day—containing the same concentration of lactobacilli found in supermarket acidophilus milk and some yogurts. The investigators measured how active the carcinogen catalysts were in the intestines in both cases.

Changes were dramatic. During the time the subjects drank acidophilus milk, the cancer-converting enzyme activity in their colons sank by 200 to 400 percent. When they quit drinking the acidophilus milk, the enzymes' activity returned to normal carcinogen-producing levels.

This elicited an extraordinarily strong comment from the authoritative *Nutrition Reviews:* "We have the development of a new rationale for these milks, namely, protection from colon cancer for populations on Western diets. More studies of the potential . . . are clearly warranted. The yogurt connection cannot be overlooked."

Certainly not. After all, yogurt has had a successful 5000-year field test as a health food. Science is now merely giving millions of souls a multitude of new reasons to go on believing what they—and folk medicine—have long suspected to be true.

YOGURT BY ANY OTHER NAME: AN INTERNATIONAL GUIDE

Around the world, fermented milk goes by many names and owes its creation to a variety of bacteria, usually from a large family called lactobacillus. When mixed into milk, these bacterial strains proliferate, causing the milk to curdle or ferment (taking on a sour taste) and thicken or coagulate. Left to thrive in milk, these bacteria create unique metabolic compounds that both alter the chemistry of the milk and, as it turns out, inadvertently exert a dramatic beneficial impact on human physiology and disease. The strain of bacteria used determines the character of the yogurt or fermented milk and its peculiar health benefit.

MILK PRODUCT	TYPE OF BACTERIA
Acidophilus milk	L. acidophilus
Bulgarican milk	L. bulgaricus
Cheeses	L. brevis, L. bulgaricus, L. casei, L. helvetics, L. lactis
Kefir	L. caucasicus
Koumiss	L. bulgaricus
Yakult	L. casei
Yogurt (American)	L. bulgaricus, S. thermophilus, L. acidophilus (occasionally)

12.

MILK AND EGGS: A CURIOUS LOOK AT THE FUTURE

"This milk guaranteed to help fight colds, diarrhea, influenza, measles, chicken pox, salmonella, staph, herpes, hepatitis, and other common infections. Drink your milk and get your antivirus, antibacterial medicine at the same time. Approved by the Food and Drug Administration as a natural, fortified infection-fighter."

Is this the kind of food label the future will ever see? Some experts think so. At least the concept is already in the works—the ultimate in designer foods. If you accept the fact that certain foods already contain infection fighters as a part of the serendipity so pervasive in the food pharmacy, what is to keep someone from building on that to make super infection-fighting foods?

You might ask Dr. Robert H. Yolken. His investigations have plunged him into futuristic visions that could transform some of nature's humble offerings into disease-fighting superfoods, and hurtle us into a new dimension, where the line between foods and medicine vanishes. One might term it science fiction were Dr. Yolken not such a sturdy type.

Robert Yolken, M.D., is the director of pediatric infectious diseases at one of medicine's finest institutions, the Johns Hopkins University Medical School. He became fascinated by the unexpected discovery of antiinfectious agents in foods because he has a mission: to prevent infectious diarrhea, especially in developing countries, where it is a mortal wound, accounting for thirty to forty percent of all childhood deaths. Even in the United States, infectious diarrhea, although rarely fatal, puts some 50,000 youngsters in hospitals yearly and sends countless more to physicians' offices. Dr. Yolken and his colleagues are searching for cheap, safe agents to combat a particular type of virus called a rotavirus, primarily responsible for the infection.

That led him to flirtations with some novel ideas and to a surprising discovery among the milk herds of Maryland.

Perhaps only a professor keeps forward in his mind the fact that antibodies can enter a body two ways. Your immune system makes its own. These are "active antibodies"; they remember the foreign invader forever. Vaccines—which are low doses of antigens—force your body to create active antibodies.

Or you can receive a gift of antibodies created by another living creature's biology. Such "passive antibodies" may offer transient protection (they have no lifetime memories). In the nineteenth century, before antibiotics and vaccines, "passive antibody therapy" was routine.

An antibody is one of biology's most elegant creations, a guided missile that homes in on a specific target. If you are exposed to the flu, your body designs a set of antibodies to pursue only that particular flu virus. Antibodies usually are not microbial killers; they are like scouts that round up, disarm, and stick to microbe prisoners, then signal other immune-system troops to come in for the kill. Commonly, white "killer" cells rush to the scene, and envelop or literally swallow the invading microbe. Theoretically, the more antibodies on tap, the stronger the body's resistance to disease.

But antibody therapy need not be a planned medical event or even, if medical visionaries have their way, an accidental one. Controlling disease with passive antibodies is back in style. In nature, of course, it has never gone out of style. Since infants are born without antibodies, they take in oodles of passive antibodies with the first sucks at their mother's breast. That's why breast milk is considered a baby's best immunological boost.

Still, it will probably come as a monumental surprise to learn that passive antibody therapy is hardly confined to babies—in fact, is widespread in the food supply. Children and adults everywhere are unknowingly consuming passive antibodies on a grand scale. It was purely by accident that Dr. Yolken stumbled onto the evidence.

"We were looking for cows that did not have any antibodies to rotavirus for one of our experiments," he recalls, "but virtually all of them did, indicating that they had once been infected by rotaviruses. It occurred to us that if they had antibody in the serum, they might also have antibody in their milk."

But it seemed hardly of practical significance. Dr. Yolken was sure the fragile antibodies would be destroyed by pasteurization. Nevertheless, a team of Johns Hopkins researchers headed by Dr. Yolken decided to investigate. They collected raw milk samples from over 200 herds of dairy cows in Maryland. They persuaded dairy farmers to sell them just-pasteurized milk right out of milk tanks; they whisked milk cartons off the shelves of supermarkets and dairy stores in the Baltimore area. They collected infant formulas from area stores and commercial suppliers.

They then put dabs of the diluted milk samples in test tubes lined with rotavirus antigen; any antibodies present in the milk would latch on to the viral attractions, and sophisticated detection equipment could measure how many were there. As Dr. Yolken perused the printouts of the lab tests, he noticed that raw milk was full of antibodies. No surprises there. But he was startled by the numbers from the pasteurized samples. He thought it must be a mistake. The pasteurized milk showed extensive antibody activity too. Fully seventy-seven percent of the antibodies had escaped destruction. So the stuff everybody drinks was infused with rotavirus antibodies. "It's clear antibody molecules are fairly hardy and can survive processing that renders milk suitable for consumption," he reported. Furthermore, a couple of weeks in a refrigerator had slight effect on pasteurized milk's antibodies. But alas, the processing temperatures had totally annihilated antibodies in all twenty-one commercial infant formulas. Very few antibodies also survived in sterilized nonrefrigerated "shelf" milk, common in European countries.

Next question: Were the antibodies in the pasteurized milk functionally active? An impotent or damaged antibody would fail to consummate a deadly embrace with the virus, or alert white killer cells to come in for the massacre, completely failing in its responsibilities.

No need to worry. In a test mixing human cells with human rotaviruses and antibodies, the antibodies performed just fine. The viruses, doomed themselves to extinction by clinging tightly to the antibodies, defeating efforts to attach to and take over cells in their rite of reproduction. All thirteen samples of raw milk and fourteen samples of the pasteurized milk blocked the viruses from replicating. There was a little antibody activity in the shelf milk and none in the infant formulas.

Next, the scientists decided to see whether ordinary antibody-packed milk could actually combat infectious gastroenteritis in baby mice. They fed a group of five-day-old mice only the rotavirus, sure to cause diarrhea, and other infant mice a dose of rotavirus mixed with the various milks. All sixteen mice exposed only to the rotavirus developed infections. None of the eight that got the virus–raw milk concoction, with the most antibodies, showed signs of infection. And only one of eight drinking the pasteurized milk plus virus got the expected diarrhea. Clearly the milk with antibodies successfully bestowed a high degree of passive immunity. The luckless mice given the infant formula, devoid of antibodies, all got sick.

Moreover, there was a critical dose response. The milk with the most antibody activity was the most protective against infection.

So does that mean that, infants aside, everybody who is drinking ordinary pasteurized milk is getting an extra dose of unexpected "passive antibodies"? Yes. It's one of nature's bonuses. Cow's milk comes ready-made with antiinfectious agents churned out by the cow's biology, saving us some of the trouble of producing our own. This is likely to occur in cows throughout the world. Milk samples from Panama and Austria, tested by Dr. Yolken's group, had the same levels of antibodies to rotaviruses as the cows in Maryland. Cows may be naturally infected with the rotavirus; some have been vaccinated against it, forcing them to make the antibodies, which end up in milk.

Dr. Yolken's group has studied only rotavirus antibodies in milk. However, he affirms, cows transfer to us in their milk—and in their yogurt, cheese, butter, and ice cream—antibodies to all of the infections they have incurred. For example, in 1986, scientists at the University of Wisconsin's Food Research Institute at Madison reported finding antibodies to toxic shock syndrome toxins in fourteen different brands of pasteurized milk bought at grocery stores and restaurants in six states. The antibodies were so sturdy that some survived even several processings to show up in cheese.

The startling bottom line is: Every time you slurp down milk, you get not only calcium, protein, and all those other nutrients the Dairy Council tells you about, but you take in globs of antibodies just as surely as if they were injected into your arm by hypodermic needle or poured down your throat as a vaccine. The doses, albeit small, probably do have physiological activity.

To what extent, however, these inadvertent antibodies prevent human infections is unknown. Dr. Yolken says it is critical to find out how high the levels of antibodies must be to prevent human infections, and whether the antibodies really survive digestion intact enough to neutralize the microbes in the human system. Such human tests are in the beginning stages. But it is relatively certain that drinking milk with *enough* preformed antibodies can zap certain infections in humans.

Dr. Yolken has given youngsters human immunoglobulin—the protein that carries antibodies—and from twenty to fifty percent of it survives its journey through the gastrointestinal tract. Additionally, diarrhea-causing rotaviruses replicate in the small bowel, just off the stomach, so the antibodies do not have to survive long to reach their target. In fact, in gastrointestinal infections, Dr. Yolken considers ingested passive preformed antibodies more effective than those active ones created by stimulating the immune system; ingested antibodies are sure to pass through the area of the gastrointestinal tract where the viruses multiply.

Now, since there's no assurance that supermarket milk carries enough pharmacologically potent antibodies to prevent infections, you could search for cows with lots of antibodies serendipitously induced by past infections. But that seems a little silly compared with Dr. Yolken's grand plan.

Think about it: Much of our food is now manipulated by technology to boost nutritional value. Milk solids, including protein, vitamins A and D, and even calcium are plopped into dairy products. Bread would flunk its government standards unless it were enriched with a broad range of vitamins and minerals. Juice drinks are bolstered with vitamin C. Cereals are fortified with fiber, vitamins, and minerals—some which nature never put there in the first place. United States Department of Agriculture scientists have even perfected a new "super carrot," oranger and fuller of carotene than ever seen before on earth, with ten times more beta carotene than God's ordinary carrots.

Clearly, we don't trust the vagaries of nature for our vitamin and mineral needs. Then why rely on chance for adequate levels of other food constituents known to be biological barriers to disease? As science uncovers the secrets of physiologically valuable food substances other than common vitamins and minerals, it may become routine to expect more from food. Enriching foods in the future may mean incorporating pharmacological manipulations to bolster human defenses against various diseases, including infections. The distinction between foods and drugs grows fainter.

One way is to fiddle with the animal's biology, creating in a sense a living pharmaceutical supply house. Dr. Yolken suggests injecting cows with specific doses of rotaviruses to insure that they produce milk with known quantities of viral antibodies that are sufficient to fight infections. Such antibody-enriched milk, if proved effective in youngsters, might be distributed as a combination food-medicine in certain high-risk areas of the world or among vulnerable youngsters (including infants who do *not* have access to breast milk) anywhere to prevent deadly diarrhea. Dr. Yolken likes the idea because quality control is easy; research shows that you can induce cows to produce exact measures of antibodies in their milk by injecting specified amounts of microbial antigens. By immunizing cows to specifications, you could engineer the production of a new creation, an antibody milk shake containing precise quantities and types of antibodies desired to combat numerous types of infections, some that cows may not even be susceptible to naturally.

In fact, human vision and technology are pressing hard against this new frontier. German, Swiss, and Japanese scientists have already ushered in this new age of disease-fighting designer foods—giving new meaning to health foods—by modifying cow antibodies and feeding them in milk to children. Researchers at the Institute for Medicine, Microbiology, and Virology at Ruhr University, Federal Republic of Germany, vaccinated cows to deliberately generate antibodies in milk against a bacterium, Escherichia coli, another prevalent microbial cause of diarrhea in children. Then they fed the antibody-laden milk to infants. It was an enormous success. Fully eighty-four percent of the stricken infants—forty-three out of fifty-one—who drank the milk within two weeks were free of infection. In a control group of infants not fed the milk, only one out of nine (eleven percent) was free of infection.

Once you start thinking about milk and antibodies and the possibilities of using food to fight infections, there is no turning back. Dr. Yolken had other ideas. What about eggs?

If cows and humans get infected by various agents, so do chickens, and yes, they make antibodies too. Wouldn't you expect antibodies to show up in eggs? Chickens have lots of rotavirus infections and the antigen—the viral agent that provides the pattern for the antibody—is similar to that of humans. It seemed likely to Dr. Yolken that chicken eggs contain antibodies capable of controlling human rotaviruses. And in case they don't have enough, you might even inject the birds with human antigen to make them lay eggs full of the right kind of antibodies.

In the 1920s and '30s physicians commonly used egg yolk preparations to treat infant diarrhea. Dr. Yolken's father, a pediatrician, had done it. They said it worked, but nobody knew why. Could it be the eggs were inadvertently transferring protective antibodies into young intestinal tracts?

So the Johns Hopkins researchers bought eggs, extracted the yolks (that's where the antibodies reside), and tested them. Ninety-six percent had detectable antibodies. There was a wide range of antibody levels, obviously depending on the level of infection in the chickens. Once again, out came the mice, this time to dine on viruses and eggs instead of milk. Worse luck, the eggs did not have enough antibodies to save them, and many came down with diarrheal infections.

Undaunted, Dr. Yolken and his team gave up depending on chickens' chance encounters with infections for antibody yields. They inoculated chickens with a low dose of rotavirus. Then for the next two or three weeks they gathered eggs laid in the Johns Hopkins laboratories by the chickens, whipped up the yolks, extracted their immunoglobulin, and gave it along with viruses to the mice. The eggs had twenty times the antibodies that nature had provided. Not a single mouse came down with infection.

Dr. Yolken sees chickens as a virtual antibody factory. He notes that a single chicken could provide up to thirty kilograms of immunoglobulin a year. "Eggs have the potential of providing a large, economical supply of antibodies," he declares, "fit for consumption by all ages." Theoretically, the high-antibody eggs could be powdered and sent overseas, distributed as a food supplement. Or they could be incorporated into cake mixes and bread, even in this country. Or probably better yet, you would simply ship the antigen to third world countries to use in vaccinating chickens. "The antigen needed for vaccination is cheap," says Dr. Yolken. "All you need is someone to hold down the chickens and immunize them."

In the future, milk and eggs might be labeled and advertised as antiinfective. "This milk contains antibodies to the rotavirus or the bacteria E. coli, and can help prevent certain intestinal infections, especially among children."

Forced to choose, Dr. Yolken would settle on eggs as the favored vehicle for antibody distribution because they are cheaper, more commonly eaten in the world, and are less apt to cause allergic reactions. Many people in third world countries cannot tolerate milk proteins. For an extra-potent antiinfective drink, of course, you could mix milk and eggs. "The antibody effects would be at least additive," says Dr. Yolken.

This thought may transport us not only into the future but into the past to recall a zany prediction from a Woody Allen movie. In his futuristic comedy *Sleeper*, all nutrition advice preached in the twentieth century has been declared wrong. The formerly bad stuff—junk food, chocolate, fat, and cholesterol—has now been proved beneficial. After the drubbing high-cholesterol eggs and fatty milks have suffered in this decade, it may take fortitude and a sense of humor to face a future in which the new health-food cocktail might be, of all things, *eggnog!*

Surely, the crystal ball will hold many surprises as the explorations into the food pharmacy send us off in uncharted directions. But experts already predict that:

- Eating in the future will increasingly be a therapeutic experience.
- People will come to depend more on foods and less on drugs to preserve health.
- Scientists will increasingly test the pharmacological powers of whole foods in humans and compare their effectiveness and safety with those of drugs.
- The government will begin to systematically analyze foods for levels of pharmacologically active constituents, just as it does now for nutrients. At the moment, it's virtually impossible for scientists to adequately judge a food's pharmacological potential because they don't know what chemicals are in it. In the beginning it makes sense to pick out those foods most closely tied to lower disease rates in the population—such as cabbage, broccoli, spinach, and so forth—and try to find out what compounds they have in common.
- Scientists will try to establish effective and safe doses of foods. For example, experiments show that very high doses of capsaicin in chili peppers promote certain cancers, but that low doses retard cancer. Further, some food chemicals may work very selectively. As Dr. Thomas Kensler points out, a compound might help block colon cancer but not lung cancer due to smoking. Indeed, a food compound that thwarts colon cancer might even promote cancer elsewhere in the body. It's important to find out the cancer effects of whole foods—and in what quantities—so that in the future cancer-inhibiting food might be matched to combat vulnerabilities to specific cancers.
- The government will better coordinate investigations of the food pharmacy. Dr. Norman Farnsworth suggests establishing a national institute for testing foods and food compounds. We're one of only a few countries in the world without one, he says.
- More foods will be enriched or fortified with natural, nonnutrient, disease-fighting agents to make superhealthful foods.
- Foods increasingly will be promoted for their specific health-giving properties.

The last two will send officials into a tizzy over the labeling, advertising, and creation of new generations of health-promoting foods. What to say to apple growers who want to tout the cholesterol-lowering attributes of their product? To onion producers who contend the white bulb elevates good HDL cholesterol three times better than the latest wonder drug? To scientists who want to put natural soybean anticancer chemicals into the milk supply? To a professor who suggests manipulating the biology of chickens to produce eggs full of infection-fighting antibodies? To a physician on the West Coast who is breeding a super fish full of omega-3 oils designed to prevent all the ills of humankind? All this and more is already here or coming fast, and someone will have to decide the legitimate limits of health claims and how far we should go in fulfilling Hippocrates's imperative by engineering a modern fusion of foods and medicine.

It can only get more exciting as science further expands the boundaries of the food pharmacy frontier.

PART THREE

THE FOODS: A MODERN PHARMA-COPOEIA

A MODERN PHARMACOPOEIA

One must eat to live
and not live to eat
—Molière

Although science is on the threshold of enormous breakthroughs in understanding the food pharmacy, it's needless to wait for everything to be defined before using information to save your life. Clues, as we know from the past, often precede by decades establishment blessings, and waiting for more knowledge can be a mistake. Ignoring the health wisdom in lemons is a case in point. As early as the 1600s observant physicians, among them John Hall, son-in-law of William Shakespeare, prescribed watercress, juniper berries, and lemons to treat scurvy. But it was not until 1753 that Scottish naval surgeon James Lind proved in a famous controlled experiment that eating citrus fruits cured scurvy. Yet, because at the time vitamin C, the scurvy-fighting compound, had not been discovered and nobody knew exactly how citrus combated scurvy, it was not until 1795 that the British Admiralty issued an order requiring all members of the Royal Navy to be given a daily ration of lemon or lime juice. During that forty-year delay, almost 200,000 British sailors died of scurvy.

Although science has advanced far in many areas today, we still know so little about the pharmacology of foods that we are apt to overlook evidence all around us. Few of us even know what types of experiments have been done on foods. Thus, here is a current guide to the food pharmacy—the latest scientific findings about the potential therapeutic effects of fifty-five common foods, distilled from scientific journals, conferences, abstracts, computer searches of medical and

111

nutritional literature, and correspondence and interviews with the most prominent scientists in the field. Only foods on which there exists credible research are included. Folklore is noted, too, and some of it is scientifically valid.

Predictably, most of the foods listed are fruits and vegetables. For overwhelming evidence shows that vegetarians fare best in averting disease; thus, scientists are more apt to look for—and find—medicinal powers in plant foods. This does not mean everyone should be a strict vegetarian, nor that animal food is devoid of benefit (meat has many nutritional aspects), but it seems clear that eating *more* vegetables, grains, and fruits is not only intrinsically more healthful, but can also dampen some ill effects of meat diets, such as heart disease and cancer.

This pharmacopoeia is on the far side, surely the revolutionary side of conventional nutrition. For it lists a food's tested *pharmacological* attributes usually due to exotic dietary constituents quite apart from traditional nutritional values such as vitamins and minerals.

Some explanations:

- How much? Researchers deliberately test high doses to get an effect; thus, if three apples a day lowered blood cholesterol, this does not necessarily mean that many are needed, but simply that three was the lowest effective dose tested. These are also *average* medicinal doses. Just as people vary widely in their responses to pharmaceutical drugs, so do they to foods. Some get a drug benefit from small amounts of certain foods; alas, some get little or no benefit. Also critical: foods have an additive effect of unknown proportions. If you don't eat three apples to get a cholesterol-lowering effect, you may get it from one apple, some oat bran, and beans.
- Most foods listed here are thought to bestow a long-term preventive effect. Far lower doses are likely to prevent rather than cure a specific ailment.
- In most cases, it's not known how long it takes for specific foods to exert protective effects. The benefit may be immediate, as in sugar's ability to heal wounds. On the other hand, scientists find that it takes at least a couple of months for oats and onions to significantly boost beneficial HDL cholesterol.
- Foods often contain contradictory chemicals—for example, anticarcinogens and antimutagens along with mutagens and cancer promoters, or cholesterol-boosters along with cholesterol reducers. Only specific tests of the whole foods fed to humans reveal which chemicals win out in the biological system, so pay most attention to such evidence.

Next best clues come from epidemiological research, in which scientists look for links between disease and diet by doing population surveys and analyses. Animal tests that show physiological effects from eating certain foods strongly suggest the same thing happens in humans. Test-tube experiments usually offer initial indications that a food is pharmacologically active. Such tests are also extremely critical in helping spot the mechanisms by which foods work.

The Food Pharmacopoeia, by its very name, is intended to be positive and health promoting. It gives you valid justification for eating foods scientists currently have reason to believe will boost your health and prolong your life.

Saluté!

APPLE

To eat an apple going to bed
Will make the doctor beg his bread.
—Old rhyme

POSSIBLE THERAPEUTIC BENEFITS:
- A good heart medicine
- Lowers blood cholesterol
- Lowers blood pressure
- Stabilizes blood sugar
- Dampens appetite
- Packed with chemicals that block cancer in animals
- Apple juice kills infectious viruses

How Much? Eating two or three whole apples a day can lower blood cholesterol and slightly raise heart-protective HDLs. That amount can also reduce blood pressure and help keep blood sugar levels steady. Generally, the higher your blood cholesterol, the greater the benefit.

FOLKLORE

In Greek mythology, apples tasted like honey and healed all ailments. In American folk medicine, the apple is called "the king of fruits," a neutralizer of all the body's excess acids, and thus, according to a 1927 article in *American Medicine*, "therapeutically effective in all conditions of acidosis, gout, rheumatism, jaundice, all liver and gall bladder troubles, and nervous and skin diseases caused by sluggish liver, hyperacidity, and states of autointoxication."

FACTS

No doubt about it. Modern scientific investigations find apples a versatile and potent package of natural drugs that deserve their reputation for keeping doctors away.

HEART PROTECTOR

The fruit helps keep the cardiovascular system healthy. First Italian, then Irish researchers, and now the French have all confirmed that eating apples puts a dent in blood cholesterol. A team headed by R. Sablé-Amplis at the University of Paul Sabatier, Institute of Physiology, in Toulouse, was startled to find that apples precipitated a twenty-eight-point drop in cholesterol in normal hamsters and a spectacular fifty-two-point drop in animals with genetically high cholesterol.

That impelled Dr. Sablé-Amplis to ask a group of thirty middle-aged, healthy men and women at the university not to change their diet one bit—except for one thing: Eat two or three apples every day for a month, one at about ten A.M., another at four P.M. By the month's end, the apples had pushed down the blood cholesterol of twenty-four—or eighty percent—of the group. In half of them the drop was more than ten percent. One person's cholesterol dived by thirty percent. Furthermore, the apples manipulated the blood so that good HDL cholesterol went up and the destructive artery-clogging LDL cholesterol went down.

Dr. Sablé-Amplis thinks the apple's secret drug is pectin, that soluble-type fiber, the same kind of stuff that goes into jelly. Pure pectin extracted from fruits is a well-known anticholesterol agent. But pectin alone does not explain the apple's powers, for the whole apple itself is a much more powerful cholesterol depressor than all the pectin squeezed out of an apple. Dr. Sablé-Amplis speculates that the pectin as packaged in the apple interacts with other apple substances, perhaps vitamin C, that together more efficiently sweep cholesterol out of the blood. New French studies are trying to define the apple's cardioprotective mechanism.

BLOOD SUGAR

Unquestionably, apples tend to be good for diabetics and others who want to avoid steep rises in blood sugar. Apples rank near the bottom of the "glycemic index" (a measurement of how fast blood sugar rises after eating)—right along with dried beans, one of the very best regulators of blood sugar. This means that despite an apple's natural sugar content, it does not spur a rapid rise in blood sugar. The fruit keeps the throttle on insulin, and foods that do this invariably also lower blood cholesterol and blood pressure.

In fact, researchers at prestigious Yale University have found that you may have only to *smell* apples to get your blood pressure down. Dr. Gary Schwartz, director of Yale's Psychophysiology Center, reported that the aroma of spiced apples has a calming effect on many people that tends to lower blood pressure.

DIET FOOD

Because whole apples keep blood glucose levels up for a while, they also make you feel fuller than do equivalent carbohydrate calories from apple juice or apple puree, a bonus if you are dieting. The juice is much quicker at inducing a spurt of insulin and drop in blood sugar, making you hungry. Apples, then, are a far better weight-loss food than apple juice.

VIRUS AND COLD FIGHTER

Viruses don't live long in the presence of apple juice. In Canadian studies, apple juice taken right off supermarket shelves proved highly potent in inactivating polioviruses in test tubes. Tested against eighteen other commercial juices, apple juice ranked tops with grape juice and tea as being able to cause the demise of the viruses one hundred percent. Researchers also find that those who eat more apples tend to have a lower incidence of colds and upper respiratory ailments.

Indeed, researchers at Michigan State University branded apples an all-around health food. In 1961 the scientists compared health records of 1300 students with how many apples they ate and found that the most dedicated apple eaters over three years made fully one third fewer calls to the university's health centers than non–apple lovers, and had less upper respiratory infection, and less tension and sickness in general than was expected.

ANTICANCER AGENT

Whole fresh apples may help ward off cancer because they are shot through with caffeic or chlorogenic acid, which blocks cancer formation in lab animals dosed with potent carcinogens.

PRACTICAL MATTERS

- The more apples you eat—up to a point—the more likely you are to push down blood cholesterol, although individuals react differently depending on body chemistry.
- For unknown reasons, women seem to get a more pronounced lowering of blood cholesterol from eating apples than do men.
- Within the first three weeks of eating more apples, your total blood cholesterol may actually rise; then it generally settles down to lower-than-ordinary levels. Apples, however, do not work on everyone, the French studies show.
- Be sure to eat the skin; it is especially high in pectin fiber. Apple juice contains little pectin and cannot be expected to lower blood cholesterol or blood pressure or stabilize blood sugar. Apple juice also has much lower concentrations of anticancer chemicals.

CAUTIONS

- Cider, or fermented apple juice, can suppress the body's fibrinolytic, or blood-clot-dissolving system, which could make the blood more vulnerable to clotting. However, apple juice does not adversely affect the blood-clotting system.
- Apple juice, even in moderate amounts, may aggravate chronic diarrhea in some children. Two University of Connecticut investigators noted that several of their patients, ages thirteen tc thirty-one months, whose parents complained that apple juice seemed to make the diarrhea worse, did react to apple juice by developing metabolic signs of diarrhea. The reason is a mystery; researchers suggest perhaps certain children are unable to adequately absorb carbohydrates.

APRICOT

POSSIBLE THERAPEUTIC BENEFITS:
• Best recognized as a possible cancer inhibitor, especially against smoking-related cancers, including lung

FOLKLORE

When King Solomon said: "Comfort me with apples for I am sick," he meant what we now call the apricot. Apricots, not apples, grew in the Garden of Eden. In folk medicine the apricot's primary medicinal part was the *kernel* (later a source of the drug laetrile), although the fruit was reputed to be an anticancer agent. And the apricot is cherished in the Himalayan kingdom of Hunza (the land of Shangri-La in the novel and film *Lost Horizon*) as a source of health and exceptional longevity. The people eat prodigious amounts of a type of wild apricot called khubani. Scientists have seriously proposed there is truth to the apricot's mystical reputation. Indeed, Nobel-prize winner G. S. Whipple in 1934 hailed the apricot as "equal to liver in hemoglobin regeneration."

FACTS

Unfortunately, because the apricot has not been singled out for special study, its pharmacological powers are largely unexplored. Nevertheless, apricots are high on the list of fruits and vegetables likely to help prevent certain cancers, notably of the lung and possibly of the pancreas, both extremely difficult tumors to treat, and both linked to cigarette smoking.

That's because apricots, like other bright-orange fruits or vegetables, contain highly concentrated amounts of beta carotene, a form of vitamin A that is spectacularly successful in lab tests in thwarting certain cancers, including lung and skin. Surveys also indicate that people who eat lots of fruits and vegetables high in beta carotene have lower rates of these cancers as well as cancer of the larynx. Scientists, because it blocks cancer in lab animals, often credit the beta carotene in the foods as the primary protective factor, but other undiscovered agents in apricots and similar foods may also be responsible.

At this point, because of the beta carotene, apricots look good as a potential cancer preventive—especially recommended for ex-smokers. High beta carotene foods appear to have some ability to mitigate the latent cancerous effects of the noxious cigarette smoke.

PRACTICAL MATTERS

- For maximum benefit, eat dried apricots; they have much higher concentrations of beta carotene than the raw fruit.

CAUTION

- The kernel is poisonous because of its amygdalin, or laetrile, content. Eating quantities of the seeds has caused serious poisoning, especially among children.

ARTICHOKE

POSSIBLE THERAPEUTIC BENEFITS:
- Lowers blood cholesterol
- Stimulates bile and urine (diuretic)

FOLKLORE .

The globe artichoke has a long history as a diuretic, an aid to digestion, and a good way to lower blood sugar.

FACTS

In recent years scientists have neglected this edible thistle. But for many years the artichoke spurred a flurry of scientific excitement that confirmed some of its folklore reputation. Although the studies are old, they do illustrate quite striking human physiological effects.

A series of studies in 1940 by a Japanese researcher found that the artichoke lowered total cholesterol somewhat, stimulated production of bile by the liver, performed as a diuretic, and enhanced "well-being strikingly." A similar study done by Swiss investigators a few years later noted that blood cholesterol of humans dropped significantly after eating artichoke. That was followed up by tests in 1947 in Texas, where researchers fed artichokes to humans and also saw a drop in blood cholesterol.

Russian scientists in 1970 reported that the edible parts of the artichoke exerted an antiinflammatory activity in dogs. In 1969 French scientists were so successful in using artichoke extract for treating liver and kidney ailments that they took out a patent on it.

In fact, cynarin, a constituent of the artichoke, was formulated into a drug for lowering blood cholesterol. Cynarin also is well known to be "liver protective" in both animal liver cells and living animals.

BANANA AND PLANTAIN

POSSIBLE THERAPEUTIC BENEFITS:
- Prevents and heals ulcers
- Lowers blood cholesterol

FOLKLORE

Considering the widespread use of bananas (usually eaten raw and ripe) and the larger plantains (often eaten unripe and cooked), which are a staple in many South American and African countries, there is surprisingly little folklore about their therapeutic powers. Even the respected herbalist Maud Grieve noted in her 1931 book that "the banana family is more of interest for its nutrient than for its medicinal properties."

However, in India, the plantain enjoys a huge folklore reputation as a treatment for peptic and duodenal ulcers. According to the Indian *Materia Medica* (1954), flour made of green plantains and made into "chappatis" (handmade bread) is good in cases of dyspepsia and flatulence, and a "slight gruel made of banana flour mixed with milk is a nice easily digestible article of the diet in cases of gastritis."

FACTS

Observant Indians, it turns out, are being proved right. Unquestionably, plantains contain some powerful medicinal stuff that can heal the distressed cells of present ulcers and ward off the appearance of new sores. Several noted researchers in India and Great Britain have devoted years to pinning down the amazing biological changes that plantain imposes on the stomach lining of animals. They conclude that it works the same way as an antiulcer drug, carbenoxolone, but without that drug's serious side effects.

New double-blind studies in several medical centers in India find that unripe plantain banana powder induces healing of duodenal ulcers in about seventy percent of the patients. A placebo worked in only sixteen percent of the cases.

GENERATIONS OF BANANA EATING, ULCER-FREE RATS

Bananas first emerged in the medical literature as a cure for ulcers in the early 1930s. At first, researchers thought bananas neutralized stomach acid or even that ripe bananas soothed the irritation. Indeed, few mice in a British experiment that hunkered down to sliced ripe bananas for a week prior to being given ulcer-producing injections developed gastric ulcers. And researchers even isolated a chemical in ripe and unripe bananas that suppressed acid secretion, thereby blocking the development of ulcers in animals.

But recently teams of British and Indian researchers have discovered exactly why banana-eating rodents end up with about one third fewer and less severe ulcers. The plantains work just like the most sophisticated drugs. It was Professor A. K. Sanyal, College of Medical Sciences, Banaras Hindu University in Varanasi, India, who figured it out along with a team of British investigators headed by Dr. Ralph Best, Department of Pharmacy, University of Aston, in Birmingham.

If you were designing an antiulcer drug, you would probably first look for one to neutralize or suppress the destroyers of the stomach lining, acid and pepsin, a digestive enzyme. That's what common antiulcer drugs such as antacids and cimetidine (Tagamet) do. Only one drug takes a different approach, carbenoxolone, infrequently used because it also induces high blood pressure. Nevertheless, it is an idea copied from nature. The drug carbenoxolone, instead of knocking out the aggressors, builds a better defensive wall.

BANANAS BUILD A BETTER STOMACH

Wonder of wonders, that's what experts say plantains do; they strengthen the surface cells of the stomach lining, forming a sturdier barrier against noxious juices. The British experimenters were stunned to notice that the mucosa, or stomach lining, was actually *visibly* much thicker in rats fed banana powder. As a sideline experiment, they deliberately fed rats banana powder or aspirin and other chemicals to see what happened to this critical barrier. It grew considerably thicker with banana powder, decreased substantially with aspirin, and even more so with Tagamet. But in rats fed both banana and aspirin, the banana counteracted the drug's detrimental erosive effects; the lining still jumped in thickness by about twenty percent.

Thus, researchers say banana stimulates the proliferation of cells in the stomach lining, and also triggers the release of a protective layer of mucus that rapidly seals off the surface, preventing stomach hydrochloric acid and pepsin from doing further damage. The British researchers' bottom line: "The role of banana in folk medicine as an anti-ulcerogenic agent, at least against gastric ulcers, appears justified. . . ."

GOOD FOR THE BLOOD AND HEART

Other Indian investigators recently discovered that fiber from unripe plantains when fed to rats along with high doses of cholesterol dramatically counteracted the expected upsurge in destructive blood cholesterol. Fiber from *ripe* plantains didn't work. Rats fed only cholesterol had high detrimental LDL-cholesterol counts of 126 milligrams per hundred milliliters. But adding unripe plantain to the diet caused the rats' blood cholesterol to plunge to only forty-four milligrams per hundred milliliters—an astounding one third as much. Further, the plantain also raised the HDL beneficial type cholesterol by about thirty percent. The researchers mainly credited the high amount of hemicellulose fiber in unripe plantains.

It is likely that ordinary bananas also lower blood cholesterol because of their high pectin content, which on a weight basis is even higher than that of apples, a confirmed cholesterol-lowering fruit. One medium banana contains as much pectin as a medium-size apple.

PRACTICAL MATTERS

- Go for the green. Unripe, green plantains are the most potent against ulcers. And usually, the larger the plantain, the greater its protective effect. Researchers say it is unlikely the ripe fruit contains enough of the active chemical. Most of the highly successful animal and human tests have been with unripe green plantains. These are often cooked—boiled, fried, or baked—and eaten like potatoes in Africa, India, and South America.

- Best of all against ulcers is the highly concentrated powder made from dried unripe plantains.
- Although original studies found ordinary bananas—distinguished from plantains—also effective against ulcers, recent research does not bear this out.
- It appears that green unripe plantains also contain the best *heart-protective fiber.*

CONFLICTING EVIDENCE

Some studies in animals find no antiulcer activity from plantains. Dr. Sanyal attributes that to the vagaries of nature—creating more or less therapeutic potency—and not to the basic healing constituents of the fruit.

BARLEY

- Lowers blood cholesterol
- May inhibit cancer
- Improves bowel function
- Relieves constipation

> *How Much?* Eating foods made with barley products—such as flour, grits, flakes, or the grain itself—three times a day has lowered blood cholesterol by about fifteen percent. Three muffins or scones made with barley flour eaten every day can completely clear up constipation.

FOLKLORE

For about 6000 years barley has been heralded as a food for potency and vigor. Roman gladiators, called *hordearii* (barley eaters), ate the grain to build up strength. In some areas of the world, notably the Middle East, where barley is a staple as a cereal and flour grain, heart disease rates are low. In Pakistan, for example, some refer to barley as "medicine for the heart."

FACTS

Barley, true to legend, is a pharmacological package that helps ward off heart disease, constipation, and thus other digestive troubles, and possibly cancer.

CARDIOVASCULAR MEDICINE

Barley seems to work several ways to lower blood cholesterol. One method, just like the hottest new anticholesterol drug on the market, is to interfere with the liver's manufacture of cholesterol. United States Department of Agriculture researchers in Madison, Wisconsin, discovered three separate compounds in barley that throttle the liver's ability to manufacture the bad LDL-type cholesterol that damages blood vessels, leading to heart attacks and stroke. When pigs ate barley, their blood cholesterol dropped eighteen percent.

Unquestionably, barley can also drive down human blood cholesterol. Rosemary K. Newman, Ph.D., of Montana State University found dramatic reductions in blood cholesterol in men who ate a hull-less barley flour made into a nutty grain cereal, muffins, bread, and cake. For six weeks they ate three servings of barley goods a day. Their cholesterol counts sank an average of fifteen percent. The higher the blood cholesterol, the more it dropped on the barley regimen. A control group eating identical products made with wheat flour or bran showed no drop in cholesterol. Dr. Newman credits the cholesterol lowering at least partially to soluble beta glucans, a gummy fiber peculiar to barley and oats, found not in the outer coating but in the interior cell walls of the seed. Dr. Newman is now working with a group of Swedish scientists to determine which particular types of barley (cultivars) have the best cholesterol-lowering impact.

Experiments at the University of Wisconsin Medical School also show that capsules of barley oil—containing agents that clamp down on the liver's manufacture of cholesterol—lowered blood cholesterol by nine to eighteen percent in patients who had had heart bypass surgery.

CANCER ANTIDOTE

Dr. Charles Elson, nutritional scientist at the University of Wisconsin believes chemicals in the grain are anticancer agents. Dr. Walter Troll, an authority in that area, agrees. He says so-called protease inhibitors, potent chemicals in all seeds, including barley, suppress cancer-causing agents in the intestinal tract and thus may act as antidotes to cancer formation.

REGULARITY REMEDY

Israeli scientists have proposed using the barley-spent grain now wasted in beer brewing to cure constipation. They substituted barley flour for wheat flour in biscuits and scones and gave them to nineteen patients who had chronic constipation and depended on laxatives. In fifteen, or seventy-nine percent, who ate three or four barley biscuits a day, the constipation completely cleared up; they had more bowel movements, less gas and abdominal pain, and they gave up taking laxatives. As a confirming test, when they were deprived of the barley breads, virtually all of the group became constipated and went back to laxatives within a month. Dr. Newman in her studies also found barley great for regularity.

PRACTICAL MATTERS

- Generally, experts agree that the less processed the barley, the more potent its health-producing effects. Best are: whole grain barley which can be made into flour, barley grits, a cracked par-boiled product (a little like bulgur wheat), and barley flakes, similar to rolled oats—all of which can be purchased in health food stores. Scotch barley and pearled barley, commonly found in supermarkets, have less therapeutic effect, especially against constipation.
- But even the right type pearled and Scotch barley may be good for the heart. The Wisconsin scientists advocate using the least-processed barley such as whole grain or whole grain flour for the greatest effects, or blocked barley, in which only the husk and part of the seeds are removed. It's in these outer layers they find the most oil-soluble anticholesterol compounds. On the other hand, Dr. Newman finds that even denuded pearled barley, especially from the less common hull-less variety of barley, sold by a few manufacturers, has cholesterol-lowering beta glucans. Both types of barley chemicals probably help combat cholesterol.
- You can substitute barley flour for all or part of the wheat flour in recipes.
- Don't count on beer as a barley source. Virtually all the cholesterol-suppressing chemicals in the 125 million bushels (about a quarter of the United States yearly crop) that go into beer brewing is sloughed

off in the residue. Only traces get into the beer itself. Some of that "spent grain" is milled into barley flour for health food stores, cereal makers, and commercial bakers.

DR. NEWMAN'S CHOLESTEROL-LOWERING RECIPES

BARLEY TABOULI

¼ cup barley grits
½ cup water
4 chopped tomatoes
1 cup chopped parsley
4 chopped green onions
1 small diced cucumber
⅛ cup fresh mint, chopped (or 1 tablespoon dry mint leaves)
½ cup olive oil
½ cup lemon juice
Salt and freshly ground pepper

Soak barley grits in water for one hour. Squeeze dry. Set aside. Toss vegetables and mint together. Sprinkle with oil and lemon juice. Add salt and pepper to taste. Refrigerate. Makes 8–10 servings.

BANANA-BARLEY BREAD

3 cups barley flour
1 teaspoon salt
3½ teaspoons baking powder
3 ripe bananas
1 cup honey
½ cup oil
2 large eggs
1 teaspoon lemon juice
¾ teaspoon grated lemon rind

Preheat oven to 350 degrees.
Sift dry ingredients (barley flour, salt, and baking powder) together. Mash ripe bananas with a fork until smooth. In a mixer, blend

bananas, honey, and oil. Add eggs, lemon juice, and grated lemon rind. Fold dry mixture into this and blend on a slow speed for 5 minutes. Bake at 350 degrees for 35–40 minutes in a bread pan that has been greased and floured. Makes 2 loaves.

REFRIGERATOR BARLEY-BRAN MUFFINS

2 cups boiling water
6 cups bran flakes
1 cup vegetable shortening
1 cup white sugar
1 cup brown sugar
1 cup molasses
4 eggs
4 cups buttermilk
5 cups barley flour
5 teaspoons baking soda

Pour boiling water over 2 cups bran flakes; cool slightly. In mixer, on high speed, cream shortening, sugars, and molasses. Add eggs and buttermilk and mix well. Sift dry ingredients together and add to wet. Stir until well coated. Add soaked bran and remaining bran and stir well. You may refrigerate batter in covered container and bake as needed. Store up to 4 weeks. Fill well-greased muffin tins ⅔ full. Bake 18 minutes at 400 degrees. Makes 4 dozen muffins.

RIESKA—QUICK FLATBREAD

2 cups barley flour
½ teaspoon salt
1 tablespoon sugar
2 teaspoons baking powder
1 cup undiluted evaporated milk
2 tablespoons vegetable oil

Preheat oven to 450 degrees.

In a medium-size bowl stir the flour, salt, sugar, and baking powder together. Add evaporated milk and oil. Stir until all the flour is moistened and a smooth, stiff dough has formed. If dough is very stiff and all the flour isn't moistened, add more milk, one tablespoon at a time, until a cohesive dough forms. Turn the dough out onto a greased baking sheet. With the back of a spoon or your hands form the dough into a ½-inch-thick 8-inch-diameter loaf. Prick the top of the loaf with a fork. Bake at 450 degrees for 10-15 minutes, until loaf is browned. Cut into wedges and serve while warm. Makes one 8-inch round loaf.

HOW TO MAKE YOUR OWN BARLEY FLOUR

If using whole barley grains, clean the barley well of loose hulls, weeds, and other debris. Put it through the mill just as you would wheat. Vary the degree of fineness according to how you plan to use the flour. For breads or muffins, you may want to leave some texture in the grain.

If using pearled barley, you can use either a wheat mill or a blender. When using a blender, place one-half cup of pearled barley in the blender and run at high speed for one to three minutes, depending on how fine you want the flour to be. Blenders will vary, too, so experiment with your own equipment to get the fineness you need.

Keep in a cool place; barley once ground into flour has a tendency to become rancid.

BEANS

Includes black beans, black-eyed peas, chick-peas or garbanzos, fava beans, kidney beans, lentils, lima beans, split peas, pinto beans, white Great Northern, navy and white beans, and common baked beans. (See also Soybeans, page 273.)

POSSIBLE THERAPEUTIC BENEFITS:
- Reduces bad-type blood cholesterol
- Contains chemicals that inhibit cancer
- Controls insulin and blood sugar
- Lowers blood pressure
- Regulates functions of the colon
- Prevents and cures constipation
- Prevents hemorrhoids and other bowel problems

How Much? A cup of cooked dried beans every day (less if you eat other cholesterol-depressing foods) should send your bad LDL cholesterol down, control insulin and blood sugar, lower blood pressure—and keep you regular and your intestinal tract functioning in ways that may prevent gastrointestinal troubles like hemorrhoids and possibly bowel cancer.

FOLKLORE

Beans boiled with garlic are reputed to cure "otherwise incurable coughs." Beans are also believed by some to relieve depression.

FACTS

Legumes are potent medicine for the cardiovascular system. When you eat dried beans, they are not entirely digested, so the undigested material lies around in the colon, where bacteria attack it for dinner. In the process, lots of chemicals are liberated. And these chemicals act just like drugs that have beneficial effects such as telling your liver to cut down its production of cholesterol and your blood to speed up clearing out dangerous LDL cholesterol. That's one reason, experts think, that eating beans is good for your heart. The same process, called "fermentation," can also spew forth cancer-blocking chemicals. A primary therapeutic compound in dried beans is thought to be a soluble fiber.

Dr. James Anderson, at the University of Kentucky, regularly prescribes dried beans—a cup of cooked pinto or navy beans a day—to lower blood cholesterol. He has documented that cholesterol levels sink by an average of nineteen percent, even in middle-aged men with extremely high cholesterol counts—over 260 milligrams per deciliter. Simply by eating beans, one man brought his cholesterol down from 274 to 190; another lowered his from 218 to 167. Beans swept the bad kind of cholesterol—LDLs—out of the blood and bucked up the critical HDL-LDL cholesterol ratio. The bean diet improved the ratio an average of seventeen percent.

ANTIDIABETES FARE

Moreover, legumes are marvelous regulators of insulin. Type I diabetics, those who need daily insulin shots, by following Dr. Anderson's bean prescription cut their insulin needs by thirty-eight percent. Those with type II diabetes (adult onset diabetes), who do not produce enough insulin, virtually eliminated the need for any injections of insulin by adopting the bean regimen. The reason: beans produce such slow rises in blood sugar that the body needs to release much less insulin to keep the glucose under control. Beans, along with other foods high in gums and pectins, actually cause the creation of more insulin-receptor sites on cells, which means the insulin has more places to dock and is siphoned off, so less circulates in the system, which is good.

For one thing, less insulin stifles hunger and through a complicated mechanism may facilitate the excretion of sodium, thereby lowering blood pressure. Eating high fiber foods like beans does lower blood pressure substantially according to numerous studies. Vegetarians, for example, matched for age and sex, had a diastolic (lower number) blood pressure that was eighteen percent lower than that of meat eaters. Even people with normal blood pressure have brought it down another five or six percent by bucking up their intake of high fiber foods like beans.

CANCER BLOCKERS

Consider beans good bets as cancer preventers. For one reason, legumes are concentrated carriers of protease inhibitors, enzymes that can counteract the activation of cancer-causing compounds in the intestine. Cancer biologist Ann Kennedy gave lab animals a chemical known to cause oral cancer. She notes: "When protease inhibitors are brushed onto the inner cheek surfaces of hamsters, no cancers develop." Feeding animals protease inhibitors also blocked the development of colon and breast cancer.

In a series of tests, Dr. Walter Troll fed rats beans—in this case soybeans but Dr. Troll thinks other beans with protease inhibitors do the same thing. He then exposed the rodents to powerful X rays, known to cause breast cancer. Only forty-four percent of the soybean-eating animals developed the expected cancer, compared with seventy-four percent who did not eat soybeans. Dr. Troll finds that protease inhibitors can turn off oncogenes—those genetic carriers found in every normal cell that when activated may lead to cancer. He is convinced that all "seed foods," like beans, may prevent the cell division foreshadowing cancer as well as progression of the tumor. Thus, he thinks legumes are especially important, and, in fact, behave a little like chemotherapy in shutting down the cancer process. When cancer has metastasized, or spread, he does not think eating protease inhibitors will help, although they are being tested in much larger doses as possible drugs against cancer metastasis.

Beans are also rich in compounds called lignans that are anticancer on their own and are converted by colon bacteria into hormonelike substances that some scientists suggest could help fight off both breast and colon cancer.

GREAT FOR THE COLON

Although it's a subject that only scientists can discuss at conferences with a straight face, it is well established that a greater "fecal output," or large feces, is a sign of health. And such scientists urge you to eat foods that increase the fecal output. They are convinced it is a way to alleviate symptoms or reduce your chances of colon or rectal cancer, diverticular disease, hemorrhoids, and bowel irregularities.

Beans decidedly give you a much larger, softer stool, according to Sharon Fleming, Ph.D., the dean of bean researchers, at the Nutritional Sciences Department, University of California, Berkeley. Every morning she and her colleagues gave a group of young men a cup and a half of kidney beans for about three weeks. The idea was to see how the beans affected the functioning of their colons. Actually, the kidney beans were mashed into a paste, much like refried beans, which many of the men ate on a tortilla, topped with melted cheese. Some were dedicated bean lovers—they ate at least three six-ounce servings a week; others rarely touched them.

The researchers concluded that beans are good for your colon. Beans decidedly increased "fecal output," and also appeared to stimulate colonic bacteria to throw off chemicals, called volatile short chain fatty acids, that help lower blood cholesterol, blood pressure, and possibly inhibit colon cancer. These fatty acids come from fermentation of food, notably soluble fiber, in the colon, and are being intensively scrutinized for their cancer-blocking potential. Dr. Fleming highly recommends beans as a cure for constipation for people without intestinal diseases.

PRACTICAL MATTERS

- Baked beans, including canned, count too. A therapeutic daily dose of one cup is found in a seven and a half ounce can. Dr. James Anderson tested plain old canned pork and beans and found they lowered blood cholesterol an average twelve percent.

CAUTION

- However, Australian researchers recently noted that canned baked beans caused higher levels of blood sugar and insulin than baked beans first boiled and then baked at home. The researchers cautioned diabetics to avoid canned legumes.

THE FLATULENCE QUESTION

Eating beans definitely creates gas in many people, because humans generally lack the enzymes to digest certain complex bean sugars, called alpha-galactosides. The undigested sugars are then attacked by bacteria in the lower intestine, releasing various gases. But the more often you eat legumes the less likely you are to suffer discomfort from gas, because frequent bean eaters adapt physiologically. Dr. Fleming found that eaters of a cup and a half of kidney beans a day complained of gas for the first 12 to 48 hours; after that, their discomfort disappeared.

DEGASSING PROCEDURE

Proper soaking rids legumes of most of their gas-producing potential. Alfred Olson, research chemist with the United States Department of Agriculture's Regional Research Center in California, says you can eliminate ninety percent of the gas-producing sugars in beans this way: Rinse dried beans. Discard water. Then pour boiling water over the beans and let them soak for at least four hours. Again discard the water, adding fresh water for cooking. One problem: such rinsing also washes away some of the vitamins and minerals.

BEST BEANS

½ cup cooked	Soluble fiber grams
Black-eyed peas	3.7
Peas, canned	2.7
Kidney beans	2.5
Pinto beans	2.3
Navy beans	2.3
Lentils	1.7
Split peas	1.7

DR. ANDERSON'S CHOLESTEROL-FIGHTING BEAN RECIPES*

HEARTY BEAN BAKE

¼ cup finely chopped onion
1 medium garlic clove, minced
1 can (16 oz) beans in tomato sauce
1 cup cooked kidney beans
½ cup cooked baby lima beans
¼ cup ketchup
1 teaspoon prepared mustard
Dash pepper

Preheat oven to 375 degrees. Grease a one-quart casserole dish. Combine all ingredients in casserole dish. Bake 45 minutes, until hot and bubbly; stir. Makes 3 cups of 6 side-dish servings.

BEAN BURRITOS

4 cups refried beans (recipe below)
8 (9-inch) flour tortillas
½ cup chopped onion
About 4 teaspoons taco sauce
¼ cup shredded Cheddar cheese (1 oz)
To garnish: Additional taco sauce

Refried beans
2 lean bacon slices (2 oz)
1 cup chopped onions
2 (16 oz) cans pinto or red beans
2 teaspoons garlic salt

In a large skillet, fry bacon until crisp. Remove bacon; drain on paper towels. Cook onions in bacon fat until tender. Crumble bacon; add to skillet with beans and garlic salt. Mash beans with potato masher. Cook over low heat, stirring frequently, 10 minutes, or until dry.

To make burritos:
Preheat oven to 200 degrees. Add ⅔ cup refried beans to center of each

*Reprinted from Dr. Anderson's *Life-Saving Diet*, (Tucson) The Body Press, 1986.

flat tortilla. Spread onion over beans, then push down into beans. Sprinkle ½ teaspoon taco sauce over beans and onion; sprinkle each with 1½ teaspoons cheese. Fold into oblong burritos and place on an ungreased baking sheet. Heat 15 to 20 minutes, or until heated through. Add additional taco sauce on top if desired. Makes 8 servings.

HEARTY LENTIL-BARLEY DISH

1½ cups tomato juice
¼ cup water
¼ cup barley
¼ cup lentils
2 celery stalks, diced
½ medium onion, sliced
¼ cup diced carrot
½ cup diced potato
⅛ teaspoon dried leaf savory
⅛ teaspoon dried leaf chervil
¼ teaspoon dried leaf thyme
½ teaspoon dried leaf tarragon

Simmer tomato juice, water, barley, and lentils in a medium-size saucepan over medium heat 15 minutes. Add celery, onion, carrot, potato, and herbs; simmer 30 minutes, or until lentils and barley are tender. Makes 2 servings.

If you're worried about sodium in canned beans, first drain beans and rinse them with clear water; this eliminates about half the salt content.

BEER

- Prevents blockage of heart arteries
- Raises good HDL-type blood cholesterol

> *How Much?* A beer a day can modify blood, reducing the risk of coronary artery blockages. A half a pint of beer a day can boost beneficial HDL-type cholesterol.

FACTS

Disconcerting to some, pleasing to others, evidence emerges that a little drinking may be good for your cardiovascular system. Dr. Richard D. Moore, assistant professor of medicine at the Johns Hopkins University School of Medicine, recently asked twenty-eight healthy men to drink a beer a day and twenty-eight similar men to abstain. Ordinarily all drank from two to four alcoholic beverages a week.

Nothing much happened to the beer drinkers' total blood cholesterol or desirable HDLs or even detrimental LDL-type cholesterol. But—the beer drinkers showed a decided upsurge in another blood component, a protein called apolipoprotein A-1; individuals with high levels of this apo A-1 are less likely to suffer blockages in heart arteries.

139

Interestingly, the non-beer drinkers saw their protective apo A-1 levels sink slightly. Dr. Moore theorized that the beer's alcohol caused liver enzymes to make more apo A-1, and concluded that the blood changes from the beer-a-day diet "might lead to a reduced cardiovascular risk over time."

HDL PUZZLE

For years medical experts have haggled over whether drinking alcoholic beverages induces an upward spurt in that important blood component HDL-type cholesterol that transports damaging cholesterol away from artery walls to the liver, where it is destroyed. Small-scale studies have been conflicting. But scientists cannot ignore a recent very persuasive study of one hundred men and women in Great Britain, seeming to clinch the case for an HDL boost.

The subjects were asked to drink at least seven drinks a week for four weeks, and then switch back to no drinking for another four weeks. One drink was defined as a half pint of beer or cider, one glass of wine, or a measure of sherry or other spirits providing seven to nine grams of alcohol. Most drank about two drinks a day. Unquestionably, on the drinking regimen the participants had higher HDLs; up about seven percent. Their critical ratio of HDL to total blood cholesterol was also five percent better.

Most interesting to scientists is the fact that the rise occurred in the HDL-2 subfraction, which is that thought to help protect against heart disease. Previous opinion was that alcoholic beverages raised only the HDL-3 type—considered irrelevant in preventing heart disease. The authors conclude that a little alcoholic beverage may confer some protection against ischemic heart disease.

THE GERMAN EXPERIMENT

Backing up the supposition is a monumental West German prospective study by Dr. Peter Cremer and his associates in the department of clinical chemistry, University of Gottingen, who are tracking the blood biochemistry and heart disease in more than 4000 men and women until 1991. A preliminary report in 1986 from a country where beer is the national drink found drinkers had better blood profiles than nondrinkers. The nondrinkers averaged HDL cholesterol of only forty-two milligrams per deciliter compared with a more protective fifty milligrams per deciliter for those who drank one and a half to two drinks a day. The imbiber's blood also carried less bad LDL-type cholesterol.

However, Dr. Cremer notes that drinking conveyed benefits only on people with mild or moderate levels of blood cholesterol; drinking alcohol did not benefit those with high cholesterol, that is, over 230 milligrams per deciliter.

Similarly, six out of seven large-scale studies, encompassing some 55,000 people around the world, suggest that people who drink a little alcohol suffer lower rates of heart attacks. That is, light drinkers have less heart disease than teetotalers; however, alcoholics have much more.

POSSIBLE ADVERSE EFFECTS

- Gout. Beer is high in purine, which the body converts into uric acid, and too much uric acid can bring on gout, a type of arthritis. It causes pain in the elbows, feet, and hands, and classically in the big toe. Indeed, British researchers in a dietary study of men with gout tagged heavy beer drinking as the most critical difference between those who got it and those who did not. Forty-one percent of the gout sufferers, compared with only seventeen percent of healthy men, drank more than 2.5 liters (about seven twelve-ounce cans) a day.
- Blood pressure. Beer with alcohol compared with beer without alcohol pushed up both diastolic and systolic blood pressure in people with normal blood pressure.
- Cancer. Alcohol raises the risk of colon and rectal cancer in women and men. Another study showed that beer drinkers in particular had more cancer of the lower urinary tract—and they were more likely to develop this cancer the more beer they drank. Those who drank spirits also had a higher risk, but, interestingly, those who drank wine did not.
- Beer drinking has also been linked to rectal cancer. One study showed a risk three times higher in beer drinkers who consumed more than fifteen liters a month.
- Another distressing note for beer drinkers. Even when cigarette smoking is not considered, a study found that alcohol consumers, particularly beer drinkers, have a higher rate of lung cancer.
- A large-scale French study found that women who drank alcoholic beverages with meals, notably beer and wine, were more likely to

have breast cancer, and the risk increased with the amount of beer, wine, and total alcohol consumed. The drinkers had a one and a half times greater risk. A mere three drinks a week has been linked to a higher risk of breast cancer among women, notably those under age fifty.

CONFLICTING EVIDENCE ON HEART DISEASE

A recent look at the incidence of heart disease and the consumption of wine and beer in twenty-seven countries found that people in nations where beer drinking was high tended to have more ischemic heart disease; nations with more wine drinkers had less.

A major study of 2170 men with first-time heart attacks, all under age fifty-five, when compared with healthy men did not find any protective effect from beer, wine, or liquor. The researchers concluded that "moderate alcohol consumption does not reduce the risk of nonfatal myocardial infarction."

PRACTICAL MATTERS

- To drink or not to drink. In view of the dangers of beer drinking, as well as the higher risk of alcoholism, cirrhosis of the liver, pancreatitis, high blood pressure, heart arrhythmia, and fetal alcohol syndrome tied to alcohol in general, it seems folly to deliberately take up beer or alcohol in hope of avoiding a heart attack.
- However, some heart protection from moderate drinking (one or two drinks a day) may be an inadvertent bonus. So if you're already a moderate drinker, you can weigh the benefits and risks. For heavy drinkers, any slight benefit to the heart is bound to be far overshadowed by the health dangers.

BLUEBERRY

POSSIBLE THERAPEUTIC BENEFITS:
- Combats diarrhea
- Kills infectious viruses
- Blocks damage to blood vessels
- Acts as a laxative in some persons

FOLKLORE

Blueberries are a common Swedish folk remedy for diarrhea, and the belief that blueberries fight infections is widespread. Dr. Amr Abdel-Fattah Ismail, formerly a plant physiologist with the United States Department of Agriculture and now vice-president of the Maine Wild Blueberry Company, says blueberry soup is popular on European ski slopes as a cold remedy. And, Rodale's *Encyclopedia of Natural Home Remedies* notes that the "blueberry diarrhea cure" thrives in the western hemisphere. A Quebec resident claims her father suffered bloody diarrhea for many years until someone alerted him to blueberries. "Whenever someone in my family suffers from diarrhea," she says, "I treat it with blueberries. It really works."

FACTS

In Sweden, dried blueberry soup has long been used by physicians to treat childhood diarrhea. The typical dose according to Finn Sandberg, professor of pharmacognosy at Uppsala Biomedical Center in Sweden, is five to ten grams of dried blueberries, about one third of an ounce.

Undeniably, blueberries contain high concentrations of compounds that can kill both bacteria and viruses. In Canadian tests, crushed blueberries destroyed nearly one hundred percent of polioviruses within twenty-four hours, even when the berries were diluted ten times. The researchers credited tannins in the fruit with killing the microbes.

More to the point, the blueberry, just like the black currant, is full of chemicals that have been proved antidiarrheal in tests in Sweden. In fact, a powder made from the skins of black currants is marketed in Sweden and for export as a natural antidiarrheal drug. Of all fruits, the blueberry and the black currant are highest in these therapeutic agents called anthocyanosides, proved lethal to bacteria, namely E. coli, often a cause of infectious diarrhea. The antidiarrheal drug is called Pecarin. (See Currant, page 184.)

BRAIN-CHOLESTEROL BARRIER

These same blueberry-currant compounds, others have discovered, may protect blood vessels from the destructive deposits that characterize atherosclerosis, or hardening of the arteries. Thus, they may protect against heart disease and stroke.

A collaborative team of scientists at the University of Paris and the Semmelweis Medical University in Budapest extracted anthocyanosides from blueberries and injected them in rabbits eating a high cholesterol diet. The blueberry chemicals counteracted some of the ill effects of the atherosclerosis brought on by the high cholesterol diet. Rabbits fed high cholesterol *plus blueberry chemicals* had less severe calcium-fat deposits in their aortas and less-diseased small blood vessels in the brain than animals fed only cholesterol.

Investigators speculate that the anthocyanosides blocked the ability of cholesterol to penetrate vessel walls, especially in the brain, thereby reducing the amount of disease damage. A cholesterol-rich diet, they say, makes blood vessel walls more permeable. The blueberry chemicals, thus, may have interacted with collagen in both large and micro blood vessels to create a tougher wall that cholesterol could not breach. Thus, these natural chemicals may be partial antidotes to "hardening of the arteries," by keeping cholesterol away from the blood, so it flows freely through the heart and brain.

Other French researchers, using anthocyanosides from black currants instead of from blueberries, found essentially the same protection in blood vessels of monkeys, those laboratory animals closest to humans in physiology. There, too, the fruit chemicals blocked some arterial and small-vessel damage inflicted by high fat diets.

German scientists have also found that fresh blueberries in some individuals have a pronounced laxative effect.

BROCCOLI

POSSIBLE THERAPEUTIC BENEFIT:
- Lowers risk of cancer

How much? An extra half cup of broccoli a day may help protect against several cancers, notably colon and lung cancer.

FACTS

Broccoli appears to be a versatile cancer fighter. As a dark-green vegetable, it emerges high in numerous lab tests designed to identify foods with cancer-counteracting potential. It also tops the food lists of people who have lower rates of all cancers, and, in particular, cancer of the esophagus, stomach, colon, lung, larynx, prostate, oral cavity, and pharynx. As a member of the cruciferous family, it ranks high against colon cancer. In fact, in some tests broccoli looks even better than its close cousin, cabbage, which is an acknowledged superstar in this area.

Broccoli, like other cruciferous vegetables, is rich in known cancer antidotes such as indoles, glucosinolates, and dithiolthiones. Broccoli, also like spinach and kale, is endowed with carotenoids, which may give it added powers against cancers such as lung. Probably due to its abundance of chlorophyll, broccoli is extraordinarily potent in blocking cell mutations foreshadowing cancer.

146

BROCCOLI IN BUFFALO

When Dr. Saxon Graham, in a ground-breaking study, compared the diets of several hundred Buffalo, New York, residents with and without colon and rectal cancer, he found that the risk was cut among those eating more broccoli, cabbage, and brussels sprouts. And there was a dose response; the risk decreased the more broccoli eaten. For example, in general those eating broccoli (and other cruciferous vegetables) never or up to ten times a month were nearly twice as likely to have colon cancer as those eating broccoli more than twenty-one times a month.

Tests done in the early 1950s by the army found that broccoli kept guinea pigs from succumbing to otherwise lethal doses of irradiation. Cabbage worked, too, but the researchers concluded that "broccoli was even more effective." Of experimental animals given meals of broccoli and then showered with 400 rads of radiation, sixty-five percent survived; all guinea pigs irradiated but not fed broccoli died. In comparison, cabbage kept alive fifty-two percent of the animals.

Broccoli may even help block cervical cancer. In a 1983 study, Dr. James R. Marshall and his colleagues working with Dr. Graham at the Roswell Park Memorial Institute in Buffalo found that although eating lots of cruciferous vegetables in general—more than four times a week—strangely seemed linked to higher rates of cervical cancer, an exception was broccoli. Women who ate more broccoli were less prone to cancer of the cervix.

Broccoli, along with other dark-green vegetables, in a study of New Jersey men with lung cancer, protected both current smokers and smokers who had quit within the past five years. Three-times-a-week eaters of dark-green vegetables had double the risk of lung cancer in the five years following their stopping smoking as men who ate the green stuff every day. The theory: compounds in the green vegetables (and in dark-orange vegetables) act as antidotes to a cancer process that continues years after exposure to carcinogens such as smoke.

BRUSSELS SPROUTS

POSSIBLE THERAPEUTIC BENEFIT:
• A good bet to inhibit cancer, especially colon and stomach

FACTS

Brussels sprouts look exceptionally good as a way to boost the body's defenses if you're worried about cancer, notably colon cancer. The sprouts are of the brassica, or cruciferous family that along with cabbage and broccoli are tops in the diets of people with low rates of cancer in general, and colon and stomach cancer in particular.

If you ask people around the world with low rates of cancer what they eat, green vegetables like brussels sprouts are mentioned consistently. Of the world's seven large-scale diet and colon cancer studies done, fully six of them (two in the United States, one in Japan, one in Greece, one in Norway, one in Israel) point to green vegetables, including brussels sprouts, as formidable cancer preventers.

Of those, brussels sprouts emerged (along with cabbage and broccoli) as particularly outstanding in saving men from colon cancer in Dr. Saxon Graham's 1978 landmark study in Buffalo. Eating more cruciferous vegetables, including brussels sprouts, may even suppress the precancerous growths in the colon called polyps, from which cancer springs, according to another recent landmark study in

Norway. Surveys find that brussels sprouts and other cruciferae may also cut the risk of rectal, stomach, lung, bladder, and esophageal cancer.

PACKED WITH ANTICANCER CHEMICALS

Scientists have discovered specific chemicals in the green globes that retard cancer in laboratory animals, including chlorophyll, indoles, dithiolthiones, carotenoids, and glucosinolates. Animals that eat such foods or compounds and then are exposed to potent cancer-causing chemicals are less likely to develop cancers than those fed no brussels sprouts or their active compounds. For example, Dr. Lee Wattenberg found that animals eating brussels sprouts and then subjected to the potent carcinogen benzopyrene not only developed fewer cancers, but showed conclusive evidence of greater liver enzyme activity known to ward off cancer formation. In fact, of several vegetables tested—cabbage, turnip greens, broccoli, cauliflower, spinach, and alfalfa—that helped rev up cancer defenses, brussels sprouts were the most potent—twice as protective as next in line, cabbage.

In other tests brussels sprouts detoxified one of the world's most virulent carcinogens, aflatoxin, a fungal mold linked to high rates of cancer, especially liver cancer. Aflatoxin frequently contaminates such foods as peanuts, corn, and rice, and is a special threat in third world countries.

First, experimenters at Cornell University fed separate batches of rats brussels sprouts, glucosinolates (the vegetable's chemicals suspected of disarming aflatoxin), and nothing. Then the rats got doses of aflatoxin guaranteed to produce liver tumors. But rats fed either brussels sprouts or the pure glucosinolates remained relatively free of malignancy; their livers spewed out high concentrations of enzymes that neutralized the cancer potential of the aflatoxin. The brussels sprouts compounds also immunize animals against other cancer-causing chemicals.

PRACTICAL MATTERS

- Cruciferous vegetables, including brussels sprouts, because they contain chemicals thought to harm thyroid functions, are usually regarded as potential causes of goiter. However, in a recent test, humans eating five and a half ounces of cooked brussels sprouts a day for four weeks showed no sign of disturbed thyroid functioning. The investigators concluded that cooking neutralized the antithyroid chemicals.

CABBAGE

POSSIBLE THERAPEUTIC BENEFITS:
- Lowers the risk of cancer, especially of the colon
- Prevents and heals ulcers (juice especially)
- Stimulates the immune system
- Kills bacteria and viruses
- Fosters growth

> *How Much?* Eating cabbage raw, cooked, or as sauerkraut only once a week may cut your chances of colon cancer by sixty-six percent! Since there appears to be a dose response, eating cabbage more often is likely to boost its anticancer potency.

FOLKLORE

Cabbage has an ancient and esteemed place in medical folklore. Cato the Censor (234–149 B.C.) wrote: "It will purge wounds full of pus, and cancers, and make them well when no other treatment can accomplish it. . . ." In ancient Rome, cabbage was regarded as a panacea. To quote a sixteenth-century historian: "The old Romans having expelled physicians out of their commonwealth, did for many years maintain their health by the use of cabbages, taking them for every disease."

In the twentieth century, according to A. M. Liebstein, M.D.

(*American Medicine*, January 1927), "cabbage is therapeutically effective in conditions of scurvy, diseases of the eyes, gout, rheumatism, pyorrhea, asthma, tuberculosis, cancer, gangrene. . . . Cabbage is excellent as a vitalizing agent, blood purifier, anti-scorbutic." Modern folk medicine also hails cabbage as an antiulcer remedy.

FACTS

Cabbage, unquestionably, is one of the unassuming, unappreciated true stars of the food pharmacy. Cabbage looks to be a virtuoso of pharmacological powers, a concentrated package of several known therapeutic compounds. Cabbage's main claim to fame currently is its potential for preventing cancer, notably of the colon.

CABBAGE SAVES IRRADIATED RATS

The first modern scientific clues came in 1931; a German scientist experimenting with deadly radiation discovered that rabbits survived an otherwise lethal dose of radiation if they ate cabbage leaves prior to exposure. French scientists in 1950 found the same thing. In extensive experiments in 1959, two United States Armed Forces researchers fed diced raw cabbage (as well as broccoli and beets) to guinea pigs before and after giving them 400 rads of deadly whole body X radiation. As expected, one hundred percent of the guinea pigs fed no vegetables died within fifteen days. Over fifty percent of those *prefed* cabbage survived. Those eating cabbage *after* irradiation also lived longer. Most likely to survive: guinea pigs that ate cabbage (or broccoli) both before and after the irradiation. (Beets provided no protection.)

LONGEVITY FOOD

In studies to ferret out the most potent anticancer foods in humans, cabbage in remarkable regularity turns up at the top. Large population surveys in Greece, Japan, and the United States link cabbage to formidable protection against colon cancer. In fact, one large year-long survey in five areas of Japan published in 1986 concluded that those who ate the most cabbage had the lowest death rates from *all causes*, lifting cabbage to new status, along with yogurt and olive oil, as potential life extenders.

FIRST AGAINST COLON CANCER

Recently, Greek physicians, comparing the diets of one hundred colorectal cancer patients with those of noncancer patients of the same age and sex found that cancer victims ate far fewer vegetables, in particular cabbage, spinach, lettuce, and beets. The risk soared eight times for those eating the least vegetables compared with those eating the most. Dr. Saxon Graham, dissecting the diets of hundreds of patients, identified vegetables as protective agents against colon and rectal cancer. On further analysis, cabbage surfaced as the number one protector; men who ate cabbage once a week had one third the risk of colon cancer. (For more details, see page 57.) Worldwide, six out of seven large-scale population analyses conclude that cruciferous vegetables, including cabbage, shave the risk of colon cancer.

REASONS WHY

What makes the cabbage connection so fascinating is that in the lab, scientists can match and explain the human findings in chemical terms. In the 1970s Dr. Lee Wattenberg isolated chemicals from the cabbage family, called indoles, that blocked cancer formation in animals. He and others meticulously worked out precisely how these and other chemicals in cabbage, including dithiolthiones suppress the activation of cancer-causing substances in animals. Cabbage and its cousins, brussels sprouts, broccoli, and cauliflower, appear to guard cells against the very first onslaughts that progress to full-fledged cancer.

A STRING OF NEW RESEARCH

Cabbage's popularity as an anticancer agent routinely spurs news that someone has squeezed a new anticancer chemical out of cabbage. In test tubes cabbage juice suppresses precancerous cell changes leading to cancer. Thus cabbage is classified as a "desmutagen," a chemical cancer antagonist. The Japanese found cabbage such a potent desmutagen that in 1980 they patented two techniques for isolating the cancer-fighting amino acid from cabbage juice.

The cruciferous family, of which cabbage is the most famous member, claims more known anticancer agents than any other vegetable genus. Cabbage's known anticancer compounds include chlorophyll, dithiolthiones, certain flavonoids, indoles, isothiocyanates, phenols such as caffeic and ferulic acids, and vitamins E and C.

INFECTION FIGHTER?

Cabbage can destroy bacteria and viruses in test tubes. Romanian scientists searching for foods that might correct an immune system gone awry found in 1986 that cabbage boosted the immune functioning of animal cells growing in test tubes. The vegetable stimulated the production of more antibodies. Guinea pigs fed cabbage grew faster, leading researchers to conclude that cabbage contains an unknown "growth factor." Eating cabbage also helps speed up the metabolism in the body of pharmaceutical drugs, namely acetaminophen.

> *Expert Example:* Jim Duke, Ph.D., chief of the medicinal plants section at the United States Department of Agriculture, eats cabbage every day—usually a big bowl of coleslaw for lunch—to help prevent colon cancer, prevalent in his family.

THE ULCER CONNECTION

In the 1940s a prominent American physician got the notion that fresh cabbage is a natural antiulcer drug. Dr. Garnett Cheney, a professor at the Stanford University School of Medicine, fed eyedropper amounts of fresh cabbage juice to guinea pigs, then tried to induce ulcers; not a single one developed the expected stomach damage.

Extrapolating from his animal studies, Dr. Cheney figured that a quart of cabbage juice daily for the average ulcer sufferer should do the trick. He tested it on fifty-five patients with gastric, duodenal, and jejunal ulcers. All but three felt better, and X rays confirmed the ulcers had healed. He announced that the cabbage reduced healing time of gastric ulcers by eighty-three percent and of duodenal ulcers seventy-two percent compared with standard treatment.

Later, using a cabbage juice concentrate, he did a double-blind study at San Quentin prison. Reportedly, of forty-five patients, ninety-two percent who daily got the cabbage concentrate for three weeks were cured of their ulcers. That compared with only thirty-two percent of ulcer sufferers who got a placebo. And when the unhealed were switched to a cabbage regimen, their ulcers, too, cleared up in three weeks.

Since the consumption of such large amounts of cabbage juice was cumbersome, Dr. Cheney dreamed of turning the magic ingredients into a drug. But the idea faltered. A drug company trying to market the cabbage derivative had trouble producing cabbage extract that was uniformly potent. With the advent of more reliable antiulcer drugs, drug companies lost interest in cabbage.

CABBAGE CATCHES ON

Proving it wasn't such a crazy idea, scientists in other countries picked up the quest. In the 1960s Hungarian scientists compressed a cabbage factor into tablets, claiming it cured peptic ulcers in human patients. German and Indian scientists also healed ulcers with cabbage. A team of respected Indian researchers headed by Dr. G. B. Singh at the Central Drug Research Institute in Lucknow elucidated cabbage's healing mechanism. In extensive studies on guinea pigs, Dr. Singh's group induced ulcers and then cured them with cabbage juice. They examined and photographed cell changes of the ulcer at various stages of healing. This revealed that ulcerated cells rejuvenated in direct proportion to the level of stomach mucins, substances that shield the lining from acids. Their analysis of cabbage found it full of mucinlike compounds, which they credited with the prevention and the rapid healing of ulcers in animals.

In 1973, scientists investigating modern antiulcer drugs noted an interesting connection. One drug called gefarnate is found in white-headed cabbages. In animal tests gefarnate does stimulate the cells of the stomach lining to lay down a shield of mucus against noxious agents such as acid. Thus, this may be a natural constituent, that helps account for cabbage's reputed ulcer healing powers. A problem: cabbage's ulcer-fighting capabilities apparently vary greatly, depending on the season and soil conditions, but the studies generally agree that the cabbage's healing factors are present only when taken raw and usually as juice. For those interested, here is Dr. Cheney's advice:

DR. CHENEY'S ANTIULCER CABBAGE COCKTAIL

- Use only fresh green cabbage heads; best are spring and summer cabbages. Fall cabbages are less effective, winter ones the least potent.
- Put the cabbage through a juicer or grinder. It takes about four to five pounds of summer and spring cabbage to make a quart of juice—twice that amount for winter cabbages, which give less juice.
- To make it more palatable, you can use seventy-five percent cabbage juice and twenty-five percent celery juice (from both stocks and greens). Celery, too, contains the antiulcer factor.

- For extra flavor, add to each glass of cabbage juice a couple of tablespoons of tomato, pineapple, or citrus juice.
- Chill. Drink a quart a day.
- You should feel results within three weeks if not sooner.

Adapted from Dr. Cheney's instructions: *Journal of the American Dietetic Association,* September 1950.

PRACTICAL MATTERS

- Don't forget cabbage includes not only the typical head cabbage common in the United States, but also bok choy, a white stalk with green floppy leaves, and celery, or Chinese cabbage, an elongated bundle of leaves and core. All are of the cruciferous vegetable family that contains anticancer chemicals.
- Advice: Eat at least some of your cabbage raw. Some therapeutic compounds are partly destroyed by heat. Some studies found protection, especially for stomach cancer, from raw cabbage (red as well as green) and coleslaw.

CONFLICTING EVIDENCE

Although most scientists view cabbage as a possible cancer fighter, a 1985 Japanese study came up with opposite findings, out of step with most current research, showing that those who ate cabbage often— four times a week—had a relatively higher risk of both colon and stomach cancer. One explanation offered by authorities: cabbage in Japan is often pickled, fermented, and aged, introducing potential cancer-producing compounds. However, that does not explain other studies showing that cabbage-eating Japanese have less colon cancer.

In other recent studies, mice and hamsters fed cabbage and simultaneously given a carcinogen had more cancers of the pancreas. Mice fed cabbage developed more skin cancers.

CARROT

Sowe Carrets in your Gardens, and humbly praise God for them, as for a singlar and great blessing.
—Richard Gardiner, circa 1599

POSSIBLE THERAPEUTIC BENEFITS:
- A prime bet for blocking cancer, especially smoking-related cancers, including lung
- Lowers blood cholesterol
- Prevents constipation

> *How much?* A single carrot or a mere half cup of carrots once a day appears to cut the risk of lung cancer at least in half, even among former heavy smokers. Two and a half raw medium-size carrots a day have lowered blood cholesterol an average eleven percent.

FOLKLORE

Carrots, according to American folk medicine, are therapeutic against general nervousness, asthma, dropsy, and especially skin disorders.

FACTS

The most thrilling aspect of carrots is their enormous promise in curtailing some of the most virulent, incurable cancers, notably of the lung and pancreas. Exciting studies show that intakes of modest amounts of carrots and specifically the beta carotene in carrots may retard cancer progression as well as disrupt the cancer mechanism that first turns cells into growing malignancies.

With amazing regularity, carrots turn up in studies pinpointing specific foods that ward off cancer. For example, a well-constructed 1986 Swedish study designated carrots as one of two prominent dietary barriers to pancreatic cancer, a particularly dangerous smoking-related tumor. (The other was citrus fruits.) Eating carrots "almost daily" substantially trimmed the chances of cancer of the pancreas.

The research tying beta carotene vegetables and fruits to less lung cancer is formidable and extensive. Ten of eleven international dietary surveys document that people who eat the least carrots and other beta carotene foods are more likely to develop lung cancer. Marilyn Menkes, Ph.D., determined that individuals with the lowest blood levels of beta carotene compared with those with the most were four times more likely a decade later to develop squamous cell carcinoma of the lung, the most common cancer due to cigarette smoking.

Similarly, a State University of New York team in Buffalo found that men eating the most high carotene foods, including carrots, were about half as likely to develop squamous cell lung cancer. They figured that the daily difference in beta carotene between the high risk and low risk lung cancer candidates is contained in *one carrot*! Eating just an extra carrot a day might prevent, Dr. Menkes said, 15,000 to 20,000 lung cancer deaths annually in the United States. Even after years of smoking, carrots may ameliorate the cancer threat by retarding the disease process.

EX-SMOKERS' SALVATION

Richard Shekelle, Ph.D., in a 1981 landmark study, found an even more dramatic impact on lung cancer from eating beta-carotene foods, among which the carrot is premier. He analyzed the eating habits and lung cancer risk of about two thousand men over a nineteen-year period. Male smokers, even those who had smoked for thirty years, who ate the least beta carotene–containing foods had eight times the risk of developing lung cancer as those who ate the most beta carotene–

containing foods, mainly carrots. Since cancer is a long process—typically taking three or four decades to appear—it seems that beta-carotene foods interfere with cancer development at late stages. Thus, after a person has stopped smoking, carrots may help block the expected progressive damage to cells.

In a recent study of New Jersey men by Regina G. Ziegler, a National Cancer Institute epidemiologist, three vegetables stood out in preventing lung cancer—carrots, sweet potatoes, and dark-yellow winter squash. Dr. Ziegler noted that men who ate a mere half cup of carrots a day (or sweet potatoes or winter squash) were half as likely to develop lung cancer as those who ate almost none. Even men who had stopped smoking ten years before were more likely to avoid lung cancer by eating carrots. Most vulnerable to lung cancer from a diet low in beta carotene were men who had stopped smoking within the last five years. Dr. Ziegler in a follow-up study also found that non-smoking women exposed to cigarette smoke could slash their risk of lung cancer by eating more carrots.

Additionally, high beta carotene foods, including carrots, have been linked in epidemiological studies to lower risk of cancers of the larynx, esophagus, prostate, bladder, cervix, and, in a study among elderly people in Massachusetts, of all types of cancer. In lab studies, feeding carrots to rats blocked liver tumors.

GOOD HEART FOOD

Raw carrots decidedly depress blood cholesterol. In one study, eating 200 grams of raw carrots (about two and a half medium-size carrots) every morning for breakfast cut blood cholesterol an average eleven percent. The carrots also increased the bulky weight of the stool by about twenty-five percent, which helps keep the colon healthy.

PREVENTS CONSTIPATION

Some gastroenterologists note that carrots have generally unappreci-ated colonic benefits, including constipation relief, because of their capacity to create softer, larger feces. A group of leading British fiber investigators in 1978 tested fiber from carrots as well as from bran, cabbage, apple, and guar gum on nineteen healthy male volunteers. They found that carrot fiber does increase fecal bulk, a sign of colonic health (about the same as cabbage) but only half as much as wheat bran. It takes, they concluded, about four and a half cups of whole boiled carrots to double fecal bulk; in contrast, about three fourths of a cup of wheat bran can do the same thing. Carrots, especially in combination with other high fiber foods, do promote regularity. Increasing fecal bulk also may cut the chances of colon cancer because among other things carcinogens are diluted, thereby reducing exposure of the colon wall.

PRACTICAL MATTERS

- To get the most anticancer protection, eat some carrots cooked. Cooking releases carotenes, believed to be the active agents in shielding tissue against carcinogenic attacks. You get two to five times more carotene from cooked carrots than from raw ones. But don't overdo it; carrots cooked to mushy lose much of their precious beta carotene.
- Do not eat carrots in the mistaken assumption that they will allow you to continue smoking. Carrots are not a substitute for quitting smoking; they cannot offset the continued assaults from cigarette smoke. Whereas carrots may cut your risk in half, smoking boosts it ten times as much.
- Ex-smokers, especially recent quitters, should eat carrots regularly to possibly stave off smoking-related cancers down the road. Some experts even find that current smokers may benefit somewhat from loading up on carrots and other carotene foods. However, lighter current smokers seem to get the most protection. It is unknown whether current heavy smokers get any benefit from eating more carrots.

CAULIFLOWER

POSSIBLE THERAPEUTIC BENEFIT:

- Reduces risk of cancer, especially colon and stomach

FACTS

Cauliflower is high on the list of anticancer vegetables because it is a member of the cruciferous family and a close cousin to cabbage, broccoli, and brussels sprouts—all associated with lower cancer rates notably of the colon, rectum, stomach, and, possibly, prostate and bladder.

In several surveys, cruciferous vegetables come out tops in food preferred by those least likely to have such cancers. Norwegians, who regularly eat more of their calories in cauliflower (as well as cabbage, broccoli, and brussels sprouts), were found, in a recent investigation, to have fewer and smaller precancerous polyps of the colon.

When laboratory animals eat cauliflower and then are given powerful carcinogens such as nitrosamines, they do not as readily develop cancers as those fed no cauliflower. That's what Dr. Lee Wattenberg found. Only sixty-three percent of the non-cauliflower-eating rats grew cancers compared with ninety-four percent not given cauliflower. Scientists believe the cauliflower's compounds, such as indoles, stimulate the natural defense, or detoxification system to neutralize the carcinogens so they don't get a chance to attack cells and convert them into cancerous tissue.

Cauliflower is not high in the carotenes or in chlorophyll, so seems less likely to block lung and other smoking-related cancers.

CHERRY

• Prevents cavities

FOLKLORE

In ancient Greece, physicians prescribed cherries for epilepsy. In the 1920s in the United States, physicians touted black cherries to cure kidney stones and gall bladder ailments, and red cherries to remove phlegm. In 1950 Ludwig Blau, Ph.D., writing in *Texas Reports on Biology and Medicine*, claimed that he cured his crippling gout that confined him to a wheelchair by eating six to eight cherries each day. As long as he ate cherries, he avowed, the gout stayed away. He had no scientific explanation for his discovery, but he noted that at least twelve others who ate cherries or drank cherry juice also cured their gout. *Prevention* magazine printed his advice and since then, dozens of people suffering gout have written to say red or black cherries—fifteen to twenty-five a day at first and ten a day after that—work for them too.

FACTS

The only recent scientific reference to the therapeutic value of cherries found the juice to be a potent antibacterial agent against tooth decay. In a study at Forsyth Dental Center, black cherry juice blocked eighty-nine percent of the enzyme activity leading to plaque formation, which is a prelude to decay.

CHILI PEPPER

POSSIBLE THERAPEUTIC BENEFITS:
- Excellent medicine for the lungs
- Acts as an expectorant
- Prevents and alleviates chronic bronchitis and emphysema
- Acts as a decongestant
- Helps dissolve blood clots
- Kills pain
- Induces euphoria

How Much? Ten to twenty drops of red-hot chili sauce in a glass of water daily or a hot spicy meal three times a week can help keep airways free of congestion, preventing or treating chronic bronchitis and colds. Two teaspoons of jalapeño pepper can rev up the blood-clot-dissolving mechanism, protecting against heart disease and stroke.

FOLKLORE

In 1850 the Dublin medical press recommended a drop or two of hot-pepper extract on cotton applied to a sore tooth as an instant remedy for toothache. A nineteenth-century report from Peru found capsicum pepper an excellent treatment for conjunctivitis—an inflammation of the eye. In South America hot chili peppers have long been consumed to kill intestinal parasites. In the United States hot peppers are folk medicine to ward off senility, in Japan to increase fertility, in England to bring on menstruation, in Indonesia to bring on abortion, and throughout the world as an aphrodisiac. Chili peppers are also reputed to cure arthritis, prevent cardiovascular disease, and prolong life.

FACTS

Hot spicy peppers, indigenous to Mexico and South America, discovered by Columbus and popularized throughout the world, especially in India and the Orient, are potent bundles of medicinal actions.

LUNG CLEANSERS

Indeed, hot peppers may prolong life, according to Dr. Irwin Ziment, a pulmonary expert who prescribes chili peppers in various forms for his patients with chronic bronchitis and emphysema. "Sometimes the effects are profound," he notes. Chili peppers and other spicy foods, he says, probably because of the pungent component capsaicin—the stuff that burns the mouth—are expectorants just like common drugs. Dr. Ziment calls hot spices nature's Robitussin.

If you've ever had a dose of hot pepper set your eyes to watering, just imagine the same effect in your bronchial passages and lungs. There's a sudden secretion of fluid that actually thins the mucus in the lungs, pushing it along. According to Dr. Ziment, chili peppers, being an irritant in the stomach, automatically signal the bronchial cells to pour out fluids making lung and throat secretions less sticky and thick. He is convinced eating hot chilis helps prevent the onset of chronic bronchitis and makes it easier to manage if it develops.

Indeed, in experiments in animals, Swedish researchers found that a dose of capsaicin desensitized the lungs—blocked some of the swelling damage to trachea and bronchial cells and the bronchoconstriction caused by cigarette smoke and other irritants. Thus, hot-pepper extract may also be good for people with asthma and others with hypersensitive airways. Dr. Ziment notes that eating peppers does clean out the sinuses, as many pepper aficionados confirm, and chili peppers can also act as decongestants in cases of the common cold. "If you don't want to actually swallow the hot peppers, you can sprinkle twenty drops of Tabasco sauce in a glass of water and use it as a gargle," says Dr. Ziment. That's good for a cold too.

PAINKILLER

Our ancestors were right to use hot pepper extract as a local anaesthesia for toothache and to cure conjunctivitis. Now scientists have tracked the precise neurological mechanism by which the capsaicin in the hot peppers suppresses pain. Capsaicin (from the Latin "to bite") induces a reduction in nerve cells of a neurotransmitter called substance P that relays pain sensations to the central nervous system. Thus, capsaicin short-circuits the perception of pain. Specific experiments confirm that applying capsaicin to the nerves drains dental pulp of substance P, and thus reduces pain sensation. Putting capsaicin on the eye also desensitizes it to irritants and reduces inflammation.

Chili pepper essence is being tested as an all-around analgesic–painkiller. According to Thomas Burks, Ph.D., head of the department of pharmacology at the University of Arizona Health Sciences Center in Tucson, a single injection of capsaicin combats certain types of chronic pain in guinea pigs for weeks. Rubbing an ointment of capsaicin on the skin numbs pain locally. Dr. Burks thinks capsaicin eventually might be turned into a drug to alleviate pain, especially the pain of arthritis.

HEART PEPPERS

The Thais use capsicum chili peppers as a seasoning and as an appetizer with meals; thus their blood is infused with chili pepper compounds several times a day. Noting that German researchers as early as 1965 found chili peppers good for the blood as a fibrinolytic (clot-dissolving) stimulant, Thai physicians have long credited the regular consumption of chili peppers as a reason that thromboembolism—life-threatening blood clots—are rare among Thais, particularly when compared with Americans.

To test this theory, Sukon Visudhiphan, M.D., and his colleagues at the Siriraj Hospital in Bangkok make some rice flour noodles and fortified each 200 grams (about a cup and a third) with two teaspoons of fresh ground capsicum jalapeño pepper. They fed the hot-pepper noodles to sixteen volunteers and plain noodles to four others. Decidedly, the blood-clot-dissolving activity increased almost immediately in eaters of the hot-pepper-laced noodles; no blood changes occurred in those who ate the plain noodles. However, within thirty minutes after eating, the clot-dissolving activity was back to normal. In later experiments, the Indian investigators found far greater clot-dissolving activity in eighty-eight Thais compared with fifty-five Americans living in Thailand. Americans had more blood fibrinogen—the clotting substance—and less clot-dissolving activity, making them more vulnerable to arterial blockage.

Although the chili-pepper effect is short-lived, Dr. Visudhiphan suggests that the *frequent* stimulation of the clot-dissolving mechanism by chili peppers helps keep the Thais immune to thromboembolism.

Further, studies in rabbits by other Indian biochemists at the Central Food Technological Research Institute in Mysore found that both dry red pepper and pure capsaicin lowered blood cholesterol apparently by suppressing the liver's production of cholesterol. Follow-up 1985 studies discovered that capsaicin depresses cholesterol and triglycerides even when fed to animals along with cholesterol-rich food. The capsaicin overpowered the expected damaging effect of the fatty foods.

BLOCKS PAIN, BRINGS PLEASURE

At the same time chili peppers produce pain in the mouth they send signals to the brain that kill pain. If you've ever felt a certain "high" after eating hot peppers, there may be good reason, according to Paul Rozin, a psychologist at the University of Pennsylvania. It's because the burning pain on the tongue and throat excites the brain to secrete endorphin—a natural morphine—which blocks pain sensations and induces a kind of euphoria. Endorphins are those same brain chemicals credited with so-called "runner's high." Eventually, says Dr. Rozin, who has studied spices in Mexico and the United States, some people who regularly eat chili peppers "condition" themselves to produce the pleasurable endorphins in higher and higher doses. In other words, they become addicted to the pleasure brought by the excessive endorphin.

PRACTICAL MATTERS

- Learning to like it hot. Start with small doses: If you want to get the medicinal benefits of chili peppers but can't stand the heat, try a little at a time. Experts say virtually everybody can gradually build up a tolerance to the hot taste and learn to love it.

- To stifle the burning sensation, eat cool yogurt with your hot food as the Indians do; it soothes the tongue and stomach. Or try beer with your food as the Thais do; it can help put out the fire because capsaicin and other chemicals that give peppers their bite dissolve in alcohol, according to Marianne Gillette, an expert at McCormick & Co., the spice producers. She says the hot chemicals also dissolve in fat, so a few sips of whole milk or ice cream also will help put out the fire in your mouth. Milk seems to work better than water or soft drinks. The burning sensation lasts only as long as the hot irritants bind to receptors in your mouth and throat.

POSSIBLE ADVERSE EFFECTS

- Ulcers? If you don't have ulcers, there is no evidence hot peppers harm the stomach, but red chili peppers, according to research, may stimulate gastric acid and therefore may aggravate ulcers. However, a report in the *British Medical Journal* found no clinical ill effects. A group of twenty-five people with ulcers ate a normal diet and took a prescribed antacid. Another group of twenty-five took the antacid but added red chili pepper at every meal. After a month the duodenal ulcers of eighty percent of both groups had healed equally.
- According to reports in medical journals, some people after eating lots of hot chili peppers have a burning of the anus, specially during bowel movements. It was discovered during a jalapeño-pepper-eating contest in Texas. It even has a medical name: "jaloproctitis." Such hot peppers would be ill advised for hemorrhoid sufferers.
- Cancer risk or protection? Eating high amounts of red chili powder by men in India was linked in a 1987 study to higher rates of cancer of the oral cavity, pharynx, esophagus, and larynx. Animals fed extremely high doses of red chili powder (one percent of the diet)—amounts far exceeding what humans could tolerate—exhibited more tumors. On the other hand, says researcher Dr. Terry Lawson, University of Nebraska Medical Center, *small doses* of capsaicin actually act as antioxidants to block cell damage, possibly *preventing* cancer. It's not unusual, he notes, for high doses and low doses of the same chemical to have opposite effects in combating cancer.

COFFEE

POSSIBLE THERAPEUTIC BENEFITS:
- Improves mental performance
- Relieves asthma (bronchodilator)
- Relieves hay fever
- Boosts physical energy
- Prevents cavities
- Contains chemicals that block cancer in animals
- Elevates your mood

> *How Much?* Best dose seems to be a couple of cups of regular coffee a day—one in the morning and one in late afternoon. It's the perfect amount to keep you alert and concentrated, lift your mood, and rev up physical endurance. Five cups a day or more could mean trouble, and nighttime coffee is verboten for people with insomnia.

FOLKLORE

Coffee has been hailed as good for about anything that ails you. In fact, it first came to Europe from Arabia in the 1600s as a medicine, not as a beverage. In seventeenth-century France, coffee was controlled by physicians; the bean was sold more as a drug than as a drink, and coffee sellers hawked it as a type of therapeutic panacea. Coffee's mind-stimulating powers quickly caught on. French poets, among them Voltaire, called coffee "a somber, exceedingly cerebral liquor." Coffee also developed a reputation as a respiratory treatment. For example: "One of the commonest and best reputed remedies of asthma is strong coffee," wrote Dr. Hyde Salter in the *Edinburgh Medical Journal* in 1859. For many years the treatment of choice for allergic bronchial asthma was black mocha coffee.

FACTS

Coffee is one of the world's favorite drugs, a proven pick-me-up for the brain and muscles, mainly because of its high concentration of caffeine. Coffee also relaxes the bronchial muscles, boosts your exercise endurance, and has some hazards, but not nearly all those that have been attributed to it.

MENTAL BOOSTER

"Caffeine is a mind-accelerating mood booster. This isn't just sales hype brewed up by the coffee industry; it is scientific fact," declares Judith Wurtman, a distinguished mood-food research scientist at MIT. How much ordinary doses of caffeine increase mental performance was defined by Dr. Harris Lieberman, a psychologist in the Department of Brain and Cognitive Sciences at MIT.

To mimic ordinary intake—a morning cup or mug of coffee—he gave a group of men daily caffeine in capsules of various doses: 32, 64, 128, and 256 milligrams. (Thirty-two milligrams is roughly the amount of a cola soft drink or a five-ounce cup of brewed tea; 64 milligrams in a five-ounce cup of instant coffee; 128 milligrams in a five-ounce cup of brewed coffee; and 256 milligrams in a ten-ounce mug of brewed coffee.

Every morning at eight A.M., after eating or drinking nothing for twelve hours, the volunteers downed the caffeine capsules. A little later they took a series of subtle mental alertness tests that measured reaction time, attention span, concentration, acuity, and accuracy with numbers. On other days, unknowingly, they got identical-looking placebo capsules with no caffeine.

Amazing fact: The caffeine boosted their performances on every single one of the mental tests. Even the smallest dose—thirty-two milligrams—stirred the brain to improve mental functioning, reaction speed, concentration, and accuracy. As Dr. Wurtman interprets it: "Caffeine's stimulating effect on the brain and nervous system resulted in quicker thinking and reacting, greater alertness and accuracy, and extended attention spans on the part of volunteers after they had had their morning dose of this chemical."

Furthermore, the caffeine worked the same to empower the brain whether volunteers usually drank some coffee, lots of coffee, or no coffee. It was the caffeine pure and simple that bolstered brain functioning. Another study by Dr. Lieberman found that 200 milligrams of caffeine significantly improved driving performance.

MOOD-LIFTER

At the same time caffeine can significantly bolster the mood of some people. And it's likely humans have been using caffeine drinks like coffee for centuries to fight not only the blues, but chronic mild depression. In fact, researchers have now discovered how coffee can change brain chemistry in a way that makes caffeine an antidepressant similar to modern drugs. Investigators at Johns Hopkins and the Karolinska Institute in Stockholm have found that caffeine molecules can actually latch onto brain cells, blocking the attachment of a neurotransmitter that shuts off mood-raising chemicals. (The caffeine molecule fools the cells into attaching because caffeine is shaped much like the natural neurotransmitter.) Thus, caffeine, by displacing the chemical that releases the "bad-mood" producers, actually keeps good-mood chemicals circulating in your brain, making you feel "up." In some people one cup of coffee can bring a smile to the face, lifting their mood for more than two hours. That caffeine, thus coffee, can be a powerful and safe antidepressant seems confirmed by centuries of use.

Caffeine is fast-acting. It is rapidly absorbed and shows up in tissue fluids about five minutes after consumption. It gets quickly and easily into the brain and reaches peak blood levels in about twenty to thirty minutes. After peaking, caffeine in your blood will sink to about half that in three to six hours and about one fourth in another three to six hours. Virtually all the caffeine is used by the body; only one percent is excreted nonmetabolized.

PHYSICAL BOOSTER

Caffeine is so well known in sports competition as a way to boost performance that some critics claim it is abused and is similar to "doping." It's well established that caffeine prolongs the amount of time during which an individual can perform physically exhausting work.

Thus, caffeine improves performances subject to fatigue. Well-trained competitive cyclists given 330 milligrams of caffeine pedaled seven percent harder but did not notice any increased effort and endured about twenty percent longer. In another study of eighty subjects, after taking 250 milligrams of caffeine, fifty-four percent improved in the long jump, sixty percent in the shot put, and eighty percent in the one-hundred-meter sprint. (Decaffeinated coffee actually caused severe deterioration of athletic performance in short events.) Apparently, caffeine prevents muscle fatigue and enhances the body's ability to burn fat for fuel, sparing sugar, which is then stored in tissues to be called on for sudden bursts of energy. On the other hand, caffeine may impair tasks that require finger coordination, such as threading a needle, hitting a small target, or throwing darts.

IMPROVES BREATHING

As folklore claimed, recent Canadian tests show that strong coffee is good treatment for asthma patients. The caffeine in coffee dilates bronchial tubes, making it easier for asthmatics to breathe. According to research done on both children and older adults, drinking two eight-ounce cups of strong brewed coffee should produce relief within an hour or two and last for six hours or so. Although in the 1800s caffeine was the wonder drug for asthma, it lost out to theophylline, which since 1921 has been a common drug for relief of asthma. However, in modern tests comparing caffeine and theophylline, both of which have similar chemical structures, investigators at the University of Manitoba reported in the *New England Journal of Medicine* that "caffeine is as effective a bronchodilator as theophylline in young patients with asthma." In truth, the caffeine breaks down in the body into other chemicals, including theophylline.

Similarly, caffeine may be good medicine for hay fever sufferers, according to Philip Shapiro of the Albany, New York, Medical Center. To treat his allergic rhinitis (similar to hay fever), he took either caffeine tablets or placebos for sixteen days. The tablets were coded, but he did not know which he was taking. On the days he swallowed the caffeine—equivalent to two strong cups of coffee—he recorded only a couple of sneezes and little discomfort and itching compared with twenty-seven sneezes when he took the placebo.

Caffeine also makes breathing easier by decreasing respiratory muscle fatigue. Thus, coffee seems good medicine for those with breathing difficulty, especially those with chronic obstructive lung disease. Researchers at Case Western Reserve University found that the caffeine in three cups of strong coffee (600 milligrams) made both men and women breathe easier and longer in tests designed to measure breathing muscle fatigue.

A PICK-ME-UP FOR THE ELDERLY

Some older people tend to become dizzy or even faint after eating, especially at breakfast, because their autonomic nervous system does not kick in to regulate blood pressure as it did in younger days.

To correct that, a team of Vanderbilt University School of Medicine physicians recommend two cups of caffeinated coffee (250 milligrams of caffeine) with breakfast. In tests on elderly patients vulnerable to this condition, the caffeine kept blood pressure elevated enough to normalize blood flow, preventing dizziness, and retaining equilibrium. However, they noted, if you use coffee to treat this condition, don't drink coffee with caffeine for the rest of the day because too much caffeine can blunt the effect. The doctors note that drinking the coffee *before* eating works even better.

ANTICAVITY AGENT

At the prominent Forsyth Dental Research Center, Dr. Sidney Kashket and his colleagues found that coffee, because of its tannins, can interfere with bacterial processes leading to tooth decay. Drinking coffee, even decaffeinated, washes your teeth with these tannins that prevent bacterial plaque from forming and digging holes in your teeth. Coffee, like tea and cocoa, is an anticavity mouthwash.

COFFEE AND CANCER

Despite fears that drinking coffee might induce cancer, namely pancreatic and bladder cancer, later findings generally clear coffee, and laboratory evidence shows that chemicals in coffee may actually prevent cancer. Several studies in Japan, Norway, and the United States do not incriminate coffee drinking in any cancer, and most definitively not in pancreatic cancer. In fact, Norwegian studies suggest that drinking coffee might help prevent colon cancer, especially in those eating a high fat diet. Definitively, Dr. Lee Wattenberg and his colleagues at the University of Minnesota find that green coffee beans strongly block cancer in laboratory animals. Canadian cancer expert Dr. Hans Stich also considers coffee, because of its concentration of polyphenols, a potent anticancer agent in laboratory tests.

PRACTICAL MATTERS

- For greatest mental alertness, drink a cup of regular coffee early in the morning. It's the time your brain, after a night of deprivation, is most sensitive to the arousal effects. Then lay off until late afternoon, when you need another caffeine pick-me-up. Researchers say there's no need to drink coffee during the day, because the morning dose usually lasts for several hours. Dr. Wurtman says "pouring more of the chemical into your body at that time is a little like attempting to make your car run better by stopping off for gas when the tank is almost full." However, an afternoon replenishing will keep your mind power at full speed for another six hours or so.
- If you want to boost athletic performance, drink your coffee about twenty minutes to a half hour before you begin the activity.
- You can relieve an asthma attack by drinking a couple of cups of strong black coffee. Coffee is the recommended source because it contains much higher concentrations of caffeine than colas, tea, or cocoa. Still, experts conducting the studies stopped short of recommending coffee drinking as a *routine* way to deal with asthma attacks, especially in children, or as a substitute for asthma medications. But it can do a dandy job in an emergency, they say, if the usual antiasthma drugs are not available.

MYTHS AND CAUTIONS

- Coffee and blood pressure: Contrary to popular opinion, moderate coffee drinking (less than six cups a day, according to one study) does not contribute to long-term high blood pressure, except in smokers. Combining caffeine and smoking can significantly drive up the blood pressure of those already suffering from the disease. In others, coffee does commonly raise normal blood pressure, but only temporarily. Apparently, the body usually adapts to the caffeine in a few days.

  If you already have high blood pressure, Vanderbilt University researchers see no lowering effect from giving up caffeine or coffee. And people with high blood pressure who don't drink coffee don't live longer, according to research at the University of Texas Health

Sciences Center. In fact, a 1987 Italian study of 500 male and female workers shows that habitual consumers of coffee had slightly lower blood pressure, especially nonsmokers.

- Heart disease: Heavy coffee drinking seems to promote heart disease. A major study at Johns Hopkins University School of Medicine in 1985 found that men drinking five or more cups of coffee a day were almost three times as likely to develop heart problems as non-coffee drinkers. Women, too, who drink six cups of coffee a day suffer two and a half times as many heart attacks. Coffee can raise blood cholesterol slightly in some people, but that seems to be a minor problem for most, according to a review of twenty-two international studies. However, experts advise: If your cholesterol level is very high cut out coffee for a month and see if it goes down.

- Ulcers: Coffee is known to stimulate gastric secretion, so is considered damaging to ulcer patients. However, one recent large-scale Swedish study found no connection between coffee drinking and *development* of gastric or duodenal ulcers. Note: Decaffeinated coffee also spurs production of stomach acid, so apparently caffeine is not the culprit.

- Birth defects: If you are pregnant, it's a good idea to cut out or cut down on caffeine. The Food and Drug Administration in 1980 advised pregnant women to drink no more than two cups of coffee a day because of the danger of birth defects.

- Breast disease: The evidence on whether caffeine causes fibrocystic breasts, or "benign breast disease," is a mishmash of contradictions. Dr. John Minton of Ohio State University, since 1979, after studies, has urged women to cut back on methylxanthines, including caffeine, in their diets, insisting it will make breast cysts disappear or lessen. Several studies refute his findings. Others uphold it. While scientists are deciding, there can be little harm in women who have this condition cutting out caffeine and other methylxanthines to see if it works for them.

- Anxiety and panic attacks: Undeniably, caffeine can trigger panic attacks in some susceptible persons, primarily women; panic attacks if allowed to continue can lead to full-blown agoraphobia, a fear of leaving home. As little as two cups of coffee a day have induced panic attacks, and even one cup can produce noticeable symptoms. Researchers at the National Institute of Mental Health advise cutting out caffeine if you are vulnerable to panic attacks. Apparently, some persons are ultrasensitive to the central nervous system effects of caffeine.

- Headaches: Caffeine has been known to give some people headaches. But conversely, suddenly going off caffeine can typically cause withdrawal headaches. Even drinking coffee heavily on weekdays and laying off on the weekends can bring on a caffeine withdrawal headache. The cure: a little bit of caffeine or complete abstinence.
- Sleep: If you want to go to sleep quickly and sleep well, don't drink coffee before going to bed—or much after late afternoon, according to some experts. Electroencephalogram (EEG) readings show that brain wave patterns during sleep change in response to both pure caffeine and coffee, indicating a lower quality of sleep. Caffeine can prolong the amount of time it takes to go to sleep, total amount of sleep, and produce fewer periods of deep sleep. Lots of studies show that your brain waves change in response to caffeine. Coffee drinking in excess, according to the American Psychiatric Association, can cause "restlessness, anxiety, irritability, agitation, muscle tremor, insomnia, headache, sensory disturbances, diuresis, cardiovascular symptoms, and gastrointestinal complaints."

  Unquestionably, individuals differ widely in their tolerance for caffeine, and it can lead to a long list of complaints. Physicians took a look at the coffee and tea drinking habits of 4558 Australians in 1985 and were surprised to hear a litany of complaints growing in severity with the amount of caffeine consumed. Most common symptoms for both men and women were palpitations, indigestion, tremor, headache, and insomnia. The researchers came to the startling conclusion that drinking four to five cups of coffee a day could well account for about one quarter of all the tremors, palpitations, headaches, and insomnia among Australians.
- Diarrhea: Coffee has been found to be "an offending agent" in chronic diarrhea, which cleared up after the coffee drinking stopped.

A ROYAL REASON TO PUT MILK IN COFFEE

Medical controversy over coffee is hardly anything new. In the 1600s, with the advent of the coffeehouses and cafés in France, it was a constant topic of conversation. At first physicians endorsed it, then repudiated it. As soon as the craze of the 1670s brought coffee into private homes, the medical schools reacted; some physicians objected to the stimulating aspects of coffee and forbade patients to drink it. Later, scholars wrote treatises instructing how it could be used to "avoid and treat illnesses." But in 1688, wrote one member of the royal family, "coffee is in total disgrace." Parisians, especially the royalty, hardly knew what to do.

What saved the day, according to Jean Leclant in *Food and Drink in History,* assuring coffee's continued use, was a physician's ingenuity. "Monin, a physician from Grenoble, conceived the notion that coffee could have milk and sugar added to it." This somehow neutralized the dissent, making the drug seem more like a food. From then on drinking "coffied milk" or "milky coffee" was all the rage among French royalty.

COFFEE PRESCRIPTION FOR JET LAG

Charles F. Ehret, a biologist at Argonne National Laboratory near Chicago, believes that jet lag can be lessened by proper doses of caffeine. Ehret, an expert in circadian or daily rhythms, says caffeine acts as a regulator of body clocks. Here's his advice for globetrotters:

On departure day, if you are westbound, drink three cups of black coffee in the morning. If eastbound, refrain from coffee until evening. If you abstain from caffeine for three days before the flight, the beneficial effect is more pronounced, he says.

CORN

POSSIBLE THERAPEUTIC BENEFITS:
- Contains chemicals that prevent cancer
- Lowers risk of certain cancers, heart disease, and cavities
- Oil lowers blood cholesterol

FOLKLORE

In parts of Mexico corn is used to treat dysentery. In various countries the seed has credibility in treating diabetes. It is also known in American folk medicine as a diuretic and mild stimulant.

FACTS

Evidence on the pharmacological powers of corn is scant.

However, there are suggestions that it fights cancer. Corn is one of the "seed foods" high in protease inhibitors, known to prevent cancer in laboratory animals. And one worldwide study reported in 1981 by Pelayo Correa of the Louisiana State University Medical Center found a very strong correlation between low death rates from colon, breast, and prostate cancer and heart disease and increased per capita consumption of sweet corn (maize)—as well as of beans and rice.

Another survey of forty-seven countries found that in areas where people consume starch in corn rather than in wheat or rice there are lower rates of dental cavities.

CORN OIL

It's been known for more than three decades that corn oil lowers blood cholesterol more successfully than other polyunsaturated vegetable oils. However, corn oil also lowers the HDL-type cholesterol (the good type) as well. Although corn oil was once considered a heart food, many experts now consider olive oil much better.

POSSIBLE ADVERSE EFFECTS

- In studies first done by Kenneth Carroll at the University of Western Ontario, corn oil has been shown to cause cancer in laboratory animals. This has led some authorities to recommend restriction of polyunsaturated oils, like corn oil, to not more than ten percent of total fat intake.
- Corn oil in more recent studies also lowers immunity in mice, making them less able to ward off infections and cancer.

CRANBERRY

POSSIBLE THERAPEUTIC BENEFITS:
- Prevents urinary tract infections (cystitis)
- Kills viruses and bacteria
- Prevents kidney stones
- Deodorizes urine

> *How Much?* New research finds that only half a cup of cranberry juice cocktail a day can ward off urinary tract and bladder infections in individuals at high risk of infection.

FOLKLORE

For at least a hundred years in the United States the cranberry, especially in the northeast, where it is grown, has been touted for its powers against infections of the bladder, kidneys, and urinary tract. Even most physicians recommend it.

FACTS

It's true. The advice "If you have a tendency toward bladder or urinary tract infections, drink cranberry juice" is fast leaving the realm of folklore for the realm of established science. Several studies confirm that cranberries help control urinary tract infections. The traditional reason: the berries increase the urine's acidity, notably hippuric acid, that murders the bacteria.

But new research reveals that unique cranberry chemicals also give infectious bacteria the brush-off. Cranberry agents survive digestion to end up in the urine. There they wrap bacteria or cells in a kind of Teflon coating so the germs can't stick to the surface of the urinary tract. If the bacteria cannot attach, they can't cause infection, and are flushed harmlessly away. The mechanism is ingeniously simple and is powerful against the most common bacteria known to cause infections in the bladder, kidney, prostate, and throughout the urinary tract. Credit for this discovery goes to Dr. Anthony Sobota, a microbiologist at the Youngstown (Ohio) State University. (For more details about his finding, see The Cranberry's Strange Antibiotic, page 79.)

For half a century scientists have studied the cranberry effect. In an often-quoted study, Dr. Prodromos N. Papas, professor emeritus of clinical urology at Tufts University School of Medicine, fed sixteen ounces of cranberry juice per day for three weeks to sixty patients with acute infections of the urinary tract. Fifty-three percent of the patients improved dramatically, another twenty percent moderately; and after six weeks seventeen patients were completely free of signs of infection.

A HALF A CUP A DAY

A more recent inquiry by J. P. Kilbourn, Ph.D., at a private lab in Portland, Oregon, reveals that low amounts of cranberry juice cocktail may prevent but probably not cure such infections. The test was conducted on twenty-eight elderly persons prone to urinary tract infections. They all drank a mere four to six ounces of cranberry juice cocktail (regular or low calorie) daily for seven weeks. During that time the berry "appeared to prevent urinary tract infections in nineteen of them—a sixty-seven-percent success rate," report the researchers. In another test, people took cranberry concentrate capsules equal to a twelve-ounce glass of the cocktail. The capsule worked also, but did not cure those already suffering with urinary tract infections.

There is also evidence that cranberries help retard formation of or even help dissolve calcium-type kidney stones. The mechanism of the action is unknown. One theory: Cranberries could acidify the urine enough to help dissolve the calcium oxalate that accumulates to form stones. Or the "cranberry factor" may prevent bacteria from clumping together to promote stones.

SMELLY URINE

If urinary tract odors are a problem, cranberry juice is a good bet. After extensively reviewing the medical literature, Dr. Ara H. Der Marderosian, at the Philadelphia College of Pharmacy and Science, in 1977, concluded that cranberries do help deodorize the urine. Apparently, he said, cranberries, by helping rid the urine of E. coli, prevent the bacteria from releasing the odiferous ammonia. One study found that sixteen ounces of juice a day caused the odor to disappear.

GENERAL INFECTION FIGHTER?

If cranberry juice throws up an invisible shield between cells and bacteria, wouldn't you expect it to work against other types of infections? Maybe. Dr. Sobota did find that cranberry juice prevented certain bacteria from sticking on cells of the mouth. Fascinating studies done in Canada also found that cranberry extract was a fairly potent suppressor in test tubes of several viruses common in the intestinal tract. But it remains to be seen whether the cranberry compound is potent enough or stays in contact with bacteria and viruses in other parts of the body long enough to be protective. Dr. Sobota notes that the urine, carrying the cranberry agents, is stored in the bladder for many hours, which probably helps account for cranberries' potent effect.

PRACTICAL MATTERS

- What's the best dose? Folklore and medical wisdom have generally recommended a couple of glasses of cranberry juice cocktail a day, or fifteen to sixteen ounces, although Dr. Kilbourn found that only half a cup worked as a preventive. Dr. Sobota found that two glasses a day fortified the urine with enough chemicals to flush away bacteria. He says that seems to be an effective dose.
- Cranberry juice, however, does not work on everyone all the time. A couple of possible reasons: (1) Not everyone's urine retains the "cranberry factor" in sufficient quantities, or (2) You may be hit by a urinary tract infection that is caused by a type of bacteria not susceptible to the cranberry blockade. There are hundreds of different strains of just E. coli, one of the most common bacteria causing urinary tract infections. Dr. Sobota tested the cranberry factor on about a couple of hundred isolates of bacteria and found it worked about sixty percent of the time. If you are infected by a bacterial

strain not susceptible to cranberry action, you are out of luck. The only way to find out is to try it and see if the symptoms go away or do not occur as frequently.

- Low-calorie cranberry juice is effective also, since the therapeutic agent is in the cranberry itself and has nothing to do with sugar. Pure cranberries and cranberry juice, of course, also contain concentrated amounts of the active agent.

CAUTION

- Cranberry juice is *not a substitute for antibiotic drugs;* the juice, as Dr. Sobota's work showed, is more effective than traditional antibiotics in *preventing bacteria from attaching to cells,* but cranberry juice is definitely *not as effective in killing bacteria the way antibiotics can* after an infection is in full swing. Advocates, including many physicians, think of cranberry juice as one of nature's clever ways to stop the initiation or progression of an infection at an early stage. As in . . . "a glass of cranberry juice a day keeps the doctor away."

Thus, cranberry juice is best viewed as a preventive, especially for those susceptible to recurring urinary infections. But once bacteria have gained a foothold, pharmaceutical drugs may be needed to control the infection, which, if allowed to progress, could cause severe kidney destruction. People with symptoms of urinary tract infections should seek a physician's advice. Cranberries are nature's marvelous way of keeping us healthy over the long term, but they do not match antibiotics in a crisis.

CURRANT

POSSIBLE THERAPEUTIC BENEFITS:
- Prevents and treats diarrhea
- Protects blood vessels
- Prolongs life

FOLKLORE

Black currant has long been recommended for colds, as an astringent, and as a laxative. "For a sore throat, take a tablespoonful of the black currant jam or jelly; put it in a tumbler and fill the tumbler with boiling water. This Black Currant Tea has a soothing, demulcent effect, taken several times in the day and drunk while hot." *A Modern Herbal* by Maud Grieve, 1931.

FACTS

New evidence validates some of the folklore about black currants. In fact, Swedish investigators have recently turned crushed black currants into a new antidiarrheal drug. The preparation, called Pecarin, is made by trimming off the skin and outer layer from the fruit flesh; the skins and outer layer, which comprise forty percent of the whole black currant berries, are then dried and powdered, becoming Pecarin. This portion of the black currant is full of anthocyanosides, chemicals known to thwart the growth of bacteria, especially E. coli, often a key villain in causing diarrhea. The black currant extract has proved successful in combating gastrointestinal infections in mice and humans and is sold as a pharmaceutical in both Sweden and other countries.

These anthocyanosides, which are also heavily concentrated throughout the entire blueberry (not just in the skin as with the black currant), in animal tests have helped protect blood vessels against assaults from a high cholesterol diet and are antiinflammatory.

In a fascinating bit of research published in *Experimental Gerontology* in 1982, researchers in Cardiff, Wales, to their great surprise discovered that a flavonoid-fortified black currant juice concentrate significantly prolonged the life of aging female mice. The researchers were struck by the effect, noting that it seemed real because it extended life in animals already genetically predisposed to living a long time. So whatever life stretch the currants provided was in addition to good longevity genes.

EGGPLANT

POSSIBLE THERAPEUTIC BENEFITS:
- Protects arteries from cholesterol damage
- Contains chemicals that prevent cancer in animals
- Contains chemicals that prevent convulsions

FOLKLORE

This vegetable, with its satiny violet skin, has very little medicinal history in the United States. But in Nigeria it is highly regarded as a contraceptive, an antirheumatic agent, and an anticonvulsant. In traditional Korean medicine, the dried plant, including the fruit, is consumed to treat lumbago, pain, measles, stomach cancer, alcoholism, and is applied externally to cure rheumatism, gastritis, and burns.

FACTS

Eggplant may counteract artery-damaging assaults. For example, eggplant may serendipitously help cancel some of the ill effects of the cheese in a dish like eggplant parmigiana. In 1947, studies at the University of Texas found that constituents in eggplant inhibit rises in human blood cholesterol induced by fatty foods such as cheese.

Austrian scientist Dr. G.H.A. Mitschek at the University of Graz in the 1970s did a series of animal tests and found the same thing. He fed rabbits a high cholesterol diet; some he also gave various amounts of eggplant. When he examined the animal's arteries, he noted that even small doses of the eggplant had dramatically reduced the development of fatty plaques and atherosclerosis. Interestingly, the eggplant seemed to work best when it was eaten not alone, but with high fat, high cholesterol foods. Dr. Mitschek speculated that certain eggplant chemicals bound up cholesterol in the intestinal tract, carting it off so it was not absorbed into the bloodstream.

ANTICONVULSANT

That Nigerians prize this plant to "relieve excitement in nervous diseases" also has scientific merit. In tests, mice given a seizure-producing drug were much less likely to have convulsions when also given antidotal crude extracts of eggplant. Compounds in eggplant called scopoletin and scoparone apparently blocked the convulsions. Thus, the use of eggplant against epilepsy and other causes of convulsions, as practiced in traditional medicine, makes sense.

ANTICANCER AGENT

Recent tests in Japan found that juice from eggplant significantly suppressed damage to animal cells (chromosomal aberrations) foreshadowing cancer. Furthermore, eggplant contains protease (trypsin) inhibitors, compounds believed to help counteract cancer-causing agents as well as certain viruses. Eggplant surfaced in one study as a food most eaten by those with a low rate of stomach cancer.

CONFLICTING EVIDENCE

Japanese screenings of plants show eggplant to be slightly mutagenic; that is, in test tubes it caused genetic damage associated with cancer to cells. In one Japanese population survey, eating eggplant was associated with an increased death rate.

FIG

POSSIBLE THERAPEUTIC BENEFITS:
- Fights cancer
- Juice kills bacteria
- Juice kills roundworms
- Aids digestion

FOLKLORE

The medicinal use of figs is almost as ancient as the plant itself. The Old Testament tells of an Israelite king, Hezekiah, who was "sick unto death," from "a boil," which was probably a cancerous growth. Isaiah called for "a lump of figs"; the king recovered.

For centuries figs have been recommended to treat cancer, constipation, scurvy, hemorrhoids, gangrene, liver conditions, boils, and eruptions, and to restore energy and vitality.

Pliny, the Roman naturalist (A.D. 23/24–79), wrote: "Figs are restorative, and the best food that can be taken by those who are brought low by long sickness . . . professed wrestlers and champions were in times past fed with figs." The ancient Egyptian king Mithrydates in 1551 B.C. proclaimed figs a health tonic. Reportedly Aaron Burr once had a swollen jaw, disfiguring pimples, and infected skin boils. He applied a poultice of figs and by morning the swelling had reputedly gone down.

FIG   189

FACTS

Granted, that old Hebrew folk remedy of figs to save King Hezekiah from cancer seems far-fetched, but there's modern justification for it, explaining its deeply ingrained roots in human experience. "The use of fig fruit as a traditional anticancer agent is widespread all over the world," note Japanese scientists at the Institute of Physical and Chemical Research at the Mitsubishi-Kasei Institute of Life Sciences in Tokyo, who have isolated an anticancer chemical from figs and used it to treat cancer patients.

First they implanted adenocarcinomas in mice, and then injected the animals with a distillate made from frozen figs homogenized with water. The fig injections shrunk the tumors by an average thirty-nine percent. The Japanese identified the active fig agent as benzaldehyde.

Emboldened, the scientists gave oral doses of the fig distillate to human cancer patients, with some success. Later they injected the fig chemical with dramatic results. Fully fifty-five percent of patients with advanced cancer improved when injected with doses of a benzaldehyde derivative. Seven patients went into complete remission, twenty-nine into partial remission. Patients given the fig substance generally lived longer. "This substance proved more markedly effective on human malignant tumors than on experimental tumors in mice," noted the investigators.

Scientists have isolated from figs enzymes called ficins that help digestion. Fig juice has also killed bacteria in test tubes and roundworms in dogs.

FISH

A land with lots of herring can get along with few doctors.
—Dutch proverb

POSSIBLE THERAPEUTIC BENEFITS:
- Thins the blood
- Protects arteries from damage
- Inhibits blood clots (antithrombotic)
- Reduces blood triglycerides
- Lowers bad-type blood cholesterol
- Lowers blood pressure
- Reduces risk of heart attack and stroke
- Lessens symptoms of rheumatoid arthritis
- Reduces the risk of lupus
- Ameliorates migraine headaches
- Acts as an antiinflammatory agent
- Regulates immune system
- Prevents cancer in animals
- Relieves bronchial asthma
- Combats early kidney disease
- Increases mental energy

How Much? Eating a mere ounce of fish a day—only one or two fish dishes a week—may cut your risk of heart disease in half. Three ounces of canned mackerel a day lowers your blood pressure about seven percent. Four ounces of fish stimulates brain chemicals, making you more alert.

FOLKLORE

As early as 1766 in England, physicians recommended cod liver oil to treat chronic rheumatism and gout. By the mid-1800s, according to the 1907 edition of the *Dispensatory of the United States,* cod liver oil was routinely prescribed for those diseases as well as for other "diseases of the joints and spine, carious ulcers, rickets, lupus, cutaneous eruptions and pulmonary consumption." American folk medicine has long advocated cod liver oil to "lubricate the joints" and relieve arthritis. Fish has an ancient reputation as "brain food."

FACTS

Fish and its oils, once laughed at by medical authorities as useless remedies, are now fulfilling claims beyond folk medicine's wildest fantasies by emerging as one of the most promising and diverse dietary miracles in history. Fish, notably extra-fatty fish (like herring and salmon), produce potent pharmaceuticallike reactions that may help protect against a long string of diseases dependent on immune-system responses or prostaglandins—intercellular messengers that regulate myriad physiological functions underlying disease.

It's now believed that unique fatty acids called omega-3's, concentrated in cold-water fish, help block the overproduction of hormonelike substances called prostaglandins and leukotrienes that in excess become overzealous and issue instructions to cells to begin harmful disease processes such as blood clots, inflammation, and immune reactions. Omega-3's have unique chemical structures that seem to throw a monkey wrench into these disease processes at a cellular level, blocking the dangerous metabolic overreactions that prompt prostaglandins to go on their destructive sprees.

HEART DISEASE

Fish and its omega-3 oils are most firmly linked to preventing heart disease—possibly by helping block reactions that lead to three big culprits in cardiovascular disease: the construction of dangerous plaques that narrow arteries, inhibiting blood flow; the accumulation of sticky blood cell fragments called platelets that form clots; and spasms of arteries and blood vessels, creating constrictions that stop the heart and shut off blood to the brain, causing strokes.

Experiments on animals fed fish oils and then induced to have heart attacks or strokes by tying off arteries show much less brain and heart damage than those not getting fish oil. Monkeys fed fish oils had far fewer arterial deposits than those fed saturated coconut oil. Numerous studies find that fish-oil eaters have much thinner blood, which is less apt to clot readily. Fish oils also lower blood fats called triglycerides and very low density lipoprotein-type cholesterol. It often also lowers total cholesterol, but can elevate it in others who have high cholesterol due to genetic disorders. Apparently, fish's main powers against heart disease are apart from its impact on blood cholesterol.

Undeniably, prodigious fish eaters have less heart disease. Heart attacks are virtually unknown among Eskimos who eat an average thirteen ounces of omega-3-rich seafood a day. Inhabitants of Japanese fishing villages who eat about seven ounces of seafood a day also have a rare immunity to coronary heart disease. A new Norwegian study finds that eating only three and a half ounces of mackerel every day thinned the blood significantly within six weeks. British scientists recently reported that fish eaters, in a large-scale study, have the highest concentrations of beneficial HDL cholesterol—even more than vegetarians. And a Swedish analysis notes that fish produces a "dose-response" in protecting against heart disease. At lowest risk were those who ate the *most* fish.

Eating even scant amounts of fish can ward off heart disease to a remarkable degree. A landmark 1985 study from The Netherlands found that in one town the residents who ate at least an ounce a day of fish had a fifty percent lower risk of fatal heart attack than those eating no fish. The researchers, headed by Daan Kromhout, Ph.D., at the University of Leiden, recommended eating a mere one or two fish dishes a week to cut your risk of heart disease. Interestingly, the researchers did not conclude that fish's protective power was exclusively due to the omega-3 fatty acids. In fact, they noted that the townsmen in the twenty-year study ate more lean fish low in omega-3's than fatty fish, high in omega-3's, and that lean fish, too, seemed to depress heart disease deaths. They concluded that other unknown constituents in fish are also cardioprotective.

Evidently, many other diseases subject to control by prostaglandins can also be thwarted by fish and its omega-3 oils. Any food that can cool off overproduction of these cell messengers that make a wreck of the body, experts reason, could be an antidote to a slew of prostaglandin-leukotriene-regulated diseases.

ON THE CANCER FRONTIER

It is believed that the promotion and metastasis of cancer is regulated by prostaglandins. A star researcher in the area, Dr. Rashida Karmali of Rutgers University says: "Every tumor that has been studied seems to be overproducing prostaglandin from arachidonic acid." Studies by her and others show that fish oils, presumably by squelching that overproduction, reduce breast, pancreatic, lung, prostate, and colon cancer in animals. High levels of certain prostaglandins—that may promote cancer—have been detected in the blood and tumors of cancer patients. There's also evidence that factors that block prostaglandin synthesis inhibit breast cancer. Some speculate the low rate of breast cancer in Japanese and Eskimo women is linked to their high seafood diet.

ARTHRITIS FOLKLORE VINDICATED

Both old medical texts and folklore for at least two centuries have recommended fish oil to treat inflammatory diseases like rheumatoid arthritis. Now, it turns out, omega-3 fish oils can relieve arthritis symptoms in humans. Dr. Joel M. Kremer, associate professor of medicine at the Albany, New York, Medical College, found that patients who took fish oil capsules (the equivalent of a salmon dinner or can of sardines) daily for fourteen weeks had only half as many tender joints and less pain than previously, and made it further through the day before fatigue set in. The benefits lasted for a month after the fish oil was discontinued. Dr. Alfred D. Steinberg of the National Institute of Arthritis and Musculoskeletal and Skin Diseases says that omega-3 fish oils "unquestionably are antiinflammatory agents." Dr. Kremer explains that the fatty acids in fish oil metabolically interfere with the production of leukotriene B4, which is a potent trigger of inflammation. "We saw a significant correlation between the drop in leukotriene B4 and decrease in the number of tender joints," he says.

Another immune inflammatory disease, systemic lupus erythematosis, was dramatically prevented in animals by fish oils. One Harvard researcher called it "the most striking protective effect ever seen" against inflammatory disease in animal tests.

FISH AGAINST MIGRAINES

At the University of Cincinnati, investigators successfully blocked both migraine headaches and kidney disease with omega-3 fish oils. Migraines let up in about sixty percent of those who took fish oil capsules for six weeks. The number of attacks generally dropped from two a week to two every two weeks. The migraines were also less severe. Men migraineurs seemed to get more relief from fish oils than women sufferers.

Switching from animal fat to omega-3 fish oils also slowed down the rate of kidney deterioration in those with early kidney disease. But there was no effect on patients with advanced kidney disease or those already on hemodialysis. "It seems fish oil must be used relatively early in the disease process," said Dr. Uno Barcelli, assistant professor of medicine at the University of Cincinnati. For some reason, he says, once there is extensive renal damage, the disease perpetuates itself regardless of the fish oil therapy.

ASTHMA AND PSORIASIS ANTIDOTE

Asthma appears to be an inflammatory disease in which leukotrienes get out of hand, causing bronchoconstriction. Eating fish oil has brought dramatic relief in some cases, presumably by countering the leukotrienes' overreaction.

Given omega-3 fish oils, about two thirds of psoriasis patients improved in one study. The beneficial oils flowed quickly into the blood and skin epidermis, said researchers, and the more oils got into skin cells, the more striking the improvement.

HIGH BLOOD PRESSURE

Eating mackerel can depress and keep blood pressure down. West German researchers at the Central Institute for Cardiovascular Research, Academy of Sciences in Berlin tested twenty-four men who had mild high blood pressure but received no medication for it. For two weeks half of them ate daily two seven-ounce cans of mackerel, high in omega-3 fatty acids. For the next eight months they ate three cans of the mackerel a week as a "maintenance dose." The levels of omega-3 fatty acids in their blood shot up. And their blood pressure fell.

Before the test, on their ordinary diets, their blood pressure averaged 149 over 99. It dropped to an average 136 over 88 after two weeks and remained at 140 over 92 on the two-month three-cans-per-week test. When they stopped eating the mackerel, their blood pressure rose almost to former levels within two months. The conclusion: A mere three ounces of mackerel a day over the long term lowered blood pressure about seven percent—from levels that might require medication to those that probably don't. Thus, mackerel, said the researchers, can be "recommended for borderline or mild hypertension—cases in which drug treatment is controversial."

Additionally, the investigators point out that the canned mackerel was fairly high in sodium (1300 milligrams per can). Even so, the fish's effect seemingly prevailed over sodium's blood-pressure-boosting abilities. Reducing sodium might bring an additional drop. Researchers think other fish rich in omega-3's would do the same thing.

BRAIN FOOD

Perhaps this is not quite what the ancients meant, because eating fish won't make you smarter than you already are, but it can help raise you to full mental potential when your brain power is lagging. That's what tests at MIT reveal.

Dr. Judith Wurtman, principal investigator, finds that the high protein in fish, namely the amino acid tyrosine, can give a wonderful boost to the brain neurotransmitters norepinephrine and dopamine, thus energizing your mind and making you feel more alert. The fish makes available to the brain the tyrosine, which is then used to make the brain-stimulating chemicals. This happens, though, only when the norepinephrine and dopamine are being rapidly used up and your brain can take an extra jolt. Thus, fish does not lift mental capacities further if your brain already has adequate supplies of the alertness chemicals. But if you have a special task to complete and want to be sure your mind can work at full power, choose fish for lunch or dinner.

Dr. Wurtman puts fish on her A list as a mental-energy-boosting food. She has found that the amounts needed are rather precise for most people, about three or four ounces, preferably broiled or grilled—not deep fried or doused with fat, which could ruin some of the effects.

The mental-energizing effect is caused by the way the protein is metabolized and has nothing to do with fish's omega-3 content.

PRACTICAL MATTERS

• Fish is not a panacea that can counteract damage from an otherwise dangerous high fat diet. Think of it not as a *supplement* but as a *substitute* for other polyunsaturated fatty foods (like vegetable oils) and saturated fatty foods like meat. In fact, the less total fat you eat, the more potent the fish is expected to be. The omega-3 fatty acids are much more effective in low fat diets such as those of the Japanese, who classically consume twenty percent of calories from fat as opposed to our thirty-eight percent.

Omega-3's exert power by diluting the other fats in tissues; thus, less fat means a higher concentration of the omega-3's. Best bet, advises one authority, is to cut back on both saturated fat and the traditional vegetable oils, substituting fish. This automatically decreases both the amount of total fat and saturated fat in the diet.

• Be aware that not all fish in the market have high amounts of omega-3's. Much white fish in the United States has very little. Richest are the cold saltwater fishes such as herring and mackerel.

Fish raised in fish tanks or ponds are commonly fed land-type food such as soybean or grain feeds; thus, they take on the physiological characteristics of just another land creature: they are low in omega-3-type oil. For example, catfish may be virtually devoid of omega-3's, having more the fatty composition of landlubber chicken. Cultured or pond-reared freshwater prawns and crayfish, in one test, displayed fat more like that of terrestrial animals than their wild seawater counterparts.

• Similarly, don't look to fast-food fish for your omega-3's. Dr. Norman Salem of the National Institute of Alcohol Abuse and Alcoholism in Bethesda, Maryland, measured the omega-3's in a number of fast foods and found that a fish sandwich had only one tenth the amount of omega-3's in its fat as a can of Chinook salmon. The reason: the fish sandwich is made from whitefish already low in fat and thus in omega-3's, and fried in saturated fat, which boosts its ratio of saturated to unsaturated fat to resemble a hamburger's.

WHAT ABOUT FISH OIL CAPSULES?

Although researchers use pure fish oil in tests, both capsules of concentrated omega-3's and doses of cod liver oil should be taken sparingly and cautiously. Cod liver oil has lots of vitamin D and vitamin A, fat-soluble vitamins that can be soaked up and stored in toxic amounts by the liver. Some experts worry that taking too much omega-3 in capsules could boomerang, overloading the system so that it produces not help, but harm from hyped-up prostaglandins. Too much omega-3 can also block normal blood clotting and lead to excessive bleeding. Fish oil capsules are also commonly high in cholesterol, and those that are not may promote lipid peroxidation, a process destructive to cells.

Dr. John E. Kinsella, professor of food science, Institute of Food Science, Cornell University, and a noted authority on omega-3's, suggests five grams a day of concentrated fish oil as enough.

Most important, the pure oil may not be as therapeutic as seafood. Omega-3's may interact with other substances in fish, making the fish itself rather than its isolated oil the therapeutic entity. As Dutch investigators suggested, by turning to fish oils, you may unknowingly cheat yourself of the full protection offered by seafood.

A SPECIAL WARNING TO DIABETICS

Researchers have discovered that omega-3 fish oil capsules can actually aggravate diabetes by producing a steep rise in blood sugar and a drop in insulin secretion.

CAUTION

• Be aware that some freshwater fish, such as catfish and lake trout, may be contaminated with chlorinated hydrocarbon pesticides and industrial chemicals such as PCBs, which are thought to be especially hazardous to pregnant women.

PHARMACEUTICAL FISH—THE MOST POTENT

Highest in omega-3 fatty acids:
(more than 1 gram per 3½ ounces)

Mackerel
Salmon (Atlantic, Chinook, chum, coho, pink)
Bluefish
Tuna (albacore, bluefin)
Sturgeon, Atlantic
Sablefish
Herring
Anchovy
Sardines
Trout, lake

GARLIC

Eat leeks in March and wild garlic in May
And all year after physicians may play.
—Old Welsh Rhyme

POSSIBLE THERAPEUTIC BENEFITS:
- Fights infections
- Contains cancer-preventive chemicals
- Thins the blood (anticoagulant)
- Reduces blood pressure, cholesterol, triglycerides
- Stimulates the immune system
- Prevents and relieves chronic bronchitis
- Acts as an expectorant and decongestant

How Much? A mere half a raw garlic clove a day can rev up the blood-clot-dissolving activity that helps prevent heart attacks and strokes. Only a couple of raw garlic cloves daily can keep blood cholesterol down in heart patients.

FOLKLORE

Garlic has an awesome reputation in medicinal folklore. Word of its healing properties has been handed down by priests, physicians, and other guardians of the common experience in wondrous detail for thousands of years. An Egyptian medical papyrus dating from around 1500 B.C. listed twenty-two garlic prescriptions for such complaints as headache, throat disorders, and physical weakness. (Builders of the Great Pyramid at Giza supposedly ate garlic to gain strength.) Pliny in his *Historia Naturalis* prescribed garlic recipes against sixty-one maladies including gastrointestinal disorders, dog- and snake-bites, scorpion stings, asthma, rheumatism, hemorrhoids, ulcers, loss of appetite, convulsions, tumors, and consumption. Hippocrates recommended garlic as a laxative, diuretic, and cure for tumors of the uterus. For centuries Chinese and Japanese physicians have recommended garlic to alleviate high blood pressure. In first-century India, physicians as instructed by the Charaka-Samhita, an important Indian medical manuscript, used garlic and onion to prevent heart disease and rheumatism. In Shakespearean England, garlic was acclaimed an aphrodisiac.

Garlic is a widely used antibiotic. At the turn of the century, garlic ointments, compresses, and inhalants were "the drug of choice" against tuberculosis. In World War I, garlic was used to fight typhus and dysentery. In World War II, British physicians, treating battle wounds with garlic, reported total success in warding off septic poisoning and gangrene. Even Dr. Albert Schweitzer employed garlic against typhus and cholera.

FACTS

The evidence about garlic's therapeutic potential is almost as stunning as the folklore. The National Library of Medicine, in Bethesda, Maryland, a prestigious repository of medical literature, contains about 125 scientific papers on garlic published since 1983. Dissections of garlic reveal potent compounds that appear to retard heart disease, stroke, cancer, and a wide range of infections.

ANTIBIOTIC

Undeniably, garlic destroys bacteria. In 1944 a chemist, Chester J. Cavallito, identified garlic's smelly compound, allicin, as an antibiotic. Tests even found raw garlic more powerful than penicillin and tetracycline. Literally hundreds of studies confirm garlic as a broad-spectrum antibiotic against a long list of microbes that spread diseases, including botulism, tuberculosis, diarrhea, staph, dysentery, and typhoid. A recent count listed seventy-two separate infectious agents squelched by garlic. As one researcher exclaims: "Garlic has the broadest spectrum of any antimicrobial substance we know of. It's antibacterial, antifungal, antiparasitic, antiprotozoan, and antiviral."

Allicin, the odiferous antibacterial compound, is formed when garlic is cut or crushed. If the aroma—hence allicin—is destroyed, as in cooking, garlic is no longer a microbe killer, although it can perform other therapeutic tricks.

In many countries garlic is legitimately used as an antibacterial agent. In Japan a cold-processed, odorless raw garlic substance called Kyolic serves as an antibiotic. In the Soviet Union garlic is known as "Russian penicillin," so common that reportedly, on one occasion officials imported 500 tons of garlic to combat an outbreak of influenza. The bulb is also a Soviet remedy for colds, whooping cough, and intestinal disorders. Polish children often are prescribed a garlic preparation as treatment for gastroenterocolitis, dyspepsia, pneumonia, sepsis, and nephrosis.

In a striking display of garlic's powers, Chinese physicians recently used it in high doses to cure cryptococcal meningitis, a fungal infection that is frequently fatal. In twenty-one cases of the disease over a five-year period, the physicians administered only garlic infusions; six persons were completely cured and five improved. Garlic combats fungal infections (such as tuberculosis), by killing the organism, but the Chinese investigators concluded that part of the cure was due to garlic's stimulation of the patients' immunological functions.

GARLIC EATERS BOOST IMMUNITY

That's precisely what Florida investigators documented in 1987. Tarig Abdullah, M.D., and his colleagues at the Akbar Clinic and Research Center in Panama City, Florida, revealed that both raw garlic and the Japanese garlic extract, Kyolic, dramatically augmented the powers of the immune system's natural killer cells—the first line of defense against infectious disease and perhaps cancer. Nine people, including the investigators, ate large amounts of raw garlic—Dr. Abdullah ate twelve and fifteen cloves a day; nine others took Kyolic and nine others did neither. Then the natural killer cells from the various bloods were mixed with cancer cells. The killer cells derived from the blood of those eating garlic or taking the garlic drug destroyed from *140 to 160 percent more cancer cells* than did killer cells from non–garlic eaters.

Dr. Abdullah says the discovery has implications for not only infections and cancer, but also for AIDS, in which immune functioning fails. Garlic, he says, might rev up immune defenses in AIDS patients; it also may directly combat the many fungal-type infections AIDS patients fall prey to. Dr. Abdullah is convinced *lower doses* of garlic boost immunity, too, but he deliberately used a big dose to make sure he got an effect. He is planning tests using garlic on AIDS patients.

Expert example: Dr. Abdullah eats a couple of raw garlic cloves every day and reports he has not had a cold since he started the garlic regimen—in 1973.

HEART FOOD

Medical journals are full of research showing that eating garlic does wonders for the cardiovascular system. Garlic decidedly lowers blood cholesterol in humans and creates other blood changes protective against heart disease—such as thinning the blood and preventing embolisms (internal blood clots). Indian researcher Arun K. Bordia of the Bombay Hospital Research Centre, found that one gram of raw garlic per day per kilogram of weight (about eighteen average garlic cloves for a 120-pound person) reduced the tendency of blood to form dangerous clots even in patients with coronary heart disease. The blood's clot-dissolving system (fibrinolytic activity) persistently rose in healthy people by 130 percent and in heart patients by 83 percent during three months. It became sluggish after the garlic treatment ended.

In lowering blood cholesterol, garlic proved far more effective in animals than the standard drug, clofibrate. In human tests in India, fresh garlic juice (about one-eighth cup for a 120-pound person) taken every day drastically reduced blood cholesterol; it dropped on the average from 305 to 218 in two months.

In 1987 Dr. Benjamin Lau and his colleagues at California's Loma Linda University got dramatic results from Japan's Kyolic concentrated garlic extract. About a gram a day (which Dr. Lau figures is about an ounce of whole garlic or nine cloves) lowered unfavorable LDL blood cholesterol and triglycerides in about sixty to seventy percent of volunteers. Good HDL cholesterol went up. Generally, cholesterol reduction was about ten percent, but in some it sank as much as fifty percent. Interestingly, in Dr. Lau's experiment, cholesterol actually rose in the first few months of garlic treatment and then dropped after four to six months. He thinks this initial rise reflects the shipping of cholesterol out of tissues into the blood to be excreted.

Amazingly low doses of garlic have helped fix up highly vulnerable arteries. Indian investigator Dr. M. Sucur fed fresh-peeled garlic to 200 patients with extra-high blood cholesterol. After twenty-five days cholesterol sank in virtually all. The dose: a mere fifteen grams daily—about five medium cloves. Dr. Sucur concluded that once cholesterol got down, only a couple of raw cloves a day worked as a "maintenance dose" to keep it depressed.

It took only two cloves a day to keep blood in tiptop shape among a group of vegetarians in the Jain community of India. Such committed garlic eaters had blood cholesterol readings of an average 159 compared with 208 for those eating no garlic. Even eaters of three garlic cloves per week had lower blood cholesterol than the garlic abstainers. (The garlic eaters also ate more onions; whether onions and garlic interacted to create greater benefits than either alone is unknown.) Blood tests revealed the most ardent garlic and onion eaters also displayed the least fibrinogen (clot factor) and their blood took longest to clot, factors protecting against heart disease.

In attempts to create new anti–heart disease drugs, Dr. Eric Block, head of chemistry at State University of New York at Albany, has discovered a garlic chemical he calls ajoene ("ajo" is Spanish for garlic) that in laboratory tests interferes with the clotting process just as effectively as one of the world's oldest and most respected blood-thinning drugs: aspirin. "As an antithrombotic agent, ajoene is at least as potent as aspirin," he notes. (Aspirin is endorsed by medical experts as a potent blood-clot inhibitor thought to prevent heart attack and stroke.) When Dr. Block fed rabbits a single dose of ajoene, platelet aggregation was shut down one hundred percent and stayed that way for an entire twenty-four hours. Dr. Block sees the garlic compound as a promising anticoagulant drug with few side effects.

HIGH BLOOD PRESSURE MEDICINE

Garlic has achieved a legendary reputation as an antihypertensive medication. It's been used in China for centuries for that purpose, and the Japanese government officially recognizes garlic as a blood-pressure depressor. American scientists first tried garlic against high blood pressure in 1921. Garlic consistently lowers blood pressure in laboratory animals. That it also works on humans was shown by tests reported in the British medical journal, *Lancet,* as well as by extensive clinical studies done for many years in Russia and Bulgaria. A well-known researcher in this area, Dr. V. Petkov, a physiologist at the Bulgarian Academy of Sciences, after numerous trials reports that garlic in humans produces a systolic blood pressure drop of twenty to thirty points and a diastolic drop of ten to twenty.

LUNG GUARD

Dr. Irwin Ziment regularly prescribes garlic as a decongestant and expectorant for common colds and as a "mucus regulator" for chronic bronchitis. He finds truth in the persistent folklore garlic remedy for colds and pulmonary problems. Dr. Ziment, an expert on pharmaceuticals, reasons that garlic works the same way as expectorants and decongestants sold commercially. The pungent property of garlic irritates the stomach, which then signals the lungs to release fluids that thin the mucus, enabling the ordinary lung mechanisms to expel it.

Regular doses of garlic (as well as other pungent spices), Dr. Ziment believes, help keep some susceptible persons from developing debilitating chronic bronchitis. "It acts as a prophylactic," he notes, "by keeping mucus moving normally through the lungs." (For more details, see page 43.)

Further, Polish physicians have used extract of garlic to cure children suffering from recurrent acute and chronic bronchitis and bronchial asthma.

ANTICANCER BULB

Garlic is one of the stars in cancer research circles. As long ago as 1952, Russian scientists successfully used garlic extracts against human tumors. Numerous animal tests show that fresh garlic can immunize animals against tumor development or reverse it, once under way. In one case, Japanese scientists injected mice with tumor cells twice, a week apart. Mice that also received fresh garlic extract were much more resistant to the second injection of tumor cells. The fresh garlic completely wiped out breast cancers in the mice. Experimenters credited garlic's allicin.

Somewhat to their amazement, Japanese scientists also found garlic extract acted as a powerful antioxidant against so-called "lipid peroxidation" that can insert inappropriate oxygen molecules into cells, causing their destruction. In fact, in mice, garlic proved a better antioxidant than vitamin E, one of the best, in reversing liver damage.

United States experiments in 1987 found that garlic in animals was more effective in warding off bladder cancers than a well-known cancer "vaccine" called BCG.

Evidence that people who eat garlic are more apt to escape cancer comes from a comparison of garlic eating in two Chinese counties in Shandong province. Gangshan County residents eat about twenty grams of garlic a day (about seven cloves) and have a gastric cancer death rate of 3.45 per 100,000 population. In nearby Quixia County, the residents care little for garlic and eat it rarely; they die of gastric cancer at the rate of 40 per 100,000; the non-garlic eaters have an almost twelve times greater risk of deadly gastric cancer.

At the M. D. Anderson Hospital and Tumor Institute in Houston, Texas, investigators testing sulfur compounds from garlic (and onions) find that the substances saved mice from colon cancer by blocking the conversion of chemicals to powerful carcinogens. The National Cancer Institute puts sulfur compounds from garlic extremely high on its list of potential natural "chemopreventives."

PRACTICAL MATTERS

- The breath problem: Unless everybody is eating garlic, the person who does can easily be identified by his or her breath. Scientists have debated for at least fifty years on how to get rid of garlic mouth odors. Some recommend strong coffee, honey, yogurt, or a glass of milk. The French call red wine an effective deodorizer. Cloves are also supposed to do it. Most commonly recommended is chewing parsley—the herb's chlorophyll is supposed to douse the garlic smell. To get rid of garlic odors on your hands, clean them with lemon or wash in cold water, then rub with salt, rinse again, and finish with a wash of warm soapy water, according to *Natural History* magazine.
- Use garlic that is as fresh as possible; growing your own is the best. Unfortunately, also, garlic varies widely in its therapeutic chemicals depending on soil conditions. That is one reason researchers say test results of garlic's therapeutic capabilities vary.
- Raw or cooked? Garlic has to be raw to kill bacteria, boost immune functioning, and probably help prevent cancer. But cooked garlic can lower blood cholesterol and help keep blood thin and perform as a decongestant, cough medicine, mucus regulator, and bronchitis preventive. Best advice: eat it both ways.

• What about garlic oils, capsules, pills, special preparations? Many of them, experts warn, have none or very little of the active garlic compounds. Dr. Abdullah's search yielded only one effective commercial therapeutic garlic preparation—Japan's Kyolic—that contained the active ingredient needed to raise immunological function. In a 1985 comprehensive international survey of medical research on garlic, two British authors in *CRC Critical Reviews in Food Science and Nutrition* concluded: "There is no evidence to suggest that . . . garlic preparations are in any way superior to the fresh or cooked vegetable."

CAUTION

▪ Garlic triggers allergic reactions in some persons.

5000 YEARS OF GARLIC AND ONION CURES

In ancient cultures, no foods were so esteemed for their magic and health qualities as garlic and its cousin onion, which are both members of the allium family. These two vegetables are nearly as old as agriculture, and are among the first cultivated food plants. Evidence of garlic and onion use as food, as part of religious rites, and as a healing potion shows up in ancient Sumeria (4000 B.C.). Garlic bulbs are pictured on the walls of tombs in ancient Egypt (3200 B.C.), and have been unearthed around the royal palace at Knossos, in Crete, and in the ruins of Pompeii and Herculaneum (A.D. 100). For centuries garlic and onions have been used as:

> anticoagulants
> antiseptics
> antiinflammatory agents
> antitumor agents
> carminatives
> diuretics
> sedatives
> poultices
> vermifuges
> hair restorers
> aphrodisiacs

Among the common ailments they have been purported to cure are:

arthritis
arteriosclerosis
asthma
athlete's foot
baldness
bronchitis
cancer
catarrh
chicken pox
cholera
common cold
constipation
dandruff
diabetes
dogbites
dropsy
dyspepsia
dysentery
epilepsy
eye burns
fits
gangrene
hypertension

influenza
intestinal gas
jaundice
laryngitis
lead poisoning
leprosy
lip and mouth disorders
malaria
measles
meningitis
phthisis
piles
rheumatism
ringworm
scorpion stings
scurvy
septic poisoning
smallpox
splenic enlargement
tobacco poisoning
tuberculosis
typhoid

GINGER

- Prevents motion sickness
- Thins the blood
- Lowers blood cholesterol
- Prevents cancer in animals

> *How Much?* About half a teaspoon of powdered ginger root prevents motion sickness.

FOLKLORE

Ginger was mentioned in Chinese medical books 2000 years ago, and is incorporated in about half of all multiitem prescriptions in Oriental medicine. Fresh ginger, among Oriental physicians, is reputed to be a good remedy for vomiting, coughing, abdominal distension, and fever, whereas the processed (steamed and dried) ginger is used for abdominal pain, lumbago, and diarrhea. Africans drink ginger root as an aphrodisiac; women in New Guinea eat the dried root as a contraceptive. In India children are given fresh ginger tea for whooping cough.

FACTS

Ginger has several medicinal qualities; as the ancients suspected, it definitely is an antinausea drug.

DIZZYING ACCOMPLISHMENT

Researchers proved that ginger is better even than Dramamine—a common motion-sickness drug—at suppressing motion-induced nausea. As a test, the researchers put people highly prone to motion sickness into a spinning tilted chair, a maneuver that brings on the stomach-turning sensations. Twenty minutes before the test, investigators gave the groups one of three undisclosed capsules. One type contained a placebo (with no pharmacological potency), another, 940 milligrams of powdered ginger root, and a third, one hundred milligrams of Dramamine.

Not a soul who took the Dramamine or placebo lasted in the spinning chair for six minutes without becoming extremely nauseated or vomiting. But fully half—six of twelve subjects—managed to survive the rotating test after taking the ginger root. It was clearly a more potent antidote to motion sickness than the oft-used drug. Another plus: unlike Dramamine, ginger does not make you drowsy, because it works in the gut and not in the brain.

Albert Leung, Ph.D., an independent consultant in plant pharmacology, says the anti–motion sickness qualities of ginger have been recognized for centuries in the Orient. "It's quite common," he says, "to see people on boats around Hong Kong munching on preserved ginger." The dose used in the above study was about half a teaspoon of ground ginger.

FIRST-RATE ANTICOAGULANT

Danish investigator K. C. Srivastava at Odense University's Institute of Community Health proclaims ginger as a more potent anticoagulant in test tubes and in rat aortas than either garlic or onion, well-known blockers of clotting. Ginger even more efficiently than garlic or onion inhibited blood cells' synthesis of a substance called thromboxane that signals blood platelets to stick together as a first step in forming clots. And the more ginger used, the greater the effects, although even extremely small amounts also worked. This led Dr. Srivastava to conclude that either ginger's "active principle is very potent or is present in high concentrations in the ginger."

· MARMALADE SURPRISE

That ginger works in humans to deter blood clots was accidentally proved by Charles R. Dorso, M.D., at the Cornell University Medical College. His experience was similar to that of Dr. Dale Hammerschmidt, who discovered the anticlotting properties of the tree ear mushroom. Dr. Dorso, like Dr. Hammerschmidt, used his own platelet blood cells in experiments as a "normal control." One day, he, too, noticed that his blood did not coagulate as usual.

The doctor recalled that the previous evening he had eaten a large quantity of "an excellent marmalade (Ginger with Grapefruit, Crabtree and Evelyn, London) whose major ingredient (15 percent) is ginger." As a test, Dr. Dorso bought some ground ginger at the supermarket and put it into test tubes with his and several of his colleagues' blood platelets. And sure enough, the platelets refused to stick together, not even when the experimenters doubled the amount of a substance known to promote blood-cell clumping. The Cornell researchers believe the anticoagulant, or blood thinning compound, in ginger is gingerol, which has a chemical structure amazingly like that of aspirin, another potent anticlotting compound.

Indian researchers also found that ginger "brings down drastically" the blood cholesterol levels in rats over the long term. The spice, in animals, strongly offset the cholesterol-raising effects of a high fat diet.

In Japan, where ginger has been extensively studied, scientists find that both fresh and processed ginger relieves pain, prevents vomiting, tunes down gastric secretion in the stomach, reduces blood pressure, and stimulates the heart. Screenings of vegetables by Japanese scientists also show ginger to be "remarkably effective" as a desmutagen, thwarting mutational cell changes leading to cancer. Feeding ginger to mice has also blocked cancer.

PRACTICAL MATTERS

- For motion sickness you can take your ginger in capsules; health food stores often carry gelatin capsules containing powdered ginger. If not, you could ask a pharmacist to make some up in doses of 500 milligrams of ginger. Take a couple about half an hour before exposure to motion. One expert warns against swallowing a teaspoon of powdered ginger plain, noting it could burn the esophagus.

- You can also mix half a teaspoon of powdered ginger in tea or other beverages, recommends Jim Duke, United States Department of Agriculture plant expert. Dr. Duke notes that if you use fresh ginger root, you should double the dose to a full teaspoon. You can peel, cut, or grind up the root and put it into a beverage.

GRAPE

POSSIBLE THERAPEUTIC BENEFITS:
- Inactivates viruses
- Thwarts tooth decay
- Rich in compounds that block cancer in animals

FOLKLORE

"Grapes next to apples have been crowned the queen of fruits. Grapes are good for all dyspeptic conditions, febrile conditions, liver and kidney troubles, tuberculosis of the lungs and bones, hemorrhoids, varicose veins, osteomyelitis, gangrene, cancer, and a great many other malignant diseases." So New York City's Dr. A. M. Liebstein told his fellow physicians in 1927. The following year, Johanna Brandt, a South African resident, wrote a book, *The Grape Cure*, in which she claimed grapes cured her abdominal cancer. The "grape cure" was instantly popular on several continents and still is in parts of Europe.

FACTS

Alas, although grapes look promising as antiviral, antitumor agents because of their high concentration of certain polyphenols, tannins, they have found slight place in the scientific sun. Canadian investigators Dr. Jack Konowalchuk and Joan Speirs did declare grapes very powerful killers of disease-causing viruses in test tubes. The two researchers bought grapes, grape juice, and raisins (dried grapes) from local grocery stores, and red, rosé, and white wines. They then added viruses to the grape extract made from pulp and skins, to the grape juice and infusions of raisins, and to the wines. All inactivated the viruses. Grapes were potent against poliovirus and herpes simplex virus, causes of polio and herpes infections respectively.

Whether grapes can destroy viruses inside the body is unknown. Such tests in animals and humans have not been done. However, grapes contain a certain tannin thought to be a virus enemy that can be absorbed in the intestinal tract, and radioactive tannins from eaten grapes have been tracked through the digestive system and right into the bloodstreams of mice. This indicates that the grape tannins can survive digestion and circulate through the blood, perhaps attacking viruses. Grape juice is also known to kill bacteria, and in animal studies dramatically thwarted the tooth decay process.

The fruit also possesses extraordinarily high levels of caffeic acid, a polyphenol compound with strong powers to prevent cancer in animals. In a recent study, raisins (dried grapes) were linked to lower rates of cancer deaths in a group of elderly Americans.

CONFLICTING EVIDENCE

Several tests show red grape juice to have mutagenic activity, tending to change genetic material in cells, foreshadowing cancer.

GRAPEFRUIT

POSSIBLE THERAPEUTIC BENEFITS:

- Great for cardiovascular system
- Lowers blood cholesterol
- Protects arteries from disease
- Lowers the risk of cancer

> *How Much?* Eating the pectin in a couple of grapefruit a day may lower blood cholesterol by up to nineteen percent and improve the critical HDL-cholesterol ratio. Eating citrus foods every day may help guard against certain cancers, notably stomach and pancreatic.

FOLKLORE

In 310 B.C. the Greek historian Theophrastus wrote of citron: "A decoction of the pulp of this fruit is thought to be an antidote to poison, and will also sweeten the breath." Later, Pliny, the Roman naturalist, who first used the word "citrus," labeled the fruit a medicine.

FACTS

Grapefruit turns out to be an amazing medicine for the heart. It contains potent compounds that lower blood cholesterol and may even clean out some of the arterial debris known as plaque, possibly *reversing* atherosclerosis. The suspected primary therapeutic compound is a polysaccharide unique to grapefruit and found in the fruit's pectin, a type of fiber. In reducing blood cholesterol, grapefruit pectin is fully as powerful as the drug cholestyramine, "the gold-standard drug for lowering plasma cholesterol," according to Dr. James Cerda, professor of gastroenterology at the University of Florida and a leading researcher on the subject.

PEOPLE-PROOF

Dr. Cerda and his colleagues found that people with high blood cholesterol (in the mid-200's) who ate fifteen grams of grapefruit pectin a day in capsules for four months had an average drop of about eight percent in cholesterol. In one third of grapefruit-pectin eaters, blood cholesterol plummeted by ten to nineteen percent. Furthermore, in half of the volunteers, the grapefruit substance improved the critical HDL-cholesterol ratio. "When you think that each one percent reduction in cholesterol cuts the risk of heart disease by two percent, these findings are exciting," says Dr. Cerda. And eating the grapefruit pulp itself is probably more potent than pure pectin, he says, because grapefruit's other chemicals, like vitamin C, are expected to potentiate the effect. (Apples, for example, depress blood cholesterol much more than pure apple pectin.) Also the therapeutic dose may be less than the fifteen grams tested in the experiment. As for how many grapefruit it takes to get fifteen grams of pectin, "Oddly enough, nobody knows," says Dr. Cerda. Recent analyses show startlingly different figures. One found fifteen grams of pectin in only two grapefruit, another in fifteen grapefruit. Dr. Cerda's advice: "Eating a grapefruit a day could do some good."

Dr. Cerda even speculates that grapefruit chemicals may promote a *regression* in atherosclerosis—turning back the clock for the cardiovascular system—by partially dissolving plaque buildup that narrows and hardens arteries, precipitating heart attacks and strokes. In tests, pigs fed grapefruit pectin—along with an excessively high fat cholesterol diet—displayed markedly less diseased and narrowed coronary arteries and aortas at autopsy, as well as a thirty percent drop in cholesterol. Thus, grapefruit pectin dramatically counteracted the ill effects of a high fat diet.

The theory is: concentrated galacturonic acid in grapefruit chemically interacts in a peculiar fashion with destructive LDL cholesterol, a main constituent of artery-clogging plaque. Such interaction may dislodge and sweep away some cholesterol buildup, somewhat restoring arteries to health.

ANTICANCER POWERS

Citrus fruits, including grapefruit, have definite anticancer capabilities. Experts point out that people who live in areas where high amounts of citrus fruits are consumed have lower cancer rates. Some speculate it is partly due to the fruit's high content of vitamin C, which is an antioxidant and can neutralize potent carcinogens. But other grapefruit constituents probably contribute too.

In lab tests on animals, grapefruit shows a decided antagonism to cancer. In Japanese studies, when grapefruit extract was injected under the skin of mice, it stopped their tumor growth and caused a partial or complete remission of the malignancy. The Japanese find grapefruit rind to be a "remarkable antimutagen," a substance that counteracts the cellular changes that can lead to cancer.

The Swedes are famous for their studies on diet and cancer. In a meticulous 1986 analysis (a so-called case control study) of the diets of a group with and without pancreatic cancer, citrus fruits (and carrots) emerged as the most striking protective factors. People who ate citrus fruit almost daily had a substantially lower chance of getting cancer of the pancreas. The Dutch also find that eating citrus fruit reduces the risk of stomach cancer.

PRACTICAL MATTERS

- For heart benefits, be sure to eat the grapefruit pulp, including, when possible, the membranes that separate the sections and the white interior of the rind. The therapeutic pectin resides in the cell walls, or "juice sacs." So to get cholesterol-lowering benefit, you must eat the chewy stuff. Grapefruit *juice* is not high in pectin and does not depress blood cholesterol.

HONEY

POSSIBLE THERAPEUTIC BENEFITS:

- Kills bacteria
- Disinfects wounds and sores
- Reduces perception of pain
- Alleviates asthma
- Soothes sore throats
- Calms the nerves, induces sleep
- Relieves diarrhea

FOLKLORE

Honey was to the ancient Egyptians what aspirin is to modern medicine: the most popular among drugs. Honey is mentioned 500 times in 900 remedies in the Smith Papyrus, an Egyptian medical text dating between 2600 and 2200 B.C. The nectar is universally hailed as an ointment to heal wounds, sores, and skin ulcers. Honey during wartime has been smeared on wounds as an antiseptic by ancient Greeks, Romans, Egyptians, Assyrians, and Chinese as well as by Germans in World War I. Hippocrates advised mixing honey, water, and other various medicinal substances to treat fever.

According to the 1811 edition of *The Edinburgh New Dispensatory* "From the earliest ages, honey has been employed as a medicine . . . it forms an excellent gargle and facilitates the expectoration of viscid phlegm; and it is sometimes employed as an emollient application to abscesses, and as a detergent to ulcers."

Honey is often mixed with lemon juice or vinegar as a soothing cough syrup. Vermont folk physician D. C. Jarvis in his best-selling book, *Folk Medicine* (1958), recommends honey for coughs, muscle cramps, burns, stuffy nose, sinusitis, hay fever, bed wetting in children, and insomnia. "A tablespoon of honey at the evening meal," he says, makes you look forward to bedtime.

FACTS

Folk medicine is entirely right in dubbing honey a potent killer of bacteria, an antiseptic, and a disinfectant. Numerous modern scientists have watched honey-touched bacteria disintegrate. In one interesting experiment, surgeon and medical historian Guido Manjo, author of *The Healing Hand*, tested the formula of a wound salve from the ancient Egyptian Smith Papyrus; it called for one-third honey, or *byt*, mixed with two-thirds fat. He was apprehensive: "I thought at first that this would be dreadful stuff to put on an open wound. . . . Instead, the bacteria in the fat tended to disappear and when pathogenic bacteria were added, like *Escherichia coli* or *Staphylococcus aureus*, they were killed just as fast."

HONEY IN THE WOUND

Physicians, especially in developing countries, routinely smear honey on wounds and sores as a disinfectant ointment, according to Dr. P. J. Armon, a physician in South Africa. Writing in a medical journal, he related excellent success in using honey to treat infected wounds at the Kilimanjaro Christian Medical Center. The honey, he says, hastens healing and keeps the wound sterile, eliminating the need for conventional antibiotics.

Indeed, in 1970 a prominent British surgeon surprised colleagues by announcing that he regularly used honey on open wounds after vulvectomies (cancer surgery). He found that the honey-covered wounds healed faster and had less bacterial colonization than wounds treated with ordinary antibiotics. As confirmation, he and his colleagues put honey in test tubes with a wide range of infectious organisms. The honey killed them all.

DIARRHEA CURE

Additionally, South African researchers found that honey squelched the growth of such germs as Salmonella, Shigella, E. coli, and V. cholerae, which cause diarrhea, a deadly curse in the third world. Most important, the honey *when eaten* retained its power against bacteria in the intestinal tract, and helped curb diarrhea.

As an experiment, Drs. I. E. Haffejee and A. Moosa, at the Department of Pediatrics and Child Health at the University of Natal, Durban, South Africa, fed one group of youngsters with acute gastro-enteritis fluids with sugar and another group fluids with honey. Those with *bacteria-caused* diarrhea who got the honey recovered forty percent faster. The researchers' inescapable conclusion: honey's antibacterial activity in the intestinal tract helped cure the diarrhea.

How honey disables bacteria is not agreed upon. Some experts say the sugar in honey sucks moisture out of bacteria, causing them to die. But that's not the entire answer. In one test of honey's antibiotic activity, the sugar was removed. The remaining sugarless distillate of honey still killed a broad range of bacteria as effectively as streptomycin did. Additionally, the germs did not develop a resistance to honey as they did to the streptomycin.

ASTHMA RATIONALE

It may seem ludicrous that honey could ward off asthma, as the ancients claimed. Still, one theory might account for it. Ingesting traces of pollen found in honey could desensitize you to allergies the same way pollen injections (allergy shots) do. But until recently it seemed doubtful that the pollen in honey would survive digestion to reach the blood stream.

However, a physician, Dr. U. Wahn of the Heidelberg University Children's Clinic, found that children who drank a pollen solution showed fewer signs of hay fever and allergy-related asthma. Seventy allergy-prone children drank a solution containing pollen daily during hay fever season and three times a week in the winter. Eighty-four percent had fewer allergic symptoms than usual. Signs of watery eyes and conjunctivitis dropped by seventy percent and bouts of runny, irritated nose fell by fifty percent. Researchers concluded that the pollen did survive digestion and get into the blood stream, somewhat desensitizing the children to their allergies and asthma. Thus, eating pollen-laden honey could produce a similar kind of desensitization to allergies and allergy-induced asthma.

And is there truth to the folk remedy that honey soothes a sore throat? Dr. Robert I. Henkin, a specialist in taste and smell disorders at the Georgetown University Medical Center in Washington, D.C., says yes. For one thing, he notes that sweets can trigger brain chemicals that dull your perception of pain.

SLEEPING POTION

Honey does tend to calm you down and put you to sleep. In the body honey is metabolized like table sugar; and it is well established that sugar leads to more serotonin in the brain, a chemical that calms down brain activity, inducing relaxation and sleep, according to experiments at MIT.

CAUTION

- Don't feed honey to infants under one year of age, cautions the Centers for Disease Control. Honey can carry bacterial botulism spores that germinate in a baby's immature intestine, colonize, and make a deadly toxin. Although infant botulism cases are rare—about one hundred were reported in the world in 1986, possibly one third involving honey—authorities say giving honey to infants is not worth the risk.

WORLD HEALTH ORGANIZATION'S RECIPE FOR TRAVELER'S DIARRHEA

Fill one glass with eight ounces orange juice, a pinch of table salt, and ½ teaspoon honey. Fill another glass with eight ounces distilled water and ¼ teaspoon baking soda. Alternate drinking from each glass.

KALE

POSSIBLE THERAPEUTIC BENEFITS:
- A good bet to block cancer of several types, especially lung

> *How Much?* An extra half cup of kale a day may help prevent cancer. Advice: Former smokers especially, load up on kale. It may boost your resistance to developing smoking-related cancers down the line.

FACTS

Kale, too little loved and eaten in the United States and other Western countries, looks like a super vegetable as a preventive of cancers of several types, in particular lung cancer. It is one of the richest of all green vegetables in carotenoids, anticancer agents. For example, raw spinach, another rich source, has thirty-six milligrams of carotenoids per 100 grams; an equal amount of kale has more than twice that much—seventy-eight milligrams.

Kale is also higher in one particular type of carotenoid, beta carotene. (Kale has twice as much as spinach.) Beta carotene, which is converted to vitamin A in the body, is singled out by some scientists as a particularly potent anticancer agent, as demonstrated by animal studies. As if that is not enough, kale is a marvelous source of chlorophyll, another constituent that some authorities label a cancer antagonist.

When diet is linked with rates of cancer, dark-green vegetables, including kale, come out tops as protective. In numerous studies, frequent eating of such vegetables is tied to lower rates of gastrointestinal, esophageal, stomach, lung, colon, oral, and throat cancer, and sometimes to cancers of all types. Being a member of the cruciferous family may give kale added powers; cruciferous vegetables are linked to lower rates of bowel, prostate, and bladder cancer.

In particular, dark-green leafy (as well as dark-orange vegetables) appear to possess unique powers to thwart the development of lung cancer, even to a mild degree among smokers and more so among former smokers. A study in Singapore singled out kale along with common dark-green leafy vegetables such as Chinese mustard greens as significantly diminishing the risk of lung cancer.

Elderly people in New Jersey who ate a little more than two servings a day of any green or yellow vegetable had only one third the cancer deaths of those who ate only three fourths of an ordinary serving a day, according to a recent five-year study.

PRACTICAL MATTERS

- Raw or cooked? Surprisingly, kale cooked in a microwave lost very little cholorophyll, according to United States Department of Agriculture analyses. However, some of its carotenoids are destroyed by heat. Nevertheless, cooking often makes more carotene available for bodily use. Truth is, it may be wise to eat both cooked and raw kale.

LEMON AND LIME

It is probable that the lemon is the most valuable of all fruit for preserving health.

—Maud Grieve: *A Modern Herbal*, 1931.

POSSIBLE THERAPEUTIC BENEFITS:
- Prevents and cures scurvy
- Contains chemicals that block cancer

FOLKLORE

In the third century A.D. the Romans believed that the lemon was an antidote for all poisons, as illustrated by the tale of two criminals thrown to venomous snakes; the one who had eaten a lemon beforehand survived snakebite, the other died. So great is the reputation of the lemon that, so the story goes, it became an accompaniment for fish in the belief that if a fishbone got stuck in the throat, the lemon juice would dissolve it.

Lemon juice has long been heralded as a diuretic, diaphoretic, an astringent, and thus a good gargle for sore throats and a lotion for sunburn, a cure for hiccoughs, and a tonic throughout the world. In India, the common "morning drink" is two tablespoons of lemon juice mixed with two tablespoons of honey and an ounce of water.

FACTS

Lemons and limes gained fame for their ability to prevent scurvy, the former curse of seamen who went for months without fresh fruits and vegetables. A little over a tablespoon of lemon juice daily prevents scurvy because of the vitamin C content. Scurvy is a dread, potentially fatal vitamin C deficiency disease. (Muscles waste away, wounds don't heal, bruises appear, gums bleed and deteriorate.) For years English ships were required by law to carry enough lemon or lime juice for each sailor to have an ounce daily after being ten days at sea. That's why the English are nicknamed "limeys."

Lately, lemons have yielded very little from scientific scrutiny. Lemon juice is an antioxidant, perhaps because of the vitamin C. And lemon peel exhibits remarkable antioxidant activity unrelated to vitamin C, according to German studies reported in 1986. Antioxidants are believed to have profound beneficial impact on human cells, including warding off cancerous changes and retarding aging. Pectin (fiber) found in the pulp of citrus fruits also lowers blood cholesterol, although it's unlikely many eat enough lemon to benefit blood chemistry.

In a screening of plants with ability to kill roundworms in humans, lemon extract was effective. Lemon oil can also kill fungi. And the Yugoslavs have found that lemon oil has a slight sedative effect on the nervous systems of fish.

MELON

POSSIBLE THERAPEUTIC BENEFITS:
- Thins the blood (anticoagulant)
- Rich in chemicals that may prevent cancer

FOLKLORE

The yellowish melon better known as muskmelon and cantaloupe is used in China to treat hepatitis. The seeds are crushed and eaten in Guatemala to expel worms, in the Philippines to treat cancer and bring on menstruation, in India as a diuretic, and in Africa they are made into a porridge and drunk to bring on abortions.

FACTS

The emerging evidence about cantaloupe makes the fruit even more important than folklore indicates. In an interesting recent experiment by Argentinian and German investigators, this melon—just like onion, garlic, black tree fungus, and ginger—proved to be an anticoagulant. The researchers, like those studying the effects of other foods in the blood, donated their platelets, then mixed them with "the sweet watery flesh of melon homogenized in a blender." Their conclusion: "The melon contains an agent that strongly inhibits human platelet aggregation." The platelet blood cells were blocked from aggregating, or clumping, and thus were not likely to form clots. Such clotting is incriminated in heart disease and stroke.

Moreover, when the donors gave blood after taking aspirin, the platelets were even less likely to clump; the melon and aspirin worked together to provide an even greater anticoagulant effect. The researchers identified the anticoagulant chemical in melon as adenosine, the same compound found in onions, garlic, and tree ears, that is believed to at least partially account for their powers as anticoagulants. It appears that melon is one more plant food that can help thin the blood, lessening the risk of heart attacks and strokes.

CANCER ANTIDOTE

Melons also reportedly guard against cancer. In epidemiological studies in which diets are compared with cancer rates, melons come out as protective along with other orange fruits and green vegetables. For example, a 1985 study found that among 1271 Massachusetts residents over age sixty-six, those who ate the most green and yellow fruits and vegetables, including fresh melon, had the lowest death rates from cancer. In fact, those who ate the absolute most had only three tenths of one percent the risk of dying of cancer as those who ate the least green and yellow fruits and vegetables. Current scientific wisdom credits the rich concentration of carotenoids in melons and other such foods as the main cancer-fighting compound.

Foods like orange melons high in beta carotene are especially linked in numerous surveys with lower rates of lung cancer.

MILK

POSSIBLE THERAPEUTIC BENEFITS:

- Prevents osteoporosis
- Fights infections, especially diarrhea
- Mollifies upset stomach from harsh foods and drugs
- Prevents peptic ulcers
- Prevents cavities
- Prevents chronic bronchitis
- Increases mental energy
- Lowers high blood pressure
- Lowers blood cholesterol
- Inhibits certain cancers

How Much? Two or three cups of vitamin D fortified skim milk a day may help ward off colon cancer; a couple of daily cups of whole milk may fend off ulcers. Only half a cup of skim or lowfat milk can give your mental energy a boost.

FOLKLORE

Milk is frequently of great advantage in . . . relieving gastro-intestinal irritation, uneasiness, unrest and insomnia.

—*King's American Dispensatory*, 1900.

FACTS

Don't underestimate milk; it's a health elixir of amazing versatility, as recent scientific inquiries document. Milk contains some amazing newly discovered biologically active chemicals, as well as the well-known calcium, that behave like curative and preventive drugs against a long list of disparate health troubles. If you can make it only one, you could do worse than to make it milk.

CANCER ANTIDOTE

Evidence that milk prevents cancer, notably colon cancer, has been snowballing for a decade. A major boost for the theory came from a study in 1985 by Dr. Cedric Garland of the University of California at San Diego. His analysis of the diets of 2000 men over a twenty-year period found that daily drinkers of about two and a half glasses of milk had decidedly healthier colons *and about one third* the colon cancer risk of those who shunned milk but otherwise ate similar foods. Consequently, Dr. Garland recommends two or three glasses of vitamin D fortified skim milk daily as a colon cancer preventive. He, like many other researchers, credits milk's high calcium and vitamin D (that promotes calcium absorption). His co-investigator, Dr. Richard B. Shekelle, however, says it has not been ascertained what in milk cuts colon cancer risk.

Bolstering the case further is a 1987 report of a massive study by the Aussies, who have high colon cancer rates. They, too, found that both men and women who drank less than 600 milliliters of milk a week—about two and a half cups—were more likely to develop colorectal cancer.

Scientists bet on calcium as the protective compound because of well-worked-out experiments showing that calcium detoxifies bile acids in the intestinal tract; bile acids can promote cancer. Impressive studies at New York's Memorial Sloan Kettering Cancer Center found that calcium "quieted" the growth rate of cancer-prone cells in the colons of those at high risk for the cancer.

Acidophilus milk, actually a liquid yogurt fermented by bacteria, also looks good as a colon cancer deterrent, and for completely different reasons. It can block cell changes in humans that lead to colon cancer, Boston researchers find. The acidophilus bacteria actually stop the conversion within the colon of natural substances into dangerous cancer-causing agents.

Everyday milk drinking is also linked to less stomach cancer in Japan. Several international surveys also reveal less lung cancer among milk drinkers and enthusiastic consumers of vitamin A foods, including milk.

SMOKER'S ALERT

In fact, Johns Hopkins University researchers recently reported the intriguing news that milk drinkers were strikingly less likely to have chronic bronchitis. And not because milk drinkers lead a more pristine life. After taking into account such things as smoking, alcohol and coffee drinking, the Johns Hopkins investigators still concluded that milk appeared to singularly guard *smokers* from bronchitis—but not non-smokers. One- or two-pack-a-day smokers who did not drink milk were about sixty percent more likely to have chronic bronchitis than milk drinkers.

"This suggests a strong effect of milk drinking," concluded the authors. The reason? Something in milk, possibly vitamin A, "may protect respiratory epithelium [cells in lung linings] offsetting to a degree susceptibility to both chronic bronchitis and lung cancer."

HEART AND BLOOD PRESSURE MEDICINE

Skim milk, unlike fatty whole milk, may benefit your arteries. Several studies show that skim milk can depress blood cholesterol in humans. Dr. George Mann of Vanderbilt University, a leading researcher on the subject, has identified a "milk factor" which he says suppresses the liver's output of cholesterol. A recent Japanese experiment documented much less cholesterol plaque and other damage in the aortas of rabbits fed skim milk, compelling the researchers to conclude that "skim milk has preventive effects on the development of hyper-cholesterolemia (high blood cholesterol) and atherosclerosis (hardened, plaque-clogged arteries)."

Mild high blood pressure also might succumb to the blandishments of milk, according to experts at Cornell University. The reason: Considerable research finds that calcium deficiencies help trigger high blood pressure in some, especially those extrasensitive to the blood-pressure-elevating effects of salt. Increased calcium may counteract the ill effects of sodium.

Although most studies have been done with calcium supplements, Dr. John Laragh, head of Cornell's Hypertension Research Center, says upping your intake of milk might work against mild high blood pressure (diastolic reading of 90 to 104). Confirming the link, a large-scale study of about 8000 middle-aged men by the National Heart, Lung and Blood Institute revealed that non–milk drinkers were twice as likely to have high blood pressure as those who drank a quart of milk a day.

IF YOU WERE A RAT, DRINKING MILK WOULD CURB YOUR ULCER

To their great surprise, researchers at the State University of New York Health Science Center at Brooklyn recently discovered that milk fat is full of biologically active prostaglandins of the E2 type. And when they fed laboratory rats whole milk and subjected them to stress, only fifty percent got ulcers compared with ninety percent fed a salt solution. To be sure it was the milk's prostaglandins that did the trick, the researchers also fed one group of rats milk with the prostaglandins removed; eighty percent came down with ulcers. A fascinating fact is that the milk prostaglandins are identical to those comprising a new antiulcer drug called Cytotec launched by G. D. Searle in 1986. In animal and human tests the pure prostaglandin E2 has proved remarkable in protecting the stomach and intestinal lining from assaults by noxious chemicals, including acid and cigarette smoke, a prime cause of ulcers. The prostaglandins apparently command stomach-lining cells to throw up an impenetrable barrier against chemical assaults. One theory: They induce cells to churn out a jellylike layer of mucus atop stomach-lining cells, just like spreading a glaze of Vaseline over the interior stomach surface.

How much milk did the rats have to drink? Only a couple of drops from an eyedropper—extrapolated to the average man, about two cups a day. The prostaglandins reside in milk fat; thus they were most concentrated in cream, followed by whole milk yogurt, whole milk, and low-fat milk. Skim milk had virtually none.

This offers a plausible explanation as to why milk drinkers seem less prone to ulcers. A large-scale survey in 1974 by Harvard and California State Department of Health investigators found that male college students who drank milk were much more likely to be ulcer free in later life than non–milk drinkers. Even men at "high risk" because of other factors appeared to be saved by milk and the protection zoomed along with the amount of milk consumed. Men who drank more than four glasses of milk daily had less than half the rate of peptic ulcers as non–milk drinkers.

However, milk may not be a good treatment for those who already have ulcers, even though it softens the pain. For years milk was standard treatment to *heal* ulcers, but the practice has fallen out of favor. It was discovered that milk stimulates gastric acid. Also, a recent study from India found that whole milk seemed to retard healing of duodenal ulcers in patients taking cimetidine (Tagamet). Ulcers of those drinking eight cups of milk a day did not heal as well as ulcers of non–milk drinkers even though milk lessened the sensation of pain. Researchers blamed milk's stimulation of stomach acid.

Some experts believe prostaglandins in milk may have enough clout to keep ulcers from forming, but not to heal them. In fact, a study at the UCLA School of Medicine noted that milk did trigger ulcer-aggravating acid secretions in stomachs already plagued by duodenal ulcers, but not in healthy non-ulcer ones.

A GUT REACTION

Milk contains antiinfectious compounds—preformed antibodies to viruses and unknown fat-residing factors that fend off intestinal microbes. Dr. Robert Yolken, professor of infectious diseases at Johns Hopkins University, who discovered the milk antibodies—immune warriors that disarm viruses and bacteria in the body—says it's unknown how well ordinary milk protects humans from gastrointestinal infections, but if antibody levels are high enough, it should work; it works in mice. Lab mice infected with a rotavirus and then fed milk did not develop infection or diarrhea; one hundred percent of infected mice deprived of milk did. (For more, see page 100.)

ANOTHER SURPRISE

Antiinfectious agents in milk *fat* help stamp out gastrointestinal diseases, especially childhood diarrhea. A major United States study of about 1200 children, aged one to sixteen, discovered that children who drank only low-fat milk were *five times* more likely to have acute gastrointestinal illnesses than those drinking whole milk. The researcher, Dr. James S. Koopman, at the School of Public Health, University of Michigan, blames about fourteen percent of all cases of medically treated gastrointestinal illness on low-fat milk consumption; at worst risk, he says, are one- to two-year-olds.

In fact, other research confirms that chronic diarrhea in young children drinking skim milk (sometimes in attempts to avoid later atherosclerosis) is quickly cured by restoring the milk fat. As for any danger to giving milk to youngsters who already have diarrhea, an excellent study from Finland disputed that old rubric. It concluded: "Cow's milk and milk products can be safely given in acute gastro-enteritis as parts of the mixed diet for children over six months of age."

The antidiarrheal factor in milk fat is still a mystery, says Dr. Koopman. One clue: Lab studies find that milk fat globules can kill bacterial toxins and also block the attachment of glues that help E. coli germs stick to the small bowel lining.

MILK FOR INSOMNIACS? NEVER

This folklore, calling for a glass of warm milk to bring on sleep, is dead wrong. At first it seemed scientifically sound. An amino acid in milk called tryptophan, when tested in high doses, at least one gram, helps induce sleep in some mild insomniacs. (A glass of milk contains about one tenth of a gram of tryptophan.) This led to the mistaken assumption that tryptophan makes milk a mild sedative. But not so, just the opposite. Milk—at least non-fat milk—perks up brain chemicals.

According to Drs. Richard and Judith Wurtman, pioneers in food-brain research at MIT, it is one of nature's minor conundrums that drinking milk, which contains tryptophan, does not get sleep-inducing tryptophan into the brain. Indeed, after drinking milk tryptophan levels in the brain tend to *decrease*. That happens because, in the fight to get into the brain, the tiny amounts of tryptophan in milk are crowded out by other more plentiful amino acid chemicals in milk. It's strange but true that eating sugar, which has no tryptophan, releases more of the calming chemical into the brain because of complicated battles over which molecules get through the brain barrier.

In any event, milk, namely skim milk or low-fat milk, actually stirs up your mental energy instead of putting it to sleep. Milk delivers tyrosine to the brain, which in turn triggers production of dopamine and norepinephrine, stimulating you to think more quickly and accurately. Whole milk, because of the fat content, tends to drag your brain's mental acuity down.

As little as half a cup of skim milk or low-fat milk can rev up your brain chemicals, according to Dr. Judith Wurtman. But if your brain is saturated with energy chemicals, drinking more milk will not further stimulate alertness chemicals, although it will provide a steady supply to keep you "up."

A YOUTH ELIXIR FOR OLD BRITTLE BONES

Milk may protect against osteoporosis (a serious bone deterioration leading to malformations and fractures in old age) in ways not totally explained by milk's calcium content. Scientists have long known that the body is better able to utilize calcium—the mineral thought to build strong bones—when it's packaged in milk than in pills. Milk also is superior to calcium supplements in helping bone tissue renew itself. Most scientists doubt that loading up on calcium—or milk—after age thirty-five or so prevents osteoporosis unless a woman also takes estrogen replacement drugs. But there is evidence that women who drank more milk *as youngsters* have denser bones at menopause, presumably making them less susceptible to the ravages of osteoporosis. In addition to calcium, there seems to be an unidentified "milk factor" that retards bone diseases.

TO CAP IT OFF

As if all the above is not enough praise to heap on a single food in nature's pharmacy, milk—and cheese—can also block cavities. A slew of studies on animal teeth find dairy products a cavity preventer, although how they work is uncertain. It may be due to milk's calcium, phosphate, casein, or to unknown substances. In a recent animal test, concentrates of milk minerals slashed cavities by up to thirty percent. Particularly effective is cheddar cheese, which has been tested in animals and humans. Substituting a special device for human mouths, researchers at the University of Toronto found that cheddar cheese extract reduced the ability of table sugar to cause cavities by fifty-six percent.

PRACTICAL MATTERS

- Best bet for adults is skim milk; it carries the same nutrients, including crucial calcium, as whole milk without the fat. Non-fat milk also tickles the brain chemicals; fatty milk may dull them.
- To get the best "brain power" boost from non-fat or low-fat milk, drink a glass *before* you eat other foods. Let the protein molecules in

the milk get the jump in creating brain-stimulating chemicals. Otherwise, competition from chemicals in other foods retards the energizing effect.

- Don't put children under age two on a low-fat diet, and that includes feeding them low-fat or skim milk. Authorities warn it may rob them of protection from gastrointestinal infections for unknown reasons and disturb their normal growth and development.
- Milk can't be relied on to lower blood pressure in everyone. Even 1000 milligrams of calcium daily in a pill, in one study, lowered blood pressure substantially in forty-four percent of those with high blood pressure. (Eight ounces of milk has about 300 milligrams of calcium.)

POSSIBLE ADVERSE EFFECTS

- Some people can't drink milk because they have lactose intolerance and suffer mild or intense stomach distress from milk but not from yogurt.
- Milk is also a prime suspect in cases of food intolerances linked to certain bowel disorders, including irritable bowel syndrome.
- Saturated fat, the type in milk, is associated with increased blood cholesterol, thus risk of heart disease, and certain cancers, notably breast, bowel, larynx, bladder, and mouth.
- Breast cancer seems particularly linked to high fat foods. A United States study correlated per capita intake of dairy foods with breast cancer risk. In a 1986 French case control study, drinking milk per se did not predispose to breast cancer, but there was a link to eating large quantities of high fat cheese and high fat milk. This suggests that it is the dairy fat—and not an intrinsic milk factor—that is linked to cancer. This is in sync with numerous studies incriminating fat in foods as a breast-cancer promoter.

CONFLICTING CANCER EVIDENCE

The large-scale Australian study found that men, but not women, drinking more than 2650 milliliters a week (about ten cups) of milk had a slightly higher risk of colon cancer.

MUSHROOM

POSSIBLE THERAPEUTIC BENEFITS:

- Thins the blood
- Prevents cancer in animals
- Lowers blood cholesterol
- Stimulates the immune system
- Inactivates viruses

FOLKLORE

In Oriental folklore, mushrooms are esteemed as a longevity tonic. In fact, the symbol for the Chinese god of longevity, Shoulau, is a walking stick capped by a mushroom ornament. The Chinese black fungus, mo-er, or tree ear, is used to treat headaches and prevent heart attacks. In Japan the basidiomycete fungus has been used as a folk remedy for cancer.

FACTS

So far few medicinal benefits are linked to the common button mushroom popular in the United States, but Oriental mushrooms contain compounds that can stimulate the immune system, inhibit blood clotting, and retard the development of cancer. The magical four with proven value: shiitake, oyster, enoki, and tree ear, also called wood ear and mo-er.

234

Japanese scientists have extensively analyzed the medicinal qualities of mushrooms, especially shiitake, increasingly cultivated and eaten
in the United States. What makes these mushrooms unusually exciting
to scientists is that some possess stimulating or potentiating properties
that may strengthen the immune system against not only a variety of
infections, but cancer and possibly autoimmune diseases such as rheumatoid arthritis, polyarthritis, and multiple sclerosis.

SHIITAKE SURPRISE

The most common edible, best-studied mushroom with the greatest
proven therapeutic powers is the shiitake. Known as "golden oaks" in
the United States or by its Latin botanical name, Lentinus edodes, this
is the big brown beefy mushroom cap (over two inches) with a slightly
smoky flavor. It was an American, Dr. Kenneth Cochran of the University of Michigan, who launched the study of the shiitake in 1960. To his
great surprise, he discovered that the mushroom possessed a strong
antiviral substance that stimulated immune system functions. The compound turned out to be lentinan, a long-chain sugar called a polysaccharide.

In follow-up Japanese tests, the compound was more effective
against influenza viruses than the powerful prescription antiviral drug
amantadine hydrochloride. Further tests found lentinan a broad-spectrum
killer of numerous viruses.

The shiitake apparently stimulates the immune system to spin out
more interferon, a natural agent of defense against both viruses and
cancer. Thus, the shiitake compound has proved amazingly successful
in fighting cancers. It has been tested in leukemia patients in China and
on human breast cancer in Japan.

Eating shiitakes may help lower blood cholesterol, even blocking
some of the bad effects of highly saturated fat. In one test, by eating
about three ounces of shiitake a day for a week, a group of thirty
healthy young women drove their blood cholesterol down by an average twelve percent. To see if the shiitake could counteract fat in the
diet, the experimenters tried another test. One group ate two ounces
of butter every day for a week; their cholesterol went up fourteen
percent; another group ate the butter but added three ounces of
shiitake. Their blood cholesterol dropped four percent.

BLOOD-THINNING TREE EAR

Only a little of the Chinese black or dark brown fungus that grows on trees (called mo-er or tree ear) is enough to inhibit blood clotting. As Dr. Dale Hammerschmidt discovered, the mushroom, in quantities commonly used in recipes, can prevent blood platelets from sticking together. (See page 24 for more details.) Such anticoagulant activity could help prevent heart disease and stroke by keeping the blood thin, much as aspirin does. Tree ears also retard cancer in animals.

Enoki is a white stringy, spaghettilike mushroom of increasing popularity in the United States. It's generally eaten raw or slightly simmered in soups. The enoki, too, stimulates the immune system of animals, and thus may help fight off viruses and tumors. In one region of Japan, where the enoki are commercially grown, and presumably eaten in large quantities, there is a lower rate of cancer.

The oyster mushroom, or Pleurotus ostreatus, is a white lilylike creation with a delicate flavor. It, too, may fight tumors, as proved in animal studies.

ANTICANCER

According to a 1986 study by the Mushroom Research Institute of Japan, several mushrooms have antitumor powers. The researchers exposed mice to carcinogens, then fed them a mixture of dried mushrooms, including button, shiitake, tree ear, enoki, oyster, and straw. Tumors in mice eating the mushrooms grew at only forty to fifty percent the rate as those of mice eating no mushrooms. The fungi apparently interfered with the late-stage growth of cancer.

CONFLICTING EVIDENCE

Common *raw* button mushrooms contain hydrazides, according to Bela Toth, Ph.D., of the University of Nebraska Eppley Cancer Research Center. Hydrazides, he says, are cancer-causing agents that are destroyed by cooking.

NUTS

POSSIBLE THERAPEUTIC BENEFITS:
- Contain chemicals that prevent cancer in animals
- Oil lowers blood cholesterol
- Regulates blood sugar

FOLKLORE

Walnuts were considered the "royal" nut of ancient Rome, credited with bringing good health and good luck.

FACTS

Nuts, although extremely nutritious (high in trace minerals), have been little tested against disease. However, all nuts—peanuts, almonds, Brazil nuts, cashews, pignolas, and so forth—contain high amounts of compounds called protease inhibitors, known to block cancer in test animals. Thus, experts like Dr. Walter Troll of New York University put nuts high on the list of possible antidotes to cancer. Dr. Troll says they are likely to interfere with the promotion and progression of cancers of various types. Nuts are also rich in certain polyphenols, other chemicals shown to thwart cancer in animals.

The oil from walnuts, like that from other vegetables, is considered healthful because it is polyunsaturated and tends to lower blood cholesterol.

237

BLOOD SUGAR REGULATOR

Peanuts ranked best on the "glycemic index," meaning they are least likely of fifty foods tested to cause sharp rises in blood sugar. They promote a steady slow rise in blood sugar and insulin, making them good foods for those worried about blood sugar and especially diabetics.

POSSIBLE ADVERSE EFFECTS

- Peanut oil, unlike other monounsaturated or polyunsaturated oils, causes severe atherosclerosis (clogged, damaged arteries) in monkeys and other laboratory animals. It is not recommended by heart-disease authorities, even though it does lower blood cholesterol.
- Peanuts, as well as peanut butter, are often contaminated by a mold called aflatoxin, which is a carcinogen. In third world countries aflatoxin is a widespread cause of liver cancer. Although the federal government regulates levels of aflatoxin contamination of foods, many experts consider the levels too high.

OATS

POSSIBLE THERAPEUTIC BENEFITS:
- An excellent heart medicine
- Lowers blood cholesterol
- Regulates blood sugar
- Contains compounds that prevent cancer in animals
- Combats inflammation of the skin
- Acts as a laxative

> *How Much?* About one-half cup of dry oat bran (a large bowlful cooked) or a cup of dry oatmeal (a couple of bowlsful cooked) a day can put a dramatic dent in your blood cholesterol. It also keeps insulin and blood sugar levels stable.

FOLKLORE

Oats have been called a stimulant, an antispasmodic, a laxative, and a nerve and uterine tonic. Tea made from oats also achieved a curious reputation in the early part of the century as being able to "cure the opium habit," and reduce the craving for cigarettes.

FACTS

Oats are a potent tonic for the heart and blood. Unquestionably, the oat seed as in oatmeal and more definitively as oat bran is for many people a powerful drug that lowers blood cholesterol. Oats have been tested on laboratory animals, and on humans with normal or high blood cholesterol who eat either a low or high fat diet. The results are almost uniformly the same: oats suppress blood cholesterol significantly, sometimes dramatically. If you're worried about blood cholesterol, there seems hardly a better food pharmaceutical than oats.

CEREAL FOR THE HEART

Most of the oats research has been done by Dr. James Anderson and his colleagues at the University of Kentucky College of Medicine. Dr. Anderson finds that about an ounce and a half of dry oat bran (about a half cup)—a large bowlful when cooked—rather quickly lowers detrimental LDL cholesterol an average twenty percent. Beneficial HDL cholesterol usually rises about fifteen percent over a period of time.

Plain oatmeal is about two thirds as potent as pure oat bran; thus you need about a cup of dry oatmeal a day to lower cholesterol. Dr. Anderson often mixes oat bran and oatmeal. Cheerios made from whole oat flour, he says, are also about as effective as oatmeal; a couple of ounces a day—or two bowlsful—should depress cholesterol. Oat-bran muffins work too. In one experiment, healthy young men who added four oat-bran muffins daily to their regular diet saw their blood cholesterol sink an average twelve percent—from 185 to 164.

Oat cereals drive down blood cholesterol of various ranges. One man had a very low cholesterol reading of 150; eating oat bran reduced it to 120. Others with dangerously high cholesterol measures of 350 got it down to 280 by eating oat bran. Dr. Anderson's own blood cholesterol dived from 285 to 175 after five weeks of eating oat bran every day. Still, oats work best, notes Dr. Anderson, in those with blood cholesterol counts between 240 and 300; they usually see a twenty-three percent reduction. It takes about three weeks for effects to show up.

> *Expert example:* Dr. Anderson usually eats a large bowl of oat bran and oatmeal combined, topped with raisins and skim milk every day, plus a couple of oat-bran muffins for lunch.

However, oat bran does not lower the blood cholesterol of about fifteen percent of the population. Nor is it successful in those with abnormally high cholesterol—in the high 300's and 400 range—who have so-called familial hypercholestermia, a genetic defect.

Eating oats also lowers blood pressure slightly and helps keep blood sugar and insulin levels steady.

LAXATIVE POWERS

Although oat bran is not as rich in insoluble fiber as wheat bran, known to relieve constipation, oats, too, work as a laxative. Dr. Anderson finds that both oat bran and oatmeal increase fecal bulk, benefiting the colon in numerous ways, including curing constipation. In a recent French study, fifty elderly people who came to a doctor with complaints of constipation were told to eat a couple of oat-bran-meal biscuits every day ("Lejfibre"). After twelve weeks the constipation disappeared, and the number of bowel movements and stool consistency improved. As a bonus, most also lost weight.

Oats also have antiinflammatory effects on certain skin problems like contact eczema. One bit of recent research dissected oat seeds and discovered they strongly inhibited the biosynthesis of prostaglandins, and heavily boiled oats were as potent as raw oats. Prostaglandin activity can lead to inflammation; thus, this seems a reasonable explanation for oats' antiinflammatory powers and the longtime reputation of oat facial packs as beneficial to the skin. Some physicians recommend oatmeal packs to treat psoriasis.

ANTICANCER AGENT

Oats, being one of the seeds that carries the genetic material, are also high in protease inhibitors, those chemicals that dampen the activation of certain viruses and cancer-causing chemicals in the intestinal tract. Thus, it's likely that oats have antiinfectious and anticancer capability, especially against hazards of intestinal origin. Their fecal-bulking activity also would tend to protect against colon cancer as well as a variety of problems such as diverticulitis and hemorrhoids.

PRACTICAL MATTERS

- For a more consistent cholesterol-lowering effect, spread out the consumption of oats throughout the day. You may want to have oat cereal both in the morning and as an evening snack.

OLIVE OIL

Italians . . . seemed never to die. They eat olive oil all day long . . . and that's what does it.

—William Kennedy: *Ironweed*

POSSIBLE THERAPEUTIC BENEFITS:

- Good for the heart
- Reduces bad LDL cholesterol
- Raises good HDL cholesterol
- Thins the blood
- Contains chemicals that retard cancer and aging
- Lowers risk of death from all causes
- Lowers blood pressure

How Much? Only one tablespoon of olive oil has wiped out the cholesterol-raising effects of two eggs. Four or five tablespoons of olive oil daily dramatically improve the blood profiles of heart attack patients. And two thirds of a tablespoon daily lowered blood pressure in men.

FOLKLORE

Olive oil has been a health potion around the Mediterranean for four thousand years. Ramses II, who ruled Egypt between 1300 and 1200 B.C., supposedly downed olive oil for every complaint.

FACTS

The residents of Crete eat more fat than any other people. About forty-five percent of their calories come from fat, and a whopping thirty-three percent of their calories come from olive oil. It should follow that Cretans have more heart disease and die earlier. Wrong. Crete is one of the anomalies on the heart disease–fat consumption charts. In fact, the population of Crete has one of the world's lowest rates of heart disease and cancer. Scientists trying to ferret out the "longevity factor" often settle on olive oil. In Crete the olive oil flows like wine. Crete consumes more olive oil per person than any other nation. Not far behind are Italians, Greeks, and others in the Mediterranean area.

OLIVE OIL EATERS DO LIVE LONGER

As if confirming author William Kennedy's observation that olive oil saves Italians, a recent study by Ancel Keys, a famous pioneer in dietary fat studies from the University of Minnesota, found that among 2300 middle-aged men from seven countries, death rates from heart disease and from *all causes* were exceptionally low in men who consumed olive oil as their major source of fat!

Several rigorously controlled scientific studies show that olive oil contains chemical components that work wonders on the blood, such as blocking the tendency of blood to clot, improving good HDL-cholesterol ratios, and combating dangerous arterial buildups of cholesterol. Consequently, some experts now "prescribe" olive oil as an excellent way to cut the risk of first time as well as subsequent heart attacks and strokes.

In Milan, a team of physicians give heart-surgery patients four to five tablespoons of olive oil per day as part of their therapeutic regimen. Within six months the patients show decidedly improved blood profiles, making them less susceptible to future heart attacks and strokes. Physicians at the University of Texas Health Science Center in Dallas, a leading center for heart disease therapy, also have found that the monounsaturated fats in olive oil dramatically lower and favorably alter blood cholesterol. In tests on middle-aged Americans, olive oil pushed down blood cholesterol by thirteen percent and dangerous LDL cholesterol by twenty-one percent. Investigator Dr. William Grundy concluded that the monounsaturated fats combated high cholesterol just as effectively as a low fat diet. Dr. Grundy advises Americans to substitute olive oil for other oils and fats to prevent cardiovascular disease.

How does the olive oil work? For one thing, olive oil is dominated by so-called monounsaturated fatty molecules, which have a more protective effect on the blood than the often recommended polyunsaturated vegetable oils like corn oil. Olive oil not only lowers total blood cholesterol, but also, unlike other vegetable oils, preserves good HDL-cholesterol levels, thus in effect improving the critical protective ratios of "good cholesterol"—HDLs—that help defeat heart disease. Other vegetable oils tend to lower *both* dangerous LDL and beneficial HDL-type cholesterol.

Until recently, that seemed the whole explanation. But new research reveals that olive oil also contains potent heart-disease-fighting agents that independently produce beneficial physiological reactions—for example, by acting as an anticoagulant (thinning the blood, cutting the chances of clots and blockages) and partially blocking the absorption of excess cholesterol in the body.

A team of Italian scientists led by Dr. Bruno Berra, a professor of biochemistry at the School of Pharmacology, the University of Milan, has identified and charted the metabolic pathways of several of about 1000 active chemical components found in olive oil. According to Dr. Berra, these chemical components can even help counteract a high fat, high cholesterol diet. One chemical in particular, called cycloarthanol, neutralizes cholesterol during the absorption cycle, helping keep it out of the bloodstream. In Dr. Berra's studies, one tablespoon of olive oil wiped out the cholesterol-raising effect of two eggs.

University of Kentucky researchers also find that olive oil lowers blood pressure. A mere two thirds of a tablespoon a day reduced blood pressure by about five systolic points and four diastolic points in men.

AN ANTIAGING, ANTICANCER AGENT?

Olive oil inserted into human cells makes cell membranes more stable and less susceptible to destruction by so-called "free radicals" roaming the body. The implication is that antioxidants in olive oil, sufficiently absorbed by human cells, could help retard aging by keeping cells alive longer, as well as fight off attacks that cause cells to become disorganized and more cancer-prone.

Olive oil also has a slight laxative effect.

PRACTICAL MATTERS

- Best type for the heart. Of the many types of olive oil, the most potent, with the most heart-disease-fighting chemicals, is extra virgin olive oil, which is extracted by merely crushing and pressing the highest quality olives. The closer the oil to the original olive source, says Dr. Berra, the greater the concentration of heart-protecting chemicals.
- How to boost the cholesterol-lowering effect. Cut down on saturated animal-type fats (in meat and dairy products) when you boost olive oil consumption. This more effectively revs up LDL receptor activity, draining off more of the detrimental stuff. Merely adding lots of olive oil on top of a high saturated fat diet won't make as big a dent in cholesterol. Too much saturated fat counteracts the beneficial impact of the olive oil.

POSSIBLE ADVERSE EFFECTS

- In rare instances, people eating high amounts of olive oil—especially at one time—have experienced temporary mild diarrhea.

ONION

My own remedy is always to eat, just before I step into bed, a hot roasted onion, if I have a cold.

—Attributed to George Washington

POSSIBLE THERAPEUTIC BENEFITS:
- Definitely a multi-faceted heart-blood medicine
- Boosts beneficial HDL cholesterol
- Thins the blood
- Retards blood clotting
- Lowers total blood cholesterol
- Regulates blood sugar
- Kills bacteria
- Relieves bronchial congestion
- Blocks cancer in animals

How Much? Only half a raw onion a day can boost your good HDL blood cholesterol by an average thirty percent. A mere tablespoon of cooked onions reverses the blood's clotting tendency after eating a high fat meal. A half a cup of onions a day—raw or cooked—can keep your blood in great shape in many ways.

FOLKLORE

Onions in soup, raw, roasted, or cooked into a syrup are centuries-old cures for the cold. The onion, like its close cousin garlic, has been cultivated for nearly 6000 years, and during that time has been reputed

246

to cure or prevent virtually every ailment known to man. In modern folklore, the onion is commonly used throughout the world against infections, in particular dysentery, as a diuretic, blood pressure reducer, expectorant, heart tonic, contraceptive, and aphrodisiac. A 1927 American medical journal calls onions "blood purifiers, sedatives, expectorants . . . beneficial in cases of insomnia, general nervous irritability, coughs, and bronchial troubles."

FACTS

The onion and its close cousin garlic are packed with similar therapeutic compounds. But onions have unique properties unseen in garlic, and are eaten in larger doses. The onion is one of the best tested miracle foods of the food pharmacy—a potent versatile bulb against a host of human ills, just as the ancients asserted.

HEARTY ONIONS

Dr. Victor Gurewich, a professor of medicine at Tufts University, has a prescription for his heart patients: "Eat onions." Dr. Gurewich finds that raw, strong onions decidedly lift critical HDL-type blood cholesterol. His typical therapeutic dose is but half a medium-size raw onion—or equivalent juice—a day. That's usually enough, he says, to "dramatically raise" HDLs an average of thirty percent in about three out of four of his heart disease patients. In a few cases the HDLs have even doubled or tripled on the onion regimen. Dr. Gurewich has not identified the HDL-boosting chemical in onions, although he has isolated about 150 onion chemicals in his vascular laboratory. However, he does know that *raw* onions work best; cooking lessens or destroys the onion's powers to raise HDLs.

Nevertheless, cooked onions are good for the cardiovascular system in other ways. As Dr. Gurewich also finds, onions act as an anticoagulant and a force to rev up the body's protective fibrinolytic (clot-dissolving) system. The body has an elaborate system of checks and balances for both clotting the blood and dissolving clots. Obstructive clots in the heart's arteries or other blood vessels can choke off oxygen supply, destroying heart muscle and brain cells. Onions both heighten the blood's tendency to dissolve clots and discourage blood cells' proclivity to stick together, forming clots. Both British and Indian scientists, during a decade of investigation, have produced striking evidence that onions can reduce the risk of heart disease in several ways.

In the early 1960s the theory that eating fat polluted the blood, causing cardiovascular disease, was just catching on. Numerous researchers had been testing compounds—drugs, nutrients, estrogens, salicylates—as potential blood-modifying anti-heart disease drugs, but most had serious drawbacks. Dr. N. N. Gupta, a professor of medicine at K. G. Medical College in Lucknow, India, had a brilliant idea. Why not try something already in the diet: onions. It was a pivotal discovery. He fed both young and middle-aged men a fat-rich meal, with and without onions, and measured changes in their blood. The test meal had 900 of its 1000 calories in fat—from butter, cream, and eggs. The experimenters knew that such a fat load would induce detrimental blood changes—elevated cholesterol and a greater tendency for the blood to clot. At first the individuals ate the fat alone; later, they consumed the fatty foods plus about two ounces of whole onions coated with chick-pea flour and lightly fried.

A startling reversal: Dr. Gupta and his colleagues were flabbergasted by the lab results of blood drawn before the meals, and again at two and four hours after. The onions unquestionably counteracted the expected detrimental blood changes from the fat. In all cases where the high fat meal had pushed up blood cholesterol, onions brought it back down. Also, especially striking was the onion's ability to restore the blood's critical clot-dissolving function to full power. A rash of studies followed showing that onion did essentially the same thing whether raw, boiled, fried, or dried.

The scant amount of onion needed to counteract fat-induced blood changes is astonishing. In one study, forty-five healthy persons in New Delhi ate a 3000-calorie-a-day diet for fifteen days—about forty-five percent of them in fat. Their blood cholesterol rose from an average 219 to 263. But when ten grams of onion per day—a mere tablespoon— were eaten with the fatty fare, the cholesterol fell to an average 237. Not quite back to pre-fat days, but still it is a mighty blow for so little onion to pack against so much fat. More onion creates steeper drops in blood cholesterol.

THE MORE THE BETTER

Dedicated onion (and garlic) eaters have better signs of cardiovascular health. A large survey—in India of a vegetarian Jain community—found that onion and garlic lovers had much better blood profiles (cholesterol, triglycerides, and HDLs) than those who ate fewer of the bulbs or shunned them altogether. There was a dose response; even those who ate *some* onions and garlic possessed more anti–heart disease factors in their blood than abstainers. The best blood showed up in those eating a pound and a third of onions a week (about three cups of cooked onions or four cups raw). Even a mere cup of onions a week kept the blood in better shape to fend off cardiovascular disease.

Onions also contain a compound that lowers blood pressure in laboratory animals. It is a prostaglandin—the first ever isolated from a plant food.

A DIABETIC DRUG?

Onions were used in ancient times to treat diabetes, and in 1923 researchers found hypoglycemic agents—blood sugar reducers—in onions. Interest waned until the 1960s when investigators isolated from onions antidiabetic compounds similar to tolbutamide (Orinase), a common antidiabetic pharmaceutical that stimulates insulin manufacture and release. Tested in rabbits, one of the onion extracts was seventy-seven percent as potent as a standard dose of tolbutamide. Other animal tests found that onion juice also lowered blood sugar.

Indian researchers discovered that onion extracts and plain raw and boiled onions did precipitate drops in blood sugar levels of humans after they had been given glucose. The conclusion: Onions helped counteract rises in blood sugar created by sugar. Recently, Egyptian pharmacists isolated a compound from onions, diphenylamine, and found it much more potent than the drug tolbutamide in lowering blood sugar in hyperglycemic laboratory rabbits.

A PUNGENT ANTIBIOTIC

Onion is a strong natural antibiotic. Pasteur first put onion to the test in the mid-1800s, and declared it antibacterial. Since then, onion and its essences have been proved to kill a long list of disease-causing bacteria, including E. coli and Salmonella. In one test against tuberculosis strains, both onions and chives were effective. Chives were declared only slightly less effective than streptomycin.

Russian scientists, for many years students of onion and garlic pharmacology, once screened 150 plants for antibacterial properties and found onions and garlic the most potent. Chief Investigator B. Tokin called onion a potent antiseptic. He noted that chewing raw onion for three to eight minutes rendered the lining of the mouth completely sterile. Vapors from onion paste were regularly used on

Soviet soldiers' wounds during World War II. Doctors reported quick obliteration of pain, and rapid healing from the onion vapor. Observing onion's antibiotic powers, one investigator commented that "eating raw onions might have a curative effect on sore throat resulting from colds."

For a different reason, pulmonary authority Dr. Irwin Ziment also dubs onions a good cold remedy. Because of their strong, pungent properties, he says, onions induce the stomach to initiate actions that release a "flood of tears" in the throat and lungs' airways, breaking up mucus congestion. That's why onions also have a reputation as expectorants—agents that prod mucus to move through the lungs and into the throat, where it is coughed up. That, too, helps the lungs in cases of colds and bronchitis.

ANTICANCER BULBS

Of late, onions are emerging as possible cancer antidotes mainly because of their concentrated sulfur compounds that can turn off cell changes preceding cancer growth. Investigators at the M. D. Anderson Hospital and Tumor Institute have isolated propylsulfide in onions that in tests blocked enzymes needed to activate a potent cancer-causing substance. Indeed, researchers at the Harvard School of Dental Medicine found that putting onion extract on cultures of oral cancer cells from animals significantly inhibited proliferation of the cancer cells and destroyed some. "Because onion extract is a nontoxic natural agent, its use as a possible cancer chemopreventive agent should be explored comprehensively," concluded the investigators. The National Cancer Institute is funding much research on sulfides in onions and garlic, calling them promising agents in fending off cancer.

PRACTICAL MATTERS

- Eat onions raw if you want to raise HDL cholesterol levels. The active compound is the one that gives onion its strong taste, so cooking onions to tastelessness destroys their effect on HDLs. Also, choose strong yellow and white onions; milder red onions without the bite are not as effective.
- Onions don't raise everyone's HDLs—there is little or no effect in one out of four persons. Allow two months of onion eating—at least a half a medium-size onion a day—for HDLs to rise substantially.
- For other heart-protective effects on the blood-clotting mechanism, both raw and cooked onions will work.

ORANGE

POSSIBLE THERAPEUTIC BENEFITS:

- Combats certain viruses
- Lowers blood cholesterol
- Fights arterial plaque
- Lowers the risk of certain cancers

FOLKLORE

"The orange is very beneficial in all bronchial and asthmatic conditions, states of emaciation, as a cardiac tonic and a stimulator of circulation. The daily use of an orange will aid in toning up the entire system, purify the blood, acting as an internal antiseptic, tonic stimulant and supportive agent."

FACTS

National Cancer Institute officials say that the year-round availability of citrus fruits is probably a major reason for the drop in stomach cancer in this country. One cancer-inhibiting agent in the fruit is vitamin C, known to counteract powerful carcinogens called nitrosamines. Further, oranges, along with other fruits, show up as foods most often eaten by those with low cancer rates. In one study, those who ate the most oranges compared with those who ate the least had about half the risk of cancer in general, and notably of the esophagus. In a recent Swedish study, citrus fruits, including oranges, ranked tops (along with carrots) as foods most favored by people with the lowest rates of pancreatic cancer.

Florida researchers also note that oranges and other citrus fruits have the power to lower blood cholesterol. Numerous findings show that pectin, a fiber in the skin and membranes of oranges (and grapefruit) can lower blood cholesterol in humans and test animals.

Scientists have also flirted with the notion that oranges, specifically orange juice, can combat viral infections. In an intriguing study, University of Florida investigators tested the therapeutic value of orange juice in humans exposed to the rubella (German measles) virus. After being infected with the virus through the nose, half the test subjects eliminated all citrus fruits from their diet as well as all vitamin supplements. The other half drank a daily liter of orange juice. The conclusion: Drinking orange juice did combat the rubella infection by lessening symptoms in the respiratory tract and accelerating the appearance of rubella-fighting antibodies in the blood. The researchers attributed the juice's therapeutic benefit to unknown natural antiviral constituents in addition to the vitamin C.

Other scientists have found that components of orange peels help kill bacteria and fungi and tend to lower blood cholesterol.

PRACTICAL MATTERS

- For maximum cholesterol-lowering and artery-protecting activity, be sure to eat the membranes and pulp of the oranges, which contains the pectin.

CONFLICTING EVIDENCE

In Canadian tests, orange juice bought at supermarkets did not display antiviral activity in test tubes.

PEA

POSSIBLE THERAPEUTIC BENEFITS:
- High in contraceptive agents
- Rich in compounds that prevent cancer in animals
- Prevents appendicitis
- Lowers blood cholesterol

FOLKLORE

In folk medicine the pea's greatest claim to fame is as an antifertility agent.

FACTS

Surprise! Plain old green peas, numerous studies show, do contain well-known antifertility agents.

Amazingly, in recent years much time, energy, and money have gone into trying to make pea chemicals into pharmaceutical contraceptives. "The population of Tibet has remained stationary for the last 200 years and the staple of the diet of the Tibetans consists of barley and peas." With that observation made in 1949, Indian scientist Dr. S. N. Sanyal of the Calcutta Bacteriological Institute undertook a lifelong mission based on his conviction that an over consumption of peas had accidentally curbed population growth in Tibet. His aim was to identify the contraceptive chemical in peas and turn it into an antifertility drug to be used in India and throughout the world. He very nearly succeeded.

The Indian government, in fact, for years had as one of its highest priorities the isolation of the pea's remarkable contraceptive secret. As far back as 1935, an Indian professor had noticed that both male and female laboratory rats which ate only "martar," or peas, were sterile. Fed peas as twenty percent of the diet, litters were reduced; at thirty percent they were nonexistent.

Dr. Sanyal managed to identify the antifertility pea chemical, m-xylohydroquinone. He synthesized it, concentrated it in capsules, and gave it to women; their pregnancy rate went down by fifty to sixty percent. When men took the antifertility pea capsule, their sperm count dropped by half. Somehow the pea compounds meddled with the reproductive hormones progesterone and estrogen. Dr. Sanyal's human trials "definitely established the oral contraceptive properties of P. sativum (pea) oil," agrees Dr. Norman Farnsworth of the University of Illinois and a leading expert on fertility-regulating drugs. But he notes, the pea chemicals never gained a place as a contraceptive because their performance could not match that of other pharmaceuticals, namely the Pill.

HEART-BLOOD FOOD

The pea, by virtue of its place in the legume family, is also good for the heart because it is rich in soluble fiber that stimulates the body to reduce its detrimental LDL cholesterol. Plain old canned peas rank right up there with kidney beans in this characteristic, containing 2.7 grams of soluble fiber per half cup. Both lentils and split peas are also exceptionally well endowed, with 1.7 grams of soluble fiber per half cup. This means that they also help control blood sugar (thus are excellent food for diabetics), and may lower blood pressure. An Egyptian study several years ago noted that injecting pea extracts into the veins of dogs caused a temporary decrease in blood pressure.

CANCER AND INFECTION FIGHTERS

Peas, being seeds, are also concentrated sources of protease inhibitors, thought to help squelch the activation of both certain viruses and chemical carcinogens in the intestine. Therefore, they may help prevent certain infections and cancers. Peas were linked in one study to slightly lower rates of prostate cancer.

Peas may also, for unknown reasons, ward off appendicitis, according to a 1986 survey in England and Wales. Researchers compared the appendicitis rates in fifty-nine areas over five years with dietary records from a national food survey and found a decided link between a few vegetables, including peas, and low rates of acute appendicitis. The researchers at the University of Southampton speculate that chemicals in the petite vegetable might suppress organisms in the appendicular wall that trigger the infection and consequent painful attack.

PRACTICAL MATTERS

- Surely, nobody should depend on peas to keep them from conceiving. On the other hand, both men and women who are having trouble with fertility may want to think twice about deliberately overconsuming peas, which unquestionably contain estrogenic chemicals considered by experts to have some contraceptive activity.

POTATO

• Contains chemicals that may block cancer

FOLKLORE

Oddly, potatoes are purported to be good for rheumatism. At one time women had special pockets in their dresses where they carried raw potatoes to ward off rheumatism. Raw potato juice and hot potato water applied to the painful area are supposed to relieve gout, rheumatism, lumbago, sprains, and bruises. Eating potatoes was once recommended by American physicians to purify the blood, cure dyspepsia, and aid digestion.

FACTS

Considering the potato's enormous popularity, scientific evidence on the nonnutritive pharmacology of this vegetable is incredibly skimpy.

ANTICANCER COMPOUNDS

The potato may have anticancer, antiviral potential although it rarely appears on lists of foods most preferred by those with low rates of cancer. White potatoes, especially when raw, have high concentrations of protease inhibitors, compounds known to neutralize certain viruses and carcinogens. In fact, investigators found recently that of several foods examined, the inhibitors extracted from the potato had the strongest antiviral powers. The potato chemicals stopped viruses even better than soybean inhibitors, considered one of the fiercest antiviral agents.

Potatoes, especially the skins, are rich in chlorogenic acid, a polyphenol, that prevents cell mutations leading to cancer. Tests in the early 1960s by investigators at Florida State University found potato skins had antioxidant activity, meaning that they could neutralize so-called "free radicals" that damage cells leading to numerous disorders, including cancer.

CAUTION

- Potatoes are high on the "glycemic index," meaning they raise insulin and blood sugar levels quickly, which could be detrimental to diabetics.

PRUNE

POSSIBLE THERAPEUTIC BENEFITS:
- Acts as a powerful laxative

> *How Much?* A mere half cup of prune juice a day produces a laxative effect in most people.

FOLKLORE

"Prunes are laxative and nutritious. . . . Imparting their laxative properties to boiling water, they serve as a pleasant and useful addition to purgative decoctions. Their pulp is used in the preparation of laxative confections. Too largely taken, they are apt to occasion flatulence, griping and indigestion." (*Dispensatory of the United States,* 1907.)

FACTS

Virtually everybody knows and always has known that prunes are an excellent laxative. Amazingly, though, the active laxative chemical in prunes has never been clearly identified. (Even though concentrated prune extract is sold over the counter as a laxative.) And scientists have spent much time searching for the active ingredient. Prunes are rich in soluble fiber, which may convey some laxative effect. Still, fiber is not the whole answer. Prune juice, practically devoid of fiber, is also a laxative.

A GOVERNMENT MATTER

In the 1950s and 1960s the United States Department of Agriculture's Western Regional Research Center devoted considerable manpower to cracking the mystery. Researchers fed countless pounds of Santa Clara California dried prunes to mice. The mice responded appropriately. There's no question, says Dr. Joseph Corse, one of the investigators, that "the laxative property of prune juice is real."

But the active agent remained elusive. After literally hundreds of experiments, the USDA's best guesses were a prune sugar or magnesium in prunes. Dr. M. Sidney Masri, USDA research biochemist who worked on the prune-mouse studies, is convinced the active ingredient is the mineral magnesium. If so, it works in an odd manner, proving once again that an isolated chemical is not the same as the food extract itself. Milk of magnesia (magnesium oxide) is a well-known laxative. But nuts also high in magnesium are not laxatives.

It proved puzzling. When USDA researchers yanked magnesium ammonium phosphate out of prunes, the fruit's laxative property dropped to almost zero. But when they fed the purified prune magnesium alone to mice, not much happened either. *It seems that the famous prune chemical works only when it is in the prunes.* Dr. Masri believes the magnesium is "chelated," or locked together, with other chemicals in prunes that potentiate the laxative effect. Peaches and apricots, high in magnesium, he says, also are mild laxatives for the same reason. He thinks prune chemicals work much the same way as epsom salt (magnesium sulfate) by squeezing water from the colon wall and dumping it into the intestinal tract, where it dilutes the contents. USDA gave up the studies in the late '60s, saying the search was not worth the time and money.

PRUNE POWER

The knowledge, though, can be a health and financial gold mine. Lest anyone doubt the power of prunes, consider the case of the Essex County Geriatric Center in Belleville, New Jersey. The center's head dietician, physician, and nutritionist conspired to take 300 elderly patients off laxatives; many were quite constipated and dependent on their daily laxative pills.

The staff started by adding about two thirds of an ounce of high-fiber bran to the morning oatmeal. It worked in sixty percent of the cases. For the remaining difficult cases, the team added up to a half cup of prune juice a day—mixing it with a little applesauce and/or bran buds.

One year later, ninety percent of the residents were off laxatives, preferring the dietary-imposed regularity. After initial complaints of gas and intestinal discomfort, they said they felt better—and there was a big cash bonus for the geriatric center: the pharmacy bills for laxatives fell by $44,000 the first year.

PRACTICAL MATTERS

- Infrequent prune eaters may at first experience a feeling of fullness, gas, and other gastrointestinal distress. But your intestinal tract usually adapts in a short time—within three weeks—and the discomfort ceases.
- Don't go overboard initially with a food laxative. Build up to it. Add a little extra each day, an ounce or so, until bowel movements are normal.

RICE

POSSIBLE THERAPEUTIC BENEFITS:
- Lowers blood pressure
- Fights diarrhea
- Prevents kidney stones
- Clears up psoriasis
- Contains chemicals that prevent cancer

FOLKLORE

"Rice forms a light and digestible food for those in whom there is any tendency to diarrhoea or dysentery. . . . A decoction of rice, commonly called rice-water, is recommended in the *Pharmacopoeia of India* as an excellent demulcent, refrigerant drink in febrile and inflammatory diseases, and in dysuria and similar affections. It may be acidulated with lime juice and sweetened with sugar."
— Maud Grieve: *A Modern Herbal,* 1931.

FACTS

Rice has a long history as a treatment for severe high blood pressure, kidney problems, and diabetes. More recent studies show that rice, especially when compared with another starch, potatoes, in non–insulin-dependent diabetics, clamps down on cholesterol synthesis and keeps blood insulin and glucose on an even keel.

Walter Kempner, M.D., of the Duke University Medical Center, pioneered the "rice diet" in the 1940s for the treatment of high blood pressure and kidney problems. And there is ample evidence that it works. However, the diet is made up for at least the first month entirely of unsalted rice and fruit. Dr. Kemper has always said he does not know what "the active principle is." It is unclear whether the rice has any physiological effects beyond crowding out other calories, restricting sodium, and inducing weight loss, all of which would be expected to lower blood pressure and take a burden off the kidneys. However, one screening of plants by Indian researchers did find rice to have specific blood-pressure-lowering capabilities.

Recently, participants on the rice diet to lose weight noticed a bonus side effect; psoriasis cleared up dramatically on the rice diet, even in cases where years of using systemic and local medications had failed.

ANTITUMOR SUBSTANCE

Rice, being a seed, contains high levels of protease inhibitors, believed to retard cancer. Further, rice bran, in animal experiments, did slash the risk of bowel cancer, but not nearly as much as wheat bran did. In 1981 Japanese scientists at Sapporo Breweries applied for patents for three antitumor substances isolated from rice bran. The rice compounds suppressed solid tumors in mice. An American professor compared the per capita consumption of various foods with certain diseases and found that eating the most rice (along with beans and sweet corn) was linked to the lowest rates of colon, breast, and prostate cancer.

DIARRHEA CURE

For centuries, boiled rice solutions were used to treat infant diarrhea. The first such advice was written in Sanskrit 3000 years ago. Only recently has the idea achieved worldwide scientific approval. For example, the International Centre for Diarrhoeal Disease Research in Bangladesh has trained mothers in villages to prepare rice-salt oral rehydration solutions to treat diarrhea. It calls for two handfuls of rice, one level teaspoon of salt, and one liter of water. Investigators report that the use of the rice solution reduces diarrhea, rehydrates, decreases stool volume, and appears to mothers to "cure" diarrhea.

KIDNEY STONE FIGHTER

If calcium kidney stones are a problem, consider this recent research. Eating rice bran, about one third of an ounce twice a day, according to Japanese investigators, is an excellent way to prevent such kidney stones. They tested rice bran on seventy patients along with a high calcium diet known to help form kidney stones. All the volunteers eating rice bran for a period of one month to three years had a significant decrease of calcium in their urine. And those who kept eating the small amounts of rice bran for one to three years clearly had fewer calcium-type kidney stones. Japanese researchers deemed the rice bran as effective as certain pharmaceuticals, but without the adverse effects. Apparently, phytic acid or phytates in the rice bran block the intestinal absorption of unwanted calcium so that it doesn't get into the urine to form stones. The patients had unusually high calcium levels in the urine to begin with, a condition known as hypercalciuria. Anyone wanting to absorb calcium for other health benefits should, of course, not eat large amounts of rice bran.

CONFLICTING EVIDENCE

One large-scale population study in Japan in 1981 found that those who ate the most rice (as well as pickled vegetables and dried salted fish) appeared to have a higher rate of stomach cancer.

SEAWEED, OR KELP*

POSSIBLE THERAPEUTIC BENEFITS:
- Kills bacteria
- Blocks cancer in animals
- Boosts immune system
- Heals ulcers
- Reduces blood cholesterol
- Lowers blood pressure
- Prevents strokes
- Thins the blood

FOLKLORE

"Kelp . . . is used in folk medicine to treat constipation, bronchitis, emphysema, asthma, indigestion, ulcers, colitis, gallstones, obesity, and disorders of the genitourinary and reproductive systems, both male and female. It is also claimed to 'clean' the bloodstream, strengthen resistance to disease, overcome rheumatism and arthritis, act as a tranquilizer, combat stress, and alleviate skin diseases, burns and insect bites." That's how Varro Tyler, Dean of the Schools of Phar-

*Kelp is an imprecise term applied generically to seaweed, but in modern-day parlance usually means brown seaweed, mainly of the Laminaria species.

macy, Nursing and Health Sciences at Purdue University, summed it up in his book *The Honest Herbal.* One thing he overlooked: In Egypt and China there is an ancient tradition of using seaweed, notably brown kelp, to treat cancer.

FACTS

Modern science confirms that seaweed is one of nature's all-around pharmaceutical miracles, full of chemicals that can accomplish everything from warding off and treating several types of cancer, lowering blood cholesterol and blood pressure, thinning the blood, preventing ulcers, killing bacteria, and even curing constipation.

ANTICANCER THESIS

In 1981 Jane Teas, at the Harvard School of Public Health, came up with an intriguing theory: Seaweed, eaten so frequently in Japan, might help explain why Japanese women have so little breast cancer. In Japan, the breast cancer rate is only one sixth that of the United States. Further, Japanese women who develop breast cancer live longer than American or British women with the disease. Seaweed is virtually absent in the American diet, ubiquitous in the Japanese. Laminaria, the long ribbonlike marine plant with ruffled fronds, is a Japanese staple eaten in salads and entrees, as a vegetable, and, most important, is the traditional seasoning in dashi, the fish-stock base for miso soup. It also flavors much Japanese food. Most Japanese eat miso soup at least twice a day. Laminaria kelp accounts for thirty-three percent of all the seaweed harvested in Japan.

Another provocative bit of evidence: In the rural areas of Japan, where seaweed consumption is increasing, breast cancer rates are lower than in urban areas, where seaweed eating is on the downswing.

Dr. Teas and her colleagues indeed discovered that feeding the brown seaweed Laminaria to rats and then giving them chemicals known to cause breast tumors partially immunized them against the malignancies. They had a thirteen percent lower cancer rate, compared with rats not pre-fed the kelp. Further, cancer in the kelp-fed animals took twice as long to appear. American Health Foundation researchers found more startling effects. The brown seaweed blocked fat-induced breast cancer in thirty percent of the animals involved. More amazing, previous Japanese experiments, in 1974, had found that Laminaria acted as not only an antidote to developing cancer but also as a chemotherapeutic agent to arrest its virulence. The kelp slowed the progression of cancer in ninety-five percent of test animals; six out of nine went into complete remission.

What is seaweed's secret: Dr. Teas notes that Laminaria contains many agents that might retard breast cancer, the most promising a chemical called fucoidan. Seaweeds, including the Laminaria, also are antibiotics, as proved both in the test tube and in animals. Thus, another possibility for fighting both breast and colon cancer: The kelp might selectively eliminate the bacteria in the colon that could produce cancer-causing substances—or affect the numbers of microorganisms in the intestine that produce hormones; hormones help control breast cancer.

AN ANTICANCER BONANZA

Numerous types of seaweed are promising cancer fighters. In a 1985 screening of edible brown seaweeds for anticancer activity, Japanese scientists, headed by Dr. Ichiro Yamamoto at the Kitasato University School of Hygienic Sciences in Kanagawa, found six species that inhibited colon cancer development in rats. Particularly potent were two species of Laminaria. The anticancer compound is fucoidan. A screening in 1986 by the same scientific team found that nine seaweeds out of eleven tested had antitumor activity. The Laminaria extracts when fed to mice were from seventy to eighty-four percent effective in suppressing intestinal cancers. They attribute the seaweed's potency to its ability to boost the animal's immune system, enabling it to better fight off cancer.

Another mouse-cancer study involved Undaria pinnantifida, called wakame, that black, stringy-looking dried stuff; rehydrated in water into long, deep-green satiny fronds, it is like a slick spinach with a mild flavor. Pharmacologists at the John A. Burns School of Medicine, University of Hawaii, in Honolulu, tested a popular health food in Japan called Viva-Natural, a dried version of wakame. Injected into mice, it helped both cure and prevent lung cancer. The scientists were especially struck by evidence that the seaweed substance enhanced immune cell activity, suggesting that the food substance carries out its antitumor work by activating the immune system.

KOMBU: A HYPOTENSIVE DRINK

According to Japan's folklore medicine, parts of the Laminaria and similar seaweeds are used as a blood-pressure-lowering drug in a preparation called kombu. One Japanese scientist confirmed that by giving people with essential hypertension a hot water drink with extract of the kelp, blood pressure went down significantly with no side effects. Others have isolated hypotensive (blood-pressure-reducing) chemicals, including histamine, from this seaweed.

In 1986 scientists also discovered that powdered brown seaweed fiber might help prevent strokes. Stroke-prone rats with high blood pressure were overfed salt; but simultaneously feeding of seaweed powder markedly reduced the incidence of strokes. In fact, all of the non–seaweed-eating rats succumbed to stroke; none of those eating seaweed did. Thus, seaweed appeared to act as an antidote to excess sodium consumption.

Seaweed, including Laminaria, reduces the blood cholesterol of rats. Researchers speculated that agents in the kelp somehow remove cholesterol from the intestine.

NORI AGAINST ULCERS

Japanese scientists have also tested an antiulcer substance from several kinds of marine algae gathered from the seaside of Japan. A definite antiulcer substance was found in porphyra ("nori" to the Japanese). The substance also had antimicrobial activity against a long list of human disease-causing bacteria, including E. coli, Pseudomonas aeruginosa, Salmonella, Staphylococcus, Aspergillus, Fusarium, and Shigella.

Some seaweed is a blood thinner. Many Japanese reports show that "brown algal-suflated polysaccharides" have anticoagulant activity similar to heparin, a popular pharmaceutical anticoagulant. One assumption is that the substances clear the blood of fatty substances the same way heparin does. For example, if you inject heparin after a fatty meal, it accelerates the disappearance of visible fats, reducing bad LDL cholesterol and raising good HDL type.'

As an experiment, scientists harvested wakame from the Shimoda Bay in Shizuoka-ken, Japan. It has been used as a typical algal marine food since ancient times. One chemical from wakame was compared with heparin in a test on rats. The wakame substance was twice as powerful as heparin in antithrombin (clot-dissolving) activity.

CONFLICTING EVIDENCE

Dr. B. S. Reddy at the American Health Foundation in New York City found that brown seaweed increased the risk of colon cancer in rodents. Carrageenin, a food additive from seaweed used often as a thickener in the United States, has also produced cancers in certain laboratory animals.

SHELLFISH

POSSIBLE THERAPEUTIC BENEFITS:
- Good food for the heart and brain
- Lowers blood cholesterol
- Slashes triglycerides
- Stimulates brain chemicals, boosting mental energy

> *How Much?* Three to four ounces of shellfish meat generally delivers enough mentally energizing chemicals to make you feel up and promote "brain power." The same amount is good for your cardiovascular system.

FOLKLORE

For centuries, oysters have been hailed as an aphrodisiac.

FACTS

You've no doubt heard that shellfish—especially oysters, clams, and crabs—are hazardous to your cardiovascular system because they elevate blood cholesterol. Banish the thought. The astounding truth is just the opposite. Far from being villains in cardiovascular disease, such shellfish actually protect arteries and blood vessels by substantially lowering bad-type blood cholesterol. They also carry high concentrations of the fabulous omega-3 fatty acids that help prevent dangerous thrombi (blood clots) in blood vessels, do other marvelous heart-protective things, and may be beneficial for a long list of diseases, including rheumatoid arthritis, asthma, allergies, headaches, psoriasis, and cancer.

Forbidding or restricting shellfish in the belief it is a heart hazard is a terrible mistake, according to Marian Childs, Ph.D., an expert in fat metabolism in the Department of Medicine, University of Washington.

Dr. Childs, too, once worried, because she and her husband love oysters. So she tested them, along with clams, crabs, shrimp, and squid. For three weeks, twice a day, male volunteers sequentially ate each of the marine creatures as a substitute for their regular sources of protein—meat, eggs, milk, and cheese. Oysters, she was delighted to find, "are just great for you. More people should eat them." Oysters, crabs, and clams lowered blood cholesterol by about nine percent. Clams also depressed triglycerides by a whopping sixty-one percent, oysters by fifty-one percent, and crabs by twenty-three percent. Neither shrimp nor squid lowered blood cholesterol, but contrary to fears, neither did they *elevate* it. "Shrimp and squid were no better or worse for blood cholesterol than eggs or meat," she says.

BAD RAP

Shellfish got its villainous reputation because it contains certain sterols that in outdated analyses were mistaken for cholesterol. Indeed, only thirty to forty percent of the sterols actually turned out to be cholesterol. And ironically, these "noncholesterol sterols" appear to be helpful, not harmful. In another test Dr. Childs and her colleagues documented that the marine sterols *blocked* cholesterol absorption. Men with normal cholesterol ate a mixture of oysters and clams or crab or chicken for three weeks. At one point they were given a dose of radioactive-tagged cholesterol which could be traced in the body. The men eating the chicken or crab absorbed about fifty-five percent of the cholesterol; the oyster-clam eaters absorbed only forty-two percent, about one fourth less. Dr. Childs says the cholesterol-lowering drug cholestyramine works on the same principle.

Even better news: The oyster-clam eaters' ratio of HDL-2 to HDL-3 cholesterol improved, a sign of heart health. Dr. Childs says new evidence shows that higher levels of blood HDL-2 in proportion to HDL-3 is *the strongest known protector against coronary heart disease*. And oysters and clams definitely boosted the beneficial ratio.

As for cholesterol content, up-to-date analyses by Dr. Childs and others find that oysters, mussels, clams, and scallops are quite low in cholesterol. Crab and shrimp have slightly more, although still modest amounts. Squid is rich in cholesterol.

BRAIN FOOD

It so happens that shellfish, along with other seafood, true to tradition, does stimulate mental energy. Dr. Judith Wurtman, a leading researcher on the subject at MIT, says that shellfish (and fish) most quickly boost your mood and mental performance. The reason: Shellfish, low in fat and carbohydrate, and almost pure protein, delivers large supplies of an amino acid called tyrosine to the brain, which then makes it into the two mentally energizing brain chemicals dopamine and norepinephrine.

Extensive research with both animals and humans proves that when the brain produces the neurotransmitters dopamine and norepinephrine, mood and energy pick up. You tend to think and react more quickly, be more attentive, motivated, and mentally energetic. As Dr. Wurtman puts it, when you're "on a mental roll, when everything just sort of clicks into place in your mind. . . . It's the dopamine and norepinephrine at work in your brain."

MIT tests also have measured fairly accurately how much protein food it takes to supply the amino acids needed to rev up the brain. For most people it is three to four ounces. Shellfish is one of the highest pure protein foods in existence.

PRACTICAL MATTERS

- Deep-frying shellfish can undo their benefits by adding sufficient fat to push up blood cholesterol. Best for the arteries are baked, broiled, steamed, and stewed shellfish.
- Eating shellfish and other high protein, low fat and low carbohydrate foods, either alone or with carbohydrates such as bread or potatoes, creates energy-boosting chemicals in the brain. But for the quickest upsurge in alertness, eat shellfish *alone*. That sends a burst of tyrosine to the brain.

- However, eating *more* than the regular dose of three or four ounces at one time will not boost mental energy further. The tyrosine works to create the alertness chemicals only when they are needed, that is, when the brain is already using them up. Shellfish will do a lot to keep your brain functioning at top level, but it cannot take it past its capabilities.

SOYBEAN

POSSIBLE THERAPEUTIC BENEFITS:

- Excellent cardiovascular medicine
- Lowers blood cholesterol
- Prevents and/or dissolves gallstones
- Reduces triglycerides
- Regulates the bowels
- Relieves constipation
- Regulates blood sugar
- Lowers cancer risk
- Replaces estrogen
- Promotes contraception

> *How Much?* One bowl of miso (soybean paste) soup a day slashes the risk of stomach cancer among Japanese by thirty percent. Eating soybean foods of any type six times a week can reduce abnormally high blood cholesterol by twenty percent.

FACTS

Soybeans promote health in numerous ways. It's a food meat eaters especially should get into their diets. Making it a point to eat soybean products somewhat regularly can dramatically improve blood profiles of those with extra-high blood cholesterol, and maybe even help reverse some damage already done to arteries. There's also evidence soybeans help regulate insulin levels, blood sugar, bowel functions, and prevent certain cancers, notably of the stomach.

HEART FOOD

Italian scientists at the Center for the Study of Hyperlipidemias of the University of Milan started studying the powers of the soybean in 1972. They found consistently that soybeans did wonders for people with genetically high, familial-type cholesterol counts, usually over 300. Eating soybeans instead of meat and dairy products for protein sent their destructive LDL cholesterol down by fifteen to twenty percent. It worked in children also.

The soybean diet even counteracted the effects of a high fat diet. When the investigators, headed by C. R. Sirtori, M.D., added 500 milligrams of cholesterol (the amount in a couple of eggs), to the diet, soybeans apparently overcame the eggs' cholesterol-raising potential and still kept blood cholesterol down. Remarkably, once blood cholesterol was down, the patients went back to their regular meat diets but ate at least six meals in a week using textured soybean protein; their cholesterol still remained low during the two years of the experiment.

Further, Dr. Sirtori contends the soybean diet after a while raised the good HDL cholesterol, and not only halted the progression of arterial heart disease but *reversed* it to an extent. One woman, after three years on the soybean diet, notes Dr. Sirtori, saw her blood cholesterol go down from 332 to 206 milligrams per deciliter, her triglycerides drop from 68 to 59 milligrams per deciliter, and the blood flow in her heart improve as documented by electrocardiograms.

Soybeans seem to work best in those with genetically controlled extra high blood cholesterol, and less so on those with borderline or normal blood profiles. However, mixing soybean fiber into an already low fat, high carbohydrate–high fiber diet can provide a substantial therapeutic bonus. In a 1985 study, Andrew P. Goldberg of Washington University gave soy fiber cookies to volunteers who were already on a cholesterol-lowering low fat diet. The soy cookies depressed their blood cholesterol further. The soy also helped correct impaired glucose tolerance and kept insulin levels down, causing the author to recommend soy fiber especially for diabetics.

For keeping blood sugar under control, you can't beat soybeans. They were second only to peanuts in a long list of foods that promote a desirable flat blood sugar response as compiled by expert Dr. David Jenkins of the University of Toronto. Beans in general are great blood sugar regulators, but soybeans were best of all legumes on Dr. Jenkins's "glycemic index."

VEGETARIAN ARTERIES

At Philadelphia's Wistar Institute, eminent investigators David Klurfeld and David Kritchevsky found that it is probably not necessary to adopt a complete vegetarian diet to rejuvenate your arteries strikingly. They found that just adding soybeans to an ordinary meat diet gave rabbits the arteries of vegetarians. First, rabbits ate all their protein from soybeans and none from meat; their blood cholesterol and their rate of atherosclerosis dropped fifty percent. But, more important, when the researchers fed the animals one half of their protein in soybeans and one half in meat or dairy products, the blood cholesterol and athero-sclerosis still went down fifty percent!

That indicates, says Dr. Klurfeld, that eating half your protein in soybean-based foods could revitalize your arteries, making them less vulnerable to heart disease and stroke. Instead of eating meat and cheese, make it tofu, soy milk, tempeh, or plain cooked soybeans.

STONE BREAKERS

Soybeans may also guard against gallstones. Drs. Klurfeld and Kritchevsky fed hamsters a diet containing either soy protein or casein, a dairy protein. Fully fifty-eight percent of the animals eating casein had gall-stones compared with only fourteen percent eating soy protein. Moreover, in a follow-up experiment, one third of the casein eaters were sacrificed after forty days; half had gallstones. Of the remaining two thirds, the investigators switched half to soy protein. It turned out that fifty-eight percent of the group kept full-time on casein had gallstones, compared with only thirty-two percent switched to the soybean diet. That meant the soy somehow reversed the gallstones— perhaps somehow dissolved them!

ANTICANCER SOUP

Japanese surveys searching for clues about which foods protect against cancers found that one apparently is miso, or soybean-paste soup. Both Japanese men and women who ate one bowl of miso a day had a one third lower risk of stomach cancer than those who never ate it. Even downing the soybean-based soup occasionally cut the stomach cancer risk among men by seventeen percent and among women by nineteen percent.

Like other legumes, soybeans are high in anticancer protease inhibitors. Rats were exposed to enough X rays to give them breast cancer. After the cancer dose, some were given soybeans and some were not. Only forty-four percent of the soybean-eating animals developed the expected cancer compared with seventy-four percent who did not get soybeans.

GOOD FOR REGULARITY

Legumes of all types are excellent in promoting healthy colons and bowel function. Soybeans, too, tend to produce softer, bulkier stools, which scientists regard favorably as protective against constipation, diverticular disease, hemorrhoids, other bowel dysfunctions, and possibly colon cancer.

A CONTRACEPTIVE PILL?

Soybeans, like peas and other legumes, are rich in natural estrogens (female hormones) and conceivably could inhibit fertility or help replace estrogen in postmenopausal women. As a test, physicians at Harvard and Duke, funded by the National Institutes of Health, are giving low daily doses of soybeans to a group of postmenopausal women to see whether their hormone levels go up.

Suspicions that natural hormones in soybeans might act as contraceptives were aroused by a study of exotic cats in the Cincinnati Zoo. Such animals are often infertile. Searching for reasons, researchers discovered that standard cat chow at the zoo was about half soybean products, loaded with plant estrogens. When the soybeans were replaced with chicken, the cats displayed signs of increased fertility and other hormone-related activity.

Although excessive estrogen has been linked to higher rates of human breast and edometrial cancer, the effect of eating legumes is unknown. One researcher notes that prolonged weak doses of food estrogens may, in fact, function as antiestrogens, helping block the ill effects of an estrogen overload that might promote breast cancer. The theory: low doses of food estrogens might desensitize breast tissue to the ravages of too much estrogen—sort of the same way tiny doses of allergens in allergy shots desensitize a person to allergic reactions. Thus, eating soybeans might be one reason for the lower breast cancer rates in vegetarian women, he says.

Although the facts are not yet in, the science establishment now recognizes that hormones in soybeans and about 300 other plants may have a profound biological impact and have set out to discover what it is.

PRACTICAL MATTERS

• Don't forget these soybean products: soy oil, soy flour, soy powder, soy milk (from cooked soybeans), soy grits, soy nuts (roasted beans), tofu (curdled soy milk), tempeh (fermented soybeans), soybean sprouts, textured vegetable protein (TVP), and soybean flakes used as a meat extender or substitute in numerous products, including imitation bacon, sausage, franks, and patties.

SPINACH

POSSIBLE THERAPEUTIC BENEFITS:
- Lowers risk of cancer
- Reduces blood cholesterol in animals

> *How Much?* Eating only a half cup of spinach a day, according to population surveys, may cut the risk of cancer, especially of the lung, nearly in half.

FOLKLORE

Spinach has been called the "king of vegetables," and "therapeutically indicated in all conditions of anemia, blood depravity, heart disturbances, kidney derangements, dyspeptic conditions and piles, and in all conditions of low vitality and marked general debility," according to a 1927 article in *American Medicine*.

FACTS

As a potential cancer-preventer, much research shows, spinach is certainly one of the international kings of vegetables. Former smokers particularly should pay attention to spinach. As a dark-green leafy vegetable, spinach tops the lists of foods—along with carrots—eaten more often by people worldwide with lower rates of all types of cancer, and specifically colon, rectal, esophageal, stomach, prostate, laryngeal, pharyngeal, endometrial, cervical, and in particular lung. Studies find consistently that people who eat the least dark-green vegetables high in compounds called carotenoids, of which spinach is one of the richest, have about double the risk of lung cancer. The studies also find that people eating a serving of spinachlike vegetables a day, even former smokers, are much less apt to develop lung cancer.

Fully ten of eleven international surveys on lung cancer bear this out. One, by Dr. Richard Shekelle, an epidemiologist at the University of Texas, found that carotene foods could help rescue smokers; those eating the least high carotene foods had eight times the chance of developing lung cancer as smokers who ate the most. Further, individuals with the highest blood levels of beta carotene are least likely to develop lung cancer, according to one analysis by Johns Hopkins University researchers. Apparently, former smokers especially can neutralize some of the damage to lung cells—blocking promotion or progression of cancer—by eating spinachlike foods.

WHY SPINACH HAS IT ALL

Spinach is hailed by scientists as a promising lung cancer antidote mainly because of its extremely high concentration of carotenoids, including beta carotene, shown in lab tests to squelch the promotion of certain cancers. A new United States Department of Agriculture analysis finds that raw spinach has thirty-six milligrams of total carotenoids per hundred grams, whereas raw carrots have fourteen milligrams per hundred grams, most of it in beta carotene. Although *beta* carotene is a confirmed cancer antagonist, spinach's panoply of other carotenoids may possess anticancer activity, and may be even more responsible than beta carotene for spinach's splendid showing in population surveys of cancer-preventive foods.

Spinach is also blessed with high amounts of chlorophyll, another potential cancer blocker. Some credit its abundance of chlorophyll for its powers to block mutations, the first steps to cancer formation. In test tubes, Italian scientists recently found spinach spectacular at blocking the formation of one of the most powerful carcinogens known, nitrosamines. Of five foods tested (carrot, cauliflower, lettuce, and strawberry were the others) spinach juice was by far the most potent.

Japanese scientists discovered in 1969 that spinach lowers blood cholesterol in laboratory animals. Follow-up studies found the leaf worked by accelerating conversion of cholesterol in the body to coprostanol, which was then washed away.

SQUASH
(INCLUDING PUMPKIN)

POSSIBLE THERAPEUTIC BENEFIT:
- Lowers risk of cancer, especially of the lung

> *How Much?* An extra half cup of squash or pumpkin a day
> may lower the risk of lung cancer by half.

FOLKLORE

Ignoring any medicinal qualities of the pulp, most practitioners prescribed the seeds of both squash and pumpkin for a variety of ailments.
Ethiopians chew the seeds as laxatives and purgatives. Common around
the world is the use of squash and pumpkin seeds to expel worms,
including tapeworms.

FACTS

Both the seeds and the pulp have pharmacological promise, both to
prevent cancer. A few years ago in Poland and at the National Institutes of Health, researchers discovered chemicals in squash seeds that
may inhibit cancer processes. They are a new squash inhibitor family of
protease trypsin inhibitors that keep both viruses and cancer-causing
chemicals from becoming activated in the intestinal tract.

More important, pumpkin and squash, notably the deep-orange winter types like Hubbards and butternuts, are full of anti-cancer carotenoids, including beta carotene.

The secret, think most scientists, is that the carotenes are antioxidants that do battle against oxygen-free radicals, rendering them harmless. Thus, these orange vegetables may help save you from all kinds of ravages due to cancer and other chronic diseases as well as from aging. On the rampage, the oxygen-free radicals can destroy blood vessel walls, accelerate aging, aggravate inflammation, and latch on to parts of cells such as DNA, causing cell alterations leading to cancer.

BROAD CANCER ANTIDOTE

Deep-orange squash appears to be a multiple-cancer preventer; as a yellow vegetable it appears in worldwide population (epidemiological) surveys to lower the risk of lung, esophageal, stomach, bladder, laryngeal, and prostate cancers, and among a group of American elderly, of deaths from all kinds of cancer.

Yellow squash was one of a triumvirate of vegetables (the others were carrots and sweet potatoes) most protective against lung cancer in a group of New Jersey men, many of whom had smoked for many years, according to a National Cancer Institute study. Those who ate the least of these vegetables had nearly double the chances of getting lung cancer. The difference in men with the highest and lowest risk was little over a half cup of squash, carrots, or sweet potatoes every day. That means men with the lowest risk ate a mere two and a half servings of any type vegetable daily.

Carrots and the other deep orange vegetables, squash and pumpkin, appear to slow down the cancer-promotion process that can continue for years in damaged cells. Nonsmokers exposed to passive smoke seem to be protected from lung cancer also by eating such vegetables.

ADVICE

Everybody, but in particular smokers, former smokers, and people who are around smokers, should make it a point to eat more deep-orange vegetables like winter squash and pumpkin.

STRAWBERRY

POSSIBLE THERAPEUTIC BENEFITS:
- Destroys viruses
- Linked to lower cancer deaths

FOLKLORE

In early pharmacopoeias, strawberries were used as a mild laxative, diuretic, and astringent. Linnaeus, according to Maud Grieve in her 1931 *A Modern Herbal*, was the first to discover and prove the efficacy of the berries as a cure for rheumatic gout. In Western folk medicine, the strawberry has been hailed as a medicant for the skin, particularly acne, ringworm, and chronic ulcerations. Grieve suggests: "A cut strawberry rubbed over the face immediately after washing will whiten the skin and remove slight sunburn."

FACTS

Modern science has paid little attention to the strawberry, thus the extent of its powers are unknown. This much is certain, however: Strawberries, as well as other fruits, when mashed up and liquified, were quite potent in disabling a number of different disease-producing viruses growing in test tubes, according to Canadian studies. The fruit destroyed the poliovirus, echovirus, reovirus, coxsackievirus, and herpes simplex virus—all common infectious agents. The greater the concentration of the fruit, the greater the potency.

Experts believe strawberries also benefit the cardiovascular system and may prevent cancer. The red berries are extra high in that super fiber pectin, found to substantially reduce blood cholesterol in a slew of animal and human studies. Italian investigators recently noted that strawberries can block the formation of one of the most potent of all cancer-causing agents, nitrosamines, which can form in the intestinal tract when the chemicals nitrite and amines react with each other. The berries are quite rich in certain polyphenols that combat cancer and are also antioxidants.

And in a cancer research first, strawberries capped a list of eight foods most linked to lower rates of cancer deaths among a group of 1271 elderly Americans in New Jersey. Those eating the most strawberries were three times less likely to develop cancer than those eating few or no strawberries.

SUGAR

In times of stress, sweeten the tea.
—Chinese proverb

POSSIBLE THERAPEUTIC BENEFITS:
- Acts as a tranquilizer
- Relieves anxiety and stress
- Induces relaxation and sleep
- Boosts concentration in some persons
- Acts as an antidepressant
- Kills bacteria
- Heals wounds

How Much? About two and a half tablespoons of white sugar, a two-ounce chocolate bar, or two ounces of gumdrops (all about thirty grams of pure carbohydrate) usually are enough to relieve mental anxiety and stress and induce relaxation and drowsiness.

FACTS

Only the ancients seemed to get the story about sugar and sweets straight. While most people think of sugar as giving an energy boost, and even producing hyperactivity in children, it generally has the opposite effect; it acts as a tranquilizer on most nervous systems, calming you down, increasing your concentration, and making you drowsy. It also does a whale of a lot in healing wounds, just as honey does.

SUGAR ON THE BRAIN

The mythology is that eating candy pumps sugar into your blood, giving you more energy. The truth is how much sugar you have in your blood has virtually nothing to do with your mood or energy. That's what hundreds of experiments done at MIT find. How you feel mentally is a matter not of blood sugar levels but of brain chemistry. And eating sugary foods sets off a process of physiological changes, generating a brain chemical that tranquilizes, not energizes.

Eating sugar or other carbohydrates forces up insulin in the blood, triggering a greater ratio of a chemical called tryptophan; tryptophan rushes to the brain, where it produces serotonin—a neurotransmitter known as "the calming chemical." And the more tryptophan available to the brain, the more serotonin it can make. "As a result, you will feel less stressed, less anxious, more focused and relaxed," says Dr. Judith Wurtman, a leading MIT researcher on the subject.

The right sugar dose, she says, is rather precise. To feel more tranquil, most people need about thirty grams of pure carbohydrate, which translates to about two and a half tablespoons of sugar or two ounces of candy. People overweight by twenty percent need slightly more—about another third to half more. Tests show that eating more than the minimum dose does not relieve stress or promote sleep any faster or better. What counts in raising serotonin levels are the first few bites of sugar.

In some persons, sugar acts as an antidepressant drug. Experts have found that people with less sugar-induced serotonin in the brain tend to be depressed and even to commit suicide. Dr. Norman Rosenthal at the National Institute of Mental Health has studied a particular group of people who suffer from a type of depression called SAD (seasonal affective disorder), apparently brought on by the decrease in daylight during winter months. Dr. Rosenthal thinks the light deprivation lowers serotonin levels in the brains of those susceptible to this disorder. In attempts, he says, to boost serotonin and fend off depression, many sufferers load up on carbohydrates during the dark days "as a form of self-medication."

Indeed, Dr. Wurtman points out that the sugar's mechanism seems similar to that of antidepressant drugs. "Maybe carbohydrates amplify serotonergic neurotransmission, just like most antidepressant drugs," she notes. In some populations, suicide rates go down as the carbohydrate consumption goes up. And autopsies on suicides often reveal lower levels of serotonin in their brains.

Contrary to popular belief, there is no substantial evidence that sugar causes hyperactivity or other untoward behaviors in children, according to carefully conducted studies by National Institutes of Health researchers. Just the opposite: The sweet stuff is more likely to sedate youngsters. Nor is there any credibility to the notion that sugary foods cause criminal behavior.

EXCEPTION–CARBOHYDRATE CRAVERS

Certain people—Dr. Wurtman counts herself as one—however, are born with brain chemistry that causes them to have an opposite reaction to sugar; sugar and other carbohydrates do not make them sleepy, but more focused, concentrated, and alert. These so-called "carbohydrate cravers," according to Dr. Wurtman, often feel low in energy, restless, and bored right before a "carbohydrate attack." After eating sugar or other carbohydrates they feel less distracted, better able to concentrate, and calmer. Furthermore, when given a drug that increases serotonin in the brain, their cravings for carbohydrates drop dramatically, proving that for some reason they lack the brain chemical.

SWEET WOUNDS

Like honey, sugar is a formidable wound-healing substance. Dr. Richard A. Knutson, a surgeon at the Delta Medical Center in Greenville, Mississippi, has applied sugar to burns, ulcers, lacerations, gunshot wounds, open fractures, and amputations on 3000 patients with "a near-perfect success rate." In many cases sugar worked when antibiotics failed, he says, and was especially effective on burns. At first he feared sugar might encourage bacterial growth, but just the opposite: sugar quickly squelched infections.

Sugar is commonly used in modern medicine to hasten wound healing—in Great Britain, Israel, Germany, and notably in Argentina. A team led by Dr. Leon Herszage in Buenos Aires used white sugar on the wounds of 120 patients when conventional treatment had failed. The success rate was ninety-nine percent.

To make sugar stick to the wounds, Dr. Knutson mixes roughly four parts of white table sugar with one part Betadine ointment, an iodine-based salve available at most pharmacies, into a peanut-butter-like consistency.

PRACTICAL MATTERS

Some tips from Dr. Wurtman:

- To get the best calming effect, take your carbohydrate straight—without protein and with as little fat as possible. Protein and fat slow down or block the process of getting serotonin into the brain.
- The sugar in fruit does not work in creating calming brain chemicals.
- Some people feel mental relief within five minutes. In general, it takes about twenty minutes for the food to be digested and the effects dispersed in the brain. Some people, however, don't feel an effect for an hour. If you're one, try drinking caffeine-free soft drinks containing sugar, or herb tea with two tablespoons of sugar, or a cup of instant cocoa made with water.
- For help with insomnia, try "one to one and a half ounces of a sweet or starch at bedtime." For most people this is "as effective as a sleeping pill, but without the side effect of morning grogginess and the potential for abuse inherent in sleep drugs," says Dr. Wurtman.

CAUTIONS

- Sugar, except for supplying calories, energy, has no nutritional value. Eating sugary foods in excess can promote weight gain, but worse, especially in children, can *replace* nutritious foods with junk foods, depriving the body of critical nutrients.
- Sugar definitely promotes cavities.
- Sugar can cause sharp spikes in insulin and blood glucose, although pure sucrose, or table sugar, ranks below certain vegetables, such as potatoes, carrots, and rice, in its ability to induce quick increases in blood sugar.
- Don't use sugar on wounds as a substitute for proper medical care. Adding sugar before bleeding has stopped or the wound cleansed could be dangerous.

SOME SUGAR MYTHS

Sugar has been cleared of these indictments. Sugar does not:

> induce hyperactivity in children
> lead to criminal behavior

cause diabetes
cause heart disease
cause acne
cause obesity. Although sugar contributes, fatty foods—often sweetened fatty foods—are the main culprit.

TEA

- Reduces cavities
- Destroys bacteria and viruses
- Fights infections
- Contains chemicals that prevent cancer in animals
- Lowers blood pressure
- Strengthens capillaries
- Retards atherosclerosis (hardening of the arteries)
- Acts as a mild sedative (decaffeinated)

FOLKLORE

Ah, the glories of tea. Plain old green and black tea has been used as a medicine in China for 4000 years. To the ancient Greeks, tea was the "divine leaf," notably good for asthma, colds, and bronchitis (hence the word theophylline, a modern bronchodilating drug derived from tea). Louis XIV's physician prescribed tea to curtail royal headaches. Nineteenth-century Russian scientists called tea "the elixir of life," capable of bestowing a parcel of benefits on "the digestion, nervous system and blood vessels, cardiovascular function, blood pressure, and the vital energy of man."

FACTS

It may seem faintly preposterous to take tea seriously as a health potion: it's so common, so ordinary, so cheap. How can a few black or green specks of a plant leaf (or root) dipped in hot water metamorphose into a health concoction of genius, as trumpeted throughout antiquity and now under scrutiny in laboratories worldwide? But scientists who investigate tea, not only exotic teas like ginseng, but the common green and black teas from India and China, the world's most popular beverage, confirm that it has formidable health powers unrecognized by most who consume it. Small wonder tea has been the number one beverage in most of the world for centuries. Tea contains various chemicals that can keep bacteria and viruses at bay, neutralize cancer-causing agents, lower blood pressure and blood cholesterol, constrict and protect blood vessels, and calm the mood. In the land of science, tea is a most serious subject.

ANTIVIRAL AGENT

Undeniably, tea, presumably because of its tannins—they give tea its astringent taste—is antibacterial and antiviral. In the 1940s, American scientists discovered that tannin controlled an influenza virus. Indian scientists recently noted that both brewed tea and its tannin "markedly inhibited" the herpes simplex virus, but only tea itself stopped a poliovirus. In Canadian test-tube experiments, tea was a potent inactivator of a number of disease-causing viruses.

A brew of green tea is commonly used in the Soviet Union to treat infections, especially dysentery. Soviet physicians also report successfully giving green tea to treat chronic viral hepatitis.

ANTICAVITY MOUTHWASH

Tea, primarily because of both its tannins and high fluoride, is a potent cavity antagonist. The idea that common tea prevents tooth decay has been around for a while, according to Dr. Shelby Kashket, a senior scientist at the Forsyth Dental Center in Boston. Japanese studies find that children drinking tea from leaves richest in fluoride have the fewest cavities. The Japanese have also developed a tannin-based toothpaste.

Compelling evidence of tea's anticavity powers come from studies done with animals. Taiwan researchers sloshed tea around in the mouths of rats and found that the "caries activity" dropped by one half to three fourths. In 1983 scientists at Ohio State University and Washington University School of Dentistry inoculated rats with cavity-producing bacteria, fed them sugar, and set out cups of four different kinds of tea made from tea leaves—Chinese green teas and Indian black teas—which the rats drank at will for five weeks. At the end of the experiment the tea-drinking rats had stained teeth but much less tooth decay than rats that drank plain water. One type of tea (Young Hyson) slashed the cavity scores in half.

Forsyth researchers have found that of several anticavity foods tested, including coffee and fruit juices, tea is by far the most protective—in this case, plain old Lipton and Salada tea bags dipped in a cup of hot water for three minutes. In tests, tea blocked ninety-five percent of the interaction between sugar and bacteria that produces the sticky stuff called dextran that attaches to the teeth and leads to cavities.

CANCER BLOCKER

Tea has rising credibility among scientists as a cancer fighter. The same tea tannins that destroy viruses and bacteria can block certain cancers. In a Japanese government search for natural cancer antidotes, tea consistently comes out tops, namely Oriental green tea. In 1985, several prominent scientists from Japan's National Institute of Genetics proclaimed "epigallo-catechin-gallate," the most common type tannin in Japanese green tea, to be a strong antimutagen and thus an antagonist to cancer. Of several hundred plants screened by the Japanese as part of a large-scale program to identify "antimutagens," the Japanese green tea (Camellia sinensis) was the most potent in laboratory tests. But-tressing their finding, said the scientists, is the fact that the tea chemical also suppressed sarcoma tumors in mice, and that habitual green-tea drinkers have dramatically lower rates of stomach cancer in Japan.

Canadian investigators at the British Columbia Cancer Research Center also document that tea counteracts the formation of nitrosa-mines, a family of powerful carcinogens that in test animals cause every type of cancer. Constituents in tea, including tannin, suppressed the nitrosamines even better than did ascorbic acid (vitamin C), commonly used for that purpose. Small amounts of brewed tea itself from Japan, China, and Ceylon in tests also countered the cancer-causing agent.

Dr. Hans Stich, head of the Center's Environmental Carcinogenesis Unit, says: "Tea—and coffee—are loaded with phenolic acids, which are anticarcinogens and antioxidants." In one study Dr. Stich found that ordinary doses of tea counteracted cancer-causing agents in a salt-preserved fermented Chinese fish called pak wik, considered largely responsible for high rates of nasal cancer in Hong Kong, South China, the Philippines, and Indonesia.

So, drinking tea might counteract the cancer?

"Right. This we have shown in animal studies and tissue cultures." Strikingly, even in humans, both tea and coffee blocked formation of a nitrosamine. Dr. Stich is so persuaded of the cancer-antagonizing properties of tea that he is using catechin capsules, extracted from tea leaves, to try to block oral cancer in snuff users and tobacco chewers in various parts of the world.

Further Russian, Indian, and Japanese tests show that tea may protect against long-term damage from radiation. Tea catechins, Japanese scientists claimed, usher strontium 90 out of the body before it can settle in bone marrow.

CARDIOVASCULAR DISEASES

Several cultures do not blush at prescribing tea for heart disease. Russian scientists, after prolific studies on patients, praise tea's ability, mainly because of its catechins, to delay atherosclerosis, strengthen capillaries, thin the blood, lower blood pressure, and "exert a favorable regulatory effect on every vital component of human metabolism." For example, Mikhail A. Bokuchava, at the Bakh Institute of Biochemistry in Moscow, reported that tea in Russian patients has been shown to relieve high blood pressure, headaches, prevent thrombosis, and strengthen blood vessels. He called tea catechins "superior to every known capillary-strengthening drug."

Indeed, other evidence substantiates tea's cardiovascular protection. In the late 1960s, scientists at the University of California's Lawrence Livermore Labs measured the degree of artherosclerosis in the coronary arteries and cerebral arteries of about 300 Caucasian coffee drinkers and 100 Chinese tea drinkers collected at autopsy over fourteen years. Tea drinkers had only two thirds as much heart artery damage and one third as much brain artery damage as coffee drinkers. As a test, researchers then gave rabbits a high fat diet and various beverages. Those drinking tea had the least-diseased aortas—much less than rabbits drinking plain water. "It is evident tea seems to protect the aorta from forming atheroma [plaques]," concluded the investigators. Tea combated atherosclerosis best when consumed at the same time as or shortly after a high fat meal.

Several studies done in the 1980s in Japan show that tea knocks down cholesterol and triglycerides in animals and humans who overdose on fat, suggesting "that tannins in green tea may be involved in the maintenance of normal blood cholesterol levels." The recent research also proclaimed tea tannins protective of the liver.

SEDATIVE AND BLOOD PRESSURE DEPRESSOR

California investigators in 1984 reported that decaffeinated green tea has a sedative action in mice. According to James P. Henry, M.D., a professor of psychiatry at Loma Linda University School of Medicine, the tea, stripped of its caffeine, seemed to relax the animals by affecting the central nervous and neuroendocrine system. The tea definitely also lowered the animals' blood pressure. What's more, mice getting the tea lived longer. Dr. Henry credits so-called bioflavonoids in tea. French scientists have found the same thing in rats eating two specific flavonoid compounds; their blood pressure dropped significantly. The French concluded that the bioflavonoids probably lower blood pressure by performing like beta blocker drugs such as Inderal.

Japanese scientists have isolated a substance from green and black tea that lowers blood sugar in rabbits.

Japan's leading researchers, too, accept a broad therapeutic value of tea, noting: "Different kinds of pharmaceutial effects such as protection of blood vessels, suppression of cancer and prolongation of life span were reported as an integrative effect. It is difficult to ascribe the effectiveness to a single ingredient." They credit four different catechins, all antioxidants that they have isolated from tea. The antioxidants are plentiful in both the tea leaf and brew made from tea leaves. Russian and Canadian scientists also endorse tea as an antioxidant.

Therein may lie a unifying theory to explain folklore's and modern science's enchantment with tea as a whole-body protector. Tea, by being an antioxidant, could have wide-ranging effects, protecting the body from numerous chronic troubles such as heart disease and cancer, even the daily cumulative insults to the body we perceive as aging. Antioxidants act as scavengers in the body, scarfing up the "free radicals" that damage cells, leading to disease.

PRACTICAL MATTERS

- The tea scientists have tested as therapeutic is traditional, ordinary *real tea,* known as Camellia sinensis, native to Asia. So-called herbal teas may also have medicinal qualities, but since they are made from a variety of plants with unknown concentrations of therapeutic chemicals, they must be evaluated one by one.
- *Green tea* appears to pack a much greater protective punch than black tea, which is allowed to oxidize, destroying some of its polyphenols, especially tannins. Green tea leaves commonly have twice the concentration of powerful catechins as black tea leaves. Instant green tea has about three times more catechin than black instant tea. The stronger the cup of tea, the greater the anticipated health benefits.
- If caffeine is a problem, buy decaffeinated tea; taking out the caffeine does not diminish the levels of other potentially therapeutic chemicals.
- Avoid drinking your tea boiling hot. There's evidence that drinking extra-hot tea (as well as other liquids) may damage the lining of the throat and esophagus, leading to cancer. For example, heavy tea drinkers in a recent Indian study were more apt to develop cancer of the esophagus. Authorities once thought that compounds in the tea itself were responsible for higher rates of esophageal cancer; they now believe the heat rather than the tea itself is responsible. The Japanese government warns against drinking very hot tea.

POSSIBLE ADVERSE EFFECTS

- Tea stains teeth.
- It contains compounds, including caffeine, alleged to promote cystic breast disease in some women, although the issue is highly controversial and unresolved. The amount of caffeine in tea leaves is quite high, but in brewed tea there is generally one third as much per cup as in coffee. Caffeine is a central nervous system stimulant.
- Tea stimulates the release of gastric acid in the stomach (so it's not recommended for those with ulcers), but this can be blunted by adding a little milk and sugar. However, adding milk also neutralizes some of the beneficial compounds, such as the tannins, diminishing their protection.
- Excessive tea drinking can severely deplete absorption of iron from plant foods, possibly causing anemia. For example, Israeli health

authorities warned against giving high amounts of tea to infants, citing high rates of anemia.

• Excessive tea drinking—two liters a day—has been incriminated in constipation.

WHY THE ENGLISH PUT MILK IN THEIR TEA

The ritual splash of milk in the British tea began as a health measure. At least until 1660 tea was considered an exotic and strong drug, full of dangerous chemicals and fit only for pharmacies in England. Tea drinking became popular only after British medical authorities said it was safe to take tea regularly if you added milk. The protein in milk binds up the tannins in tea so they supposedly can't do damage.

A few people still think the British have been saved from esophageal cancer because of this tradition, but there's no convincing evidence of it. Adding milk to tea could neutralize some of the good effects of tea, including some anticancer effects due to tannins. Milk also counteracts anticavity fluoride activity. However, milk in tea may be a good idea if you have an ulcer; the milk (skim or fat) helps block the ability of the tea tannins to stimulate secretion of stomach acids.

GINSENG: THE KING OF THERAPEUTIC TEA?

Would you believe the Russians have conducted more than 400 studies on a single type of ginseng alone! Repeatedly, they affirmed that people drinking Siberian ginseng tea appear generally healthier, feel better, withstand stress better, have more energy, and concentrate better. Dr. Norman Farnsworth, a worldwide authority on medicinal plants, had the studies translated from the Russian. He agrees that they support much of ginseng's ancient reputation as a powerful life-giving drug.

Dr. Farnsworth theorizes that ginseng functions as an "adaptogen," a medical concept foreign to most Western minds but defined by respected Russian physician Dr. I. I. Brekhman, U.S.S.R. Academy of Sciences, who performed numerous ginseng studies. An adaptogen is a harmless substance that has a normalizing action, that is, it tends to right whatever is wrong with the body. If your blood pressure is too high, it brings it down; if too low, it brings it up. Thus, adaptogen food compounds could have far-ranging physiological effects, just as antioxidants do. (Ginseng, in fact, contains antioxidants which may help account for its adaptogen capabilities.)

If adaptogen sounds like a nutty notion, consider that United States Department of Agriculture scientists recently discovered the trace mineral chromium works both ways in regulating blood sugar in humans—by raising or lowering it to correct the appropriate abnormality. It's likely that many food substances perform this biochemical yin-yang balancing act, lending new credibility to otherwise inexplicable ancient health claims for ginseng and other foods.

TOMATO

POSSIBLE THERAPEUTIC BENEFITS:
- Lowers cancer risk
- Prevents appendicitis

FOLKLORE

American folklore finds the tomato to be good for dyspepsia, liver troubles, all kidney diseases, and, according to one early twentieth-century physician, "the best of nature's remedies in conditions where there is a tendency to constipation." In Europe in the eighteenth century the bright red globe was treasured as an aphrodisiac.

FACTS

The tomato made little indelible impression on modern science until it began popping up on lists of foods preferred by people free of cancer. Tomatoes have surfaced among foods most eaten by Hawaiians with a lower risk of stomach cancer, Norwegians with lower risks of lung cancer, Americans with less prostate cancer, and elderly Americans with lower death rates from all cancers. In fact, a large group of elderly, dedicated tomato eaters were only half as likely to die of cancer as those who ate few tomatoes.

That tomatoes might protect against lung cancer came as a whopping surprise. In a study of about 14,000 American men and 3000 Norwegian men, scientists discovered that eating tomatoes (or carrots or cabbage) more than fourteen times a month in contrast with eating tomatoes or the other vegetables less than once a month cut the chances of lung cancer. Tomatoes are not extra high in beta carotene, regarded as the prime anticancer agent in vegetables. However, the tomato is distinguished for its concentration of another type of carotene called lycopene—which means that maybe beta carotene is not the only cancer protector among the carotenoid family.

In a large population study in Wales tomatoes also ranked high as a protector against acute appendicitis.

MYTHS AND CAUTIONS

- Modern folklore blames the tomato for aggravating arthritis because it is a member of the "poisonous nightshade" family, but there is no substantial evidence or logical explanation for it. The tomato is commonly incriminated in food allergies. That the tomato is an aphrodisiac is a colossal mistake in language translation.

PASSION'S MISTAKEN FRUIT

Why on earth is the tomato called the apple of love in French?

Did anybody ever get passionate from eating a tomato?

There's no scientific evidence that tomatoes increase the sexual appetite; it was probably all a mixup in translating from one language to another, writes Peter Taberner in his book, *Aphrodisiacs: The Science and the Myth*. And the tomato did have the necessary attributes. It is bright red, the symbol of passion; for a time it was also rare and expensive and that helped clinch its reputation as an aphrodisiac. But its powers came from a tangle in the language. The name for tomato in the original Latin was *mala oethopica* or "apple of the moors." That became *pomi dei mori* in Italian; it was corrupted when translated into French as *pomme d'amour*. From there it was an easy jump to English as "the love apple." By the nineteenth century, after tomatoes became popular and cheap, they lost their appeal as aphrodisiacs. The love apple became just another tomato in the spaghetti sauce.

TURNIP

POSSIBLE THERAPEUTIC BENEFIT:
- Lowers risk of cancer

FOLKLORE

Turnips are reputedly good for a variety of skin diseases, to purify the blood, and as treatment for tuberculosis of the lungs and bones.

FACTS

Turnips will not win any prizes for their vitamin and mineral content; but they excel in other nonnutrient substances, making them vegetables of importance.

Both the bulb and the greens are prime candidates as cancer preventers, because they, like cabbage and other cruciferous vegetables, contain compounds that thwart the development of cancer in laboratory animals. Rutabagas—large yellow turnips—are also chock-full of anticarcinogenic chemicals.

For example, formidable cancer fighters in the cruciferous family are compounds called glucosinolates. In laboratory animals these compounds block the development of cancer. Analyses show that both raw rutabagas and turnip greens have from 39 to 166 milligrams per hundred grams (three and a half ounces) of glucosinolates. Cooked, the concentration drops to a range of 21 to 94. That's exceptional compared even to other cruciferous vegetables, known to be high in glucosinolates. For example, in comparison, raw cauliflower ranges from 14 to 208 per three and a half ounces, watercress up to 95, kohlrabi 109, and cooked brussels sprouts from 15 to 40.

Turnip *greens*, like kale and spinach, are one of those green leafy vegetables that also tops the list of foods eaten by people with lower than average rates of cancers of various types, but in particular lung cancer. Worldwide studies consistently ferret out dark-green leafy vegetables as perhaps the single greatest dietary discouragement to the development of certain cancers. Such dark-green vegetables also are rich in carotenoids, including beta carotene, and chlorophyll, both anticarcinogens.

PRACTICAL MATTERS

- Eat at least some of your turnips and rutabagas raw. Cooking destroys some of the glucosinolates.
- How to tell a rutabaga from a white turnip: A white turnip has a white root with a purple collar around the neck. Rutabagas have a yellow to purple root and are bigger and firmer than white turnips.

WHEAT BRAN

POSSIBLE THERAPEUTIC BENEFITS:
- Relieves constipation
- Prevents diverticular disease, varicose veins, hemorrhoids, and hiatal hernia
- Improves general bowel functioning
- Linked to lower rates of colon cancer

How Much? As a laxative, a mere three tablespoons of miller's unprocessed bran or one ounce—a third of a cup of a hundred percent bran cereal—a day is usually enough to correct chronic constipation. Twice that much has produced diarrhea in some people, although research shows that individuals vary enormously in their response to wheat bran.

FOLKLORE

That wholemeal bread is a laxative was noted by Hippocrates. The idea became popular in the United States in the early 1800s, coinciding with a strong vegetarian movement and the evangelism of Sylvester Graham, namesake of the graham cracker. Nevertheless, wheat bran's benefits were regarded by much of the medical

301

profession as folklore into the 1930s. Many physicians forbade bran's use, regarding "roughage" as bad and irritating to the colon.

FACTS

Wheat bran is nature's greatest cure for constipation. And avoiding constipation, many experts contend, slashes your chances of hemorrhoids, diverticular diseases, varicose veins, hiatal hernia, and possibly colon cancer. Wheat bran, contrary to popular opinion, does not lower blood cholesterol or high blood pressure, and is not known to have specific benefits against cardiovascular disease.

Wheat bran's powers are credited to its high fiber. The bran—the outer layer or covering of the wheat kernel—is the richest dietary source of insoluble fiber known. The most crucial fact is that bran in most people dramatically increases the bulk of the stool. This, say experts, is prime in fighting constipation and other digestive and bowel problems and reducing susceptibility to colon cancer.

A MIGHTY LAXATIVE

Wheat bran is legendary in its abilities to cure constipation. Absolutely nothing else compares in its ability to produce bulkier, softer but heavier stools, push the feces more rapidly through the colon, and confer other positive metabolic effects on colonic function. Hoping to show that vegetables can be an excellent alternative source of bulking fiber, a British team of top-notch fiber experts led by Dr. John H. Cummings, Dunn Clinical Nutrition Centre, Cambridge, England, fed concentrated wheat bran (miller's bran), carrot, cabbage, and apple fibers to nineteen healthy males. They found the vegetables useful, but a very poor second to bran. Specifically, they concluded that 1.7 ounces of miller's bran (about three-fourths of a cup) a day could generally double the weight of the stool. To do the same thing it would take about fourteen slices of whole wheat bread, or four and a half cups of whole boiled carrots, or five cups of boiled cabbage, or eleven apples. So although the vegetables and fruits had an effect, wheat bran was superb!

Western populations need to at least double their stool bulk according to Britisher Dr. Denis Burkitt, the father of the bran-fiber theory. He notes that in rural Africa and India, where fiber intake is high and bowel diseases practically nonexistent, stools weigh an average 300 to 500 grams daily and transverse the alimentary tract from mouth to anus in approximately thirty to thirty-five hours. In contrast, the average daily stool weight of Westerners is slightly over one hundred grams and transit times are about three days in young healthy adults and over two weeks in the elderly.

IT WORKS

Clinics, nursing homes, and hospitals that have substituted wheat bran for laxatives have been duly rewarded. In one British test at Brighton General Hospital, physicians added fifteen grams a day—a quarter cup—of bran to cereals, milk, soup, potatoes, puddings, and other foods given to aged, disabled patients with long-standing constipation. It worked, especially in men. Similarly, in a New Jersey nursing home, a half ounce of 100 percent bran cereal a day mixed with oatmeal cured constipation in about sixty percent of the cases.

THE CANCER HYPOTHESIS

The theory is that if you eat more cereal-type fiber, as found in bran, you're less likely to develop bowel and rectal cancer. Dr. John Weisburger and his colleagues at the American Health Foundation have documented that Finnish farmers, even though they overconsume fat from dairy products, seem somewhat immunized to colon cancer by their high consumption of whole grain cereal and wheat breads. High fiber wheat cereals also appear to block cancer from high fat diets in northern Sweden. A clue to their protection, scientists believe, is their larger stools. Says Dr. Weisburger: Colon cancer is inversely associated with larger stool size.

And what does a bulkier stool from eating wheat bran have to do with malignancy? Here's the theory: Because of ordinary metabolic processes, the colon is awash in bile acids, which are regarded as cancer promoters. Passing through the colon are also other carcinogens, perhaps sloughed off from pesticide residues on foods, and so forth. If the stool is bigger and bulkier, the carcinogens are more diffused, less able to make contact with susceptible cells on the colon wall. Also, a bulkier stool moves through the colon faster, hastening the carcinogens out of the system so they can't dally and corrupt a cell. At the same time, wheat bran alters mucus in the colon, perhaps bolstering defenses against beginning tumors. Wheat bran ferments and releases metabolic compounds in the colon that may block cancer activity, including conversion of certain bile acids to carcinogens.

Fully thirty-two out of forty epidemiological studies worldwide show that eating high fiber foods, including wheat products, is linked to lower rates of human colon cancer. In experimental animals wheat bran blocks the development of colon cancer more consistently than any other fiber source—warding off the cancer in some cases even when experimenters flooded the animal colon with carcinogenic bile acid.

Indeed, wheat's secret may be a particular component of its fiber. A British physician once noticed that the colon cancer death rate among Scots was one third higher than among those living in southeast England. He set out to discover the reasons. He measured fiber intake and found no difference. But he did find that Scots ate much less pentose, a fiber sugar found mostly in wheat-based cereals. Similarly, a study by the International Agency for Research on Cancer noted that Copenhagen residents—with three times the rate of colon cancer as residents of rural Kuopio, Finland—ate only half as much pentose as the Finns. Pentose is also the stuff that mainly accounts for bran's power to produce bulkier stools.

PRACTICAL MATTERS

- If you have a history of constipation, you will probably need more bran to produce regular, acceptable bowel movements than a person who generally has a bulkier stool, studies show. Dr. Cummings's tests found enormous variation in responses to fiber. Some individuals needed six times as much fiber as others to increase stool size.
- Generally, the coarser the bran particles, the greater the effect.
- Add bran gradually to your diet, a little at a time, instead of taking on a big dose at once—and wait for the results.

POSSIBLE ADVERSE EFFECTS

- Eating too much wheat bran can cause diarrhea.
- Anyone with diverticular disease should consult a physician before loading up on bran. Eating too much fiber could cause bowel impaction.
- Extra high fiber foods, like bran, are not advised for those with Crohn's disease, an inflammatory disease of the bowels.

WINE

The most healthful and most hygienic of beverages.
—Louis Pasteur

Drink a glass of wine after your soup and
you steal a rouble from your doctor.
—Old Russian proverb

POSSIBLE THERAPEUTIC BENEFITS:
- Kills bacteria and viruses
- Prevents heart disease
- Raises good HDL blood cholesterol
- Rich in chemicals that prevent cancer in animals

How Much? A glass of wine a day will probably raise your
beneficial HDL-type blood cholesterol an average seven percent.

FOLKLORE

Wine is one of medicine's most ancient brews—administered externally
or internally, alone or combined with other natural drugs. On the
battlefield, it was an antiseptic used to cleanse the wounds of ancient
Greeks. In ancient Egypt, wine along with honey and onion was used
in medicated enemas and mixes inserted into the vagina. Among the
ancients, wine was drunk to "regulate the urine, cause purgation, kill
tapeworm, relieve anorexia, insomnia and all diseases marked by cough";
it also was a common anesthesia, especially during childbirth.

FACTS

The ancients were right. Wine is a proven and powerful but short-lived antiseptic; it kills most bacteria in short order and at low concentrations. It also knocks off viruses. Thus, it can sterilize water in a matter of minutes or hours. It raises HDL cholesterol, which experts say fights heart disease. Wine drinking is associated, for unknown reasons, with low rates of heart disease but possibly because of unknown biologically active compounds indigenous to the grape or created during fermentation of the wine.

MICROBE KILLER

Modern bacteriology has thoroughly validated wine's long-treasured place as an antiseptic. The first test came in 1892 right after an epidemic of cholera in Paris. A physician observing that wine drinkers were more apt to survive the scourge advised mixing wine into drinking water. That prompted an Austrian military doctor, Alois Pick, to test the advice. He added cholera and typhoid germs to flasks containing either water, red or white wine, or wine diluted fifty–fifty with water. The bacteria thrived in the plain water; all of the cholera germs in the pure wine and diluted wine died within ten to fifteen minutes. Within twenty-four hours all of the typhoid bacteria in the wine were also dead. Dr. Pick agreed that drinking water mixed with wine made eminent good sense during cholera and typhoid epidemics.

Every such test of wine shows the same thing with amazing consistency. Wine kills cholera germs in thirty seconds to ten minutes, E. coli in twenty-five to sixty minutes, E. typhi in five minutes to four hours.

The wine assassin was long thought to be alcohol. But take alcohol out of wine and it still kills bacteria. Leave it to the French to figure it out. J. Masquelier, a professor of pharmacology at the Faculty of Medicine and Pharmacy in Bordeaux, discovered the secret during a series of studies in the 1950s. He found that wine compounds called polyphenols—actually a subgroup called anthocyanes and in particular one called malvoside—destroy the bacteria much the same way penicillin does. He noted that red wine diluted in the ratio of one to four with water has the same potency after fifteen minutes as five units of penicillin per milliliter. Wine diluted to even a two percent level shows some bactericidal action.

Dr. Guido Manjo, a surgeon and medical historian who also tested wine against bacteria, says the Greeks were "quite right to pour wine into wounds and over dressings," even though its power is short-lived, which explains, he says, why you don't find wine in your first aid kit. In fact, the Greeks were on more solid ground than anyone could have dreamed. Says Dr. Manjo: "By cleansing wounds with wine the Greeks were actually disinfecting them with a polyphenol, a more complex version of Lister's phenol—the pioneer drug of antiseptic surgery. And the polyphenol of wine, malvoside—weight for weight and tested on *E. coli*—*is 33 times more powerful than phenol!*"

Wine works so much better than grapes or unfermented grape juice because wine's antibacterial properties, found in the grape skin pigment, are only fully chemically liberated during the fermentation, according to Dr. Masquelier's tests. Likewise, Canadian research by Dr. Jack Konowalchuk found that wine, notably red wine, inactivated viruses better than grapes or grape juice.

HEART TONIC?

Alcoholic beverages, particularly wine, may be a tonic for the cardio-vascular system. Generally, epidemiologists find a statistical correlation between a country's lower rate of heart disease and a higher rate of total alcohol consumption. However, Canadian researcher Dr. Amin A. Nanji, a pathologist at the University of Ottawa in Ontario, recently uncovered an intriguing fact when he broke down a nation's alcoholic consumption into percentages by *type* of alcoholic drink. Wine drinking emerged as the best link with low rates of fatal heart disease. In countries where more of the alcohol was consumed in wine, heart disease death rates among men sank. (The opposite showed up for beer, although, as the author notes, that conflicts with some other studies.) Countries in which more than ninety percent of the alcohol was drunk as wine had the lowest heart disease death rates. Dr. Nanji speculates wine's heart medicine is not alcohol but other unknown constituents.

Despite conflicting evidence, drinking alcoholic beverages appears to lift levels of beneficial HDL-type cholesterol. A recent impressive British study of one hundred men and women shows that drinking at least one drink a day—which in the study could be one glass of wine or sherry—did send desirable HDL-type blood cholesterol up by seven percent. When the subjects abstained, the HDLs dropped back down.

CANCER ANTIDOTE?

The antimicrobial compounds in wines also may help counteract cancer, according to Dr. Hans Stich, a noted carcinogenesis expert. "Wine, notably red wine, has high concentrations of gallic acid, one of the tannic acids that give the bouquet to the wine," says Dr. Stich. "Gallic acid is also anticarcinogenic; in tests we did, it prevented different carcinogens from inducing chromosome aberrations." Thus, it blocked mutations considered indicative of cancer-causing potential. That means wine could be anticancer, says Dr. Stich.

One analysis found red wine to have by far the most gallic acid of any beverage tested.

PRACTICAL MATTERS

▪ Wine and weight. Wine does stimulate the appetite, which is good if it is lagging. A glass of pre-dinner wine, for example, has been shown to pick up the appetite of elderly people prone to poor nutrition. But doesn't alcohol, as in wine, destroy a diet? There's fascinating new evidence on that question. The bad news is, according to tests at the Mayo Clinic, that animals on restricted-calorie diets ate more after being given alcohol, and not just because alcohol destroyed will power. Heightened appetite may be due to alcohol-induced physical changes of some sort; thus dieters should restrict pre-meal alcoholic drinks.

But the mind-boggling good news: surplus alcohol calories may not turn into fat as readily as other calories. Stanford University researchers plied middle-aged overweight men with food and an average two drinks of alcohol per day. As expected, the men consumed more calories because of the added alcohol and even ate slightly more food, compared with abstainers. But a strange thing happened: the imbiber's basal metabolism rate increased markedly after one drink per day, thereby burning off some of the excess calories. The faster metabolism offset some of the surplus alcohol calories in men who took one to three drinks a day compared with abstainers or light drinkers. Although researchers could only speculate on the reason for the paradox, their inevitable conclusion: "Alcohol use, at least at moderate levels, may not be as fattening as traditionally believed."

- Travelers in areas of the world where the water is suspect could disinfect it to a good extent by mixing half wine and half water. As far as killing bacteria, both red and white wines work equally well, with a slight edge going to the heavy southern wines like port.
- You can also let a little red wine evaporate, take the residue, and dab it on cold sores. Dr. Konowalchuk says it clears them up in a jiffy and instantly takes the pain away.

POSSIBLE ADVERSE EFFECTS

- If you are susceptible to migraine headaches, go easy on red wine. Red wine is known among headache experts as one of the most common triggers of migraine.
- Alcoholic beverages, including wine, are a hazard to those with a tendency toward gout.
- Drinking alcoholic beverages even in moderation has been linked to higher rates of certain types of cancer, including breast, colon, rectal, and lung.
- Other risks from drinking: alcoholism, cirrhosis of the liver, higher blood pressure, pancreatitis, heart arrhythmia, and fetal alcohol syndrome in infants.
- Although there may be health benefits to drinking wine in moderation, if you do not drink already, it makes little sense to take it up for that reason.

CONFLICTING EVIDENCE

A recent major study done in Great Britain finds that moderate drinking does not prevent nonfatal heart attacks in middle-aged men.

YAM

(also called Sweet Potato)

POSSIBLE THERAPEUTIC BENEFITS:
- Lowers risk of cancer
- May lower blood cholesterol

> *How Much?* Eating an extra half a cup a day can slash chances of developing lung cancer by about half, even long after you have stopped smoking. Eating more than that probably gives the lungs more anticancer ammunition, researchers believe, but they do not know precisely what the optimum dose is.

FOLKLORE

The yam in folk medicine is so often hailed as an antiarthritic agent that it is known as the "rheumatism root"—and also the "colic root." Maud Grieve in *A Modern Herbal* calls the yam "perhaps the best relief and promptest cure for bilious colic, especially helpful in the nausea of pregnant women." In some cultures the yam is also renowned as an antispasmodic, as a diuretic, as an agent to bring on menstruation, to prevent miscarriages, and to treat asthma.

FACTS

Yams, or sweet potatoes, appear to be a partial prophylactic against cancer, notably lung cancer. Several studies point to the orange threesome—sweet potatoes, winter squash, and carrots—as particularly potent in thwarting the long-stage process of lung cancer, even in ex-smokers. For example, New Jersey men with lung cancer compared with similar men without the disease in a study published in 1986 were asked what they ate and how often. The one food that showed up tops as most likely to forestall lung cancer were dark-orange vegetables—sweet potatoes, winter squash, and carrots. According to National Cancer Institute investigators, men who ate a mere half cup of sweet potatoes, carrots, or winter squash every day were only half as likely to develop lung cancer as men who ate almost none.

Since almost all the men in the study were current or former smokers, investigators conclude that sweet potatoes, among other dark-orange vegetables, can somehow interfere far down the line with processes leading to lung cancer. Most likely to suffer from not eating vegetables, including yams, were smokers who had quit within the last five years. But even those who had quit over ten years before still reduced their risk slightly by eating these and other vegetables.

Moral: It looks as if it is never too early or too late for smokers and former smokers to cut their lung cancer odds by loading up on sweet potatoes and their orange cousins. Japanese research also finds that even former *heavy* smokers come out ahead by eating orange and deep-green vegetables. However, do not count on such foods as antidotes to allow you to *continue* smoking; vegetable-eating smokers are many times more likely to come down with lung cancer than nonsmokers.

Nonsmokers fearful of cancer from passive smoking and other environmental or occupational hazards may also save themselves by loading up on yams. There's new evidence from the National Cancer Institute that deep-orange vegetables work in protecting nonsmokers as well as smokers, notably women.

Beta carotene—a well-known anticancer factor—may be the prime cancer fighter in yams, but other undiscovered yam constituents may also be responsible. Sweet potatoes also are rich in protease inhibitors, compounds that squelch cancer formation in animals. The protease inhibitors also put the kibosh on disease-producing viruses. And beta carotene in laboratory animals is potent in preventing nonmelanoma skin cancers.

Perhaps most exciting, Japanese investigators in 1984 discovered that the sweet potato has "markedly strong antioxidative activity." This makes it a potential antagonist of those scurrilous "free radicals" that ravage bodily cells, creating all kinds of disorders, including cancer and perhaps aging. The scientists attributed the antioxidant activity of sweet potato extract to a collection of polyphenols, such as chlorogenic acid.

Interestingly, the sweet potato extract itself was a much stronger antioxidant than the sum of the polyphenol compounds themselves. The investigators propose that other chemicals in the sweet potato enhance the polyphenols' natural powers.

It's possible that sweet potatoes lower blood cholesterol. In a recent test, it performed much like cholestyramine, a cholesterol-reducing drug. Of twenty-eight fruit and vegetable fibers, that of the sweet potato was the most potent in binding up cholesterol, as documented in lab experiments that simulate the human digestive system. Sweet potato fiber was nearly as good at mopping up cholesterol as cholestyramine.

THE TWIN EFFECT

Some authorities, including Dr. Percy Nylander, a professor at the University of Ibadan in Nigeria, suspect that going heavy on yams could promote the birth of twins. That's because the Nigerian Yoruba tribe he has studied has by far the highest rate of double births in the world—twice that anywhere else. And the Yorubas who eat prodigious amounts of yams, a staple of the tribal diet, have an even higher rate. The theory goes this way: yams are rich in hormone-like substances that trigger the release of other hormones, including one called follicle-stimulating hormone (FSH). This FSH, found in extremely high levels in Yoruba mothers of twins, is thought to stimulate the ovaries to release more than one ovum, setting the stage for double conception. Dr. Nylander also notes that the wealthier Yoruba people who have given up the tribal yam-dominated diet for Western fare have fewer twins.

PRACTICAL MATTERS

The darker orange the yam or sweet potato is, the higher its concentration of disease-fighting carotenoids.

ALERT

Eating loads of sweet potatoes is not dangerous as is excessive vitamin A from liver, for example. But the high levels of beta carotene could turn your skin slightly yellow or tan. The skin colorization disappears with no long-term toxic effects once you stop the sweet-potato (or carrot-squash) binge.

YOGURT

(Also known as kefir, kourmiss, yakult, yahourt, leben, acidophilus milk)

POSSIBLE THERAPEUTIC BENEFITS

- Kills bacteria
- Prevents and treats intestinal infections, including diarrhea
- Lowers blood cholesterol
- Boosts immune system
- Improves bowel functioning
- Contains compounds that prevent ulcers
- Has anticancer activity

> *How Much?* Three cups of yogurt a day have lowered blood cholesterol. A third to a half cup of skim milk yogurt daily has cured infants with severe diarrhea.

FOLKLORE

An angel is supposed to have revealed to the biblical Abraham the life-giving aspects of yogurt, accounting for his longevity. Yogurt—fermented milk with living microbes—is one of the legendary foods of all time. People around the Mediterranean have used it for centuries to ward off diarrhea and cure other troubles of the bowels. It entered modern folklore with a bang because of nineteenth-century experiments by microbiologist Dr. Elias Metchnikoff of the Pasteur Institute, who declared it a panacea against heart disease, senility, and general deterioration of the body.

314

FACTS

Yogurt has been subjected to intense scientific scrutiny in the twentieth century and found to be a versatile therapeutic agent; much of its benefit comes from the prodigious activity it stirs up in the digestive tract. Yogurt's distinguishing characteristic is its family of natural bacteria, called lactobacilli, that cause fermentation and hence a sharp taste. Yogurt's therapeutic capabilities depend on the type of bacteria present.

HOW YOGURT FIGHTS DIARRHEA

The intestinal tract is a battleground for bacteria, and which germs are winning the colonic bacterial wars helps determine the state of digestion, elimination, and general health. Disturbances in the bowel ecosystem created by an overproliferation of certain bacteria, especially E. coli in infants, can lead to diarrhea. More lactobacilli from yogurt can add enough good microorganisms to overcome the deleterious ones, thus restoring order to digestive activity.

That's why yogurt can perform two seemingly opposite functions: relieve diarrhea and act as a laxative. It does what is necessary to reinstate a normal microbial balance in the intestinal tract. A little yogurt, many researchers report, helps cure general gastrointestinal disturbances caused by food poisoning or infectious agents.

The antibacterial action of yogurt has been found notably effective against the *E.coli* germ, a frequent cause of so-called traveler's diarrhea; yogurt also alleviates diarrhea due to microbial overgrowth commonly induced by pharmaceutical antibiotics. Some physicians who prescribe pencillin also advise: "And take a little yogurt."

NATURAL ANTIBIOTICS

Much research finds that yogurt's active bacteria and by-products released in the intestinal tract are natural broad-spectrum antibiotics. Scientists have isolated *seven* natural antibiotics from yogurt and other fermented milks, some with bacteria-killing powers equal to or more effective than pharmaceutical antibiotics like terramycin. Antibiotics from cultures commonly used in American yogurt (Bulgarican) and acidophilus milk (acidophilin) can squelch common bacteria causing botulism, salmonella, and staphylococcus poisoning. Additionally, yogurt bacteria in the intestines spin off other chemicals that knock out bacteria that can cause stomach upset or infections.

Extensive research, notably in Middle European countries and Japan as well as in the United States, shows that yogurt can prevent and sometimes cure dysentery and diarrhea, especially infant diarrhea. It's routine in Italian and Russian hospitals to feed infants yogurt to ward off diarrhea. In one study done in 1963 at a New York City hospital, physicians cured infants with severe diarrhea twice as quickly with three fluid ounces (between one-third and one-half cup) of ordinary yogurt than with the standard antidiarrheal drug Neomycin kaopectate.

Yogurt appears more successful as a *prophylactic* against intestinal distress. In Japan, dysentery was completely prevented among a group of 500 servicemen eating yakult daily—a yogurt drink made with L. casei culture. Ten percent of a similar group not eating the yakult developed dysentery over a six-month period.

Polish children fed yogurt are much more resistant to influenza infections. And mice fed yogurt in United States Department of Agriculture tests were also much less apt to succumb to salmonella infections. The yogurt-fed mice also lived longer.

Particularly powerful is the acidophilus culture sometimes put in yogurt in this country (it's found in acidophilus milk) to combat deleterious bacteria. In Polish studies, it both cured and prevented diarrhea. One of the world's leading experts on fermented milks, including yogurt, Dr. Khem Shahani, at the University of Nebraska, considers yogurt a better preventive than cure of diarrhea and dysentery. He notes: "By ingesting lactobacilli through food . . . after diarrheal stress (but preferably *before*), one can reduce diarrheal incidences."

Although for years yogurt has been recognized as a microbe killer, recent research in Japan, Italy, Switzerland, and the United States finds it also boosts immune functioning in animals and human cells, causing them to spew out more antibodies and other killer cells and substances against disease. Thus, yogurt can fight infections with two distinct mechanisms: by killing bacteria and boosting immunity.

ANTICANCER AGENT?

Evidence grows that yogurt might help prevent cancer, namely, colon cancer. In the last quarter century, scientists have detected several cancer-fighting properties in yogurt. There's some evidence that humans who eat more yogurt are less susceptible to cancer. Compelling studies on the intestinal tracts of humans done by top researchers in Boston also show that the acidophilus culture can help suppress the activity of enzymes in the colon that convert harmless chemicals into cancer-causing agents. A fascinating French study published in a 1986 *Journal of the National Cancer Institute*, found that although women who ate high levels of dairy fat, such as cheese, had a higher risk of breast cancer, those who ate the most yogurt had the least risk. Dr. Shahani's group has also found that yogurt or milk with acidophilus culture inhibits cancer in mice; other researchers find the same thing in rats.

STOMACH BALM

Yogurt has gobs of natural fatty hormonal substances called prostaglandins E2 that are known ulcer antagonists and also protect the lining of the stomach against noxious agents like cigarette smoke and alcohol. Prostaglandin E has been synthesized into a new antiulcer prescription drug. Yogurt made from whole milk contains lower concentrations of biologically active prostaglandin E identical to the drug, says Dr. Samuel Money of the State University of New York Health Science Center at Brooklyn and one of the discoverers of the drug substance in yogurt and milk. Since the prostaglandins reside in milk *fat*, low-fat and non-fat skim milk yogurt carry fewer of the active agents.

Yogurt in tests on humans with normal blood cholesterol has also lowered blood cholesterol to a surprising degree—from five to ten percent within a week. The subjects ate three cups of either pasteurized or nonpasteurized yogurt and saw their cholesterol sink. Yogurt has also raised the HDL cholesterol, the good kind.

Although some reports have tagged yogurt, because of its tryptophan content, a slight sedative, authoritative studies at MIT find that yogurt actually helps tickle brain chemicals, keeping your mind more alert. Thus, skim milk or low-fat yogurt is for staying awake, not going to sleep.

PRACTICAL MATTERS

- Not all yogurts have the same therapeutic potential. The type and amount of bacteria in the yogurt determines its precise health effects on the body. Fermented milks, including yogurt, are made by adding one or more types of a family of bacteria called Lactobacilli. For example, the L. acidophilus culture is regarded as one of the most beneficial and versatile. In the United States, a few brands of yogurt contain acidophilus bacteria. Some supermarkets do carry acidophilus milk, made from that particular lactobacillus.

- The type of culture in yogurts is not required to be listed on the label in the United States; to find out, you can write the manufacturer. However, it's safe to assume that most yogurts in the United States are made from L. bulgaricus and streptococcus thermophilus, and a few with acidophilus.
- Check the label to be sure the yogurt contains "active cultures," branding it real yogurt. Yogurt in which cultures are killed by pasteurization after fermentation lose their therapeutic benefit, notably as antibacterial agents. Occasionally, milk is given the sour taste by the phony method of adding acid, then thickened and passed off as yogurt. Dr. Shahani calls this merely "acidified yogurt," without the health benefits of cultured yogurt.
- If you are allergic to milk, try yogurt. It's well established that most people who cannot tolerate milk because they lack the enzyme to break down the milk sugar (lactose) can safely eat yogurt without discomfort.

CAUTION

- Occasionally, those with lactose intolerance cannot take yogurt either without developing an upset stomach. Anyone using yogurt, especially with babies, should be alert to this possibility.

CONFLICTING EVIDENCE

Several animal and human survey studies find no effect from yogurt on blood cholesterol. One recent study on rats found more small colon tumors in rats fed yogurt than those fed plain milk.

DR. SHAHANI'S HOMEMADE YOGURT

Boil a quart of milk; let it simmer for a few minutes; cool to room temperature. Add about two or three tablespoons of old yogurt containing L. bulgaricus and streptococcus thermophilus cultures. Add a little powder of acidophilus, which you can purchase at a health food store. (In a routine check, Dr. Shahani, however, found that seventy percent of acidophilus cultures sold did not meet claims on the label. Vitaldophilus is one brand found particularly reliable.) Mix thoroughly. Cover it and put it in the oven without turning on the heat. Remove when thickened.

Add salt and pepper and/or cumin seeds.

PART FOUR

DISEASE AND FOOD

A CAPSULE GUIDE TO CURES AND PREVENTION

A man may esteem himself happy when that
which is his food is also his medicine.

—Thoreau

APPENDICITIS

Best: high fiber foods like wheat bran that keep the stool soft and
bulky. A British survey tagged peas, cabbage, cauliflower, green beans,
brussels sprouts, and tomatoes as antiappendicitis foods.

ARTHRITIS

Rheumatoid: seafood high in omega-3 fatty acids such as salmon,
sardines, lake trout, and mackerel may prevent or relieve the pain and
swelling. Fish oils dramatically prevent lupus in animals.

ASTHMA

Coffee: a couple of strong cups can thwart an asthma attack. Also good
bronchodilators—hot pungent foods, such as chili peppers, garlic, onions, mustard, horseradish. Fish oils also have dramatically relieved
bronchial asthma.

CANCER*

In general: green leafy vegetables especially the big five—broccoli, spinach, cabbage, kale, brussels sprouts. Other high-fiber vegetables, fruits, grains, and legumes. Also, milk, tomatoes, citrus fruits, dried fruits (apricots, prunes, raisins), strawberries and fish high in omega-3 fatty acids may help prevent various kinds of cancer. Garlic, onions, kelp, olive oil, tea (especially green tea), as well as seed foods, such as legumes, nuts, rice, and grains, are rich in anticancer chemicals.

Bladder: carrots, milk, broccoli, brussels sprouts, cabbage, cauliflower, coleslaw, kale, parsnips, turnips.

Breast: yogurt. Fruits and vegetables high in carotenoids.

Colon: green leafy vegetables, notably cabbage, broccoli, brussels sprouts. Also cauliflower. Acidophilus milk or yogurt, especially that made with acidophilus culture. Milk, preferably vitamin D-fortified skim milk. Wheat bran.

Esophagus: green and yellow vegetables, apples, cherries, grapes, melons, onions, peas, beans, plums, pumpkin.

Larynx: green and yellow vegetables.

Lung: carrots, kale, spinach, broccoli, dark-yellow squash, pumpkin, sweet potatoes, apricot. All dark-green and dark-orange vegetables, red and yellow fruits high in carotenoids. If you have ever smoked, load up on these foods. They may help prevent lung cancer years later.

Pancreatic: Citrus fruits, carrots.

Prostate: yellow and green vegetables. Carrots, tomatoes, cabbage, peas, broccoli, brussels sprouts, cauliflower.

Stomach: raw carrots, coleslaw, lettuce, cabbage, tomatoes, corn, eggplant, milk, onion, sweet potatoes, squash.

High fat and meat diets predispose to cancer.

CARDIOVASCULAR SYSTEM

For keeping the blood free of clots, try fatty fish, garlic, ginger, melon, tree ear mushrooms, olive oil, onion, and kelp. Green tea, beer, currants, blueberries, eggplant, and omega-3 fatty fish (salmon, sardines) appear to have special abilities to strengthen and protect arteries and capillaries from damage due to atherosclerosis or heart attack.

---

*Individual foods listed have been linked to lower rates of specific cancers in diet–cancer epidemiological studies or have induced protective changes in human physiological studies.

CAVITIES

Tea is nature's best proved anticavity mouthwash. Also tops at combating cavity-producing bacteria: grape and black cherry juice, milk, coffee, cheese (aged cheddar cheese, blue, Brie, Gouda, Monterey Jack, mozzarella, and Swiss).

CHOLESTEROL

TO REDUCE BAD LDL (LOW-DENSITY LIPOPROTEIN) CHOLESTEROL

First choice is oat bran. Next, oatmeal and dried beans, including plain old baked beans out of the can. Soybeans are great for adults and kids with genetically induced high cholesterol. Grapefruit—segments and membrane, not the juice—drives down cholesterol. Also fresh oranges, apples, yogurt, skim milk, carrots, garlic, onions, barley, ginger, eggplant, artichoke, unripe plantain, shiitake mushrooms, olive oil. Substitute seafood, including shellfish, for meat and chicken. All fruits high in pectin, which includes strawberries and bananas.

TO RAISE GOOD HDL (HIGH-DENSITY LIPOPROTEIN) CHOLESTEROL

Best bet is strong, raw onions—at least a half a medium onion a day. Substitute olive oil for other vegetable oils or saturated fats. Alcoholic drinks, such as wine, beer, spirits in moderation—one or two drinks a day—also boost HDLs.

Added advice: cut back on total fat (especially saturated fats like animal-type fat, and coconut and palm oils). This enhances the effects of the above natural cholesterol-fighters.

CONSTIPATION

Top choice: *wheat bran,* nature's most potent bulk laxative. If that doesn't work, add prune juice. Dried beans work wonders on some people. Most high fiber fruits and vegetables, like carrots, cabbage, and apples, are bulk laxatives with about one quarter the effect of wheat bran. Soluble fiber foods, like oats and barley, can help. Also kelp.

Myth: American-type rhubarb is not a laxative. Oriental-type medicinal rhubarb is.

HOW FOOD FIGHTS CHOLESTEROL*

Daily dose	Average drop in total cholesterol (percent)	Average increase in good HDL cholesterol (percent)
Apples (2 or 3)	10	
Barley (3 servings)	15	
Beans, dried (1 cooked cup)	19	
Beer (½ pint)		7
Carrot (2½ medium)	11	
Garlic, raw (9 cloves)	10	
Garlic juice (⅛ cup)	30	
Milk, skim (1 quart)	8	
Mushroom, shiitake (3 ounces)	12	
Oats and oat bran (½ cup dry oat bran)	20	15
Olive oil (40% of calories	13	
Onion, raw (½ medium sized)		30
Soybeans (1 serving soybean protein)	20	
Wine (1 glass)		7
Yogurt (3 cups)	10	

*In comparison, the cholesterol-lowering success of standard drugs is 15 to 20 percent for cholestyramine and colestipol; 5 to 15 percent for gemfibrozil, 10 to 15 percent for probucol, and 30 to 40 percent for the newest entry, lovastatin. Gemfibrozil raises HDLs about 10 percent.

DIABETES

Concentrate on foods that produce slow, steady increases instead of rapid rises in blood sugar levels. Such foods testing best on the "glycemic index"—a measure of how quickly foods raise blood sugar—are, in order: peanuts, soybeans, lentils, kidney beans, black-eyed peas, milk, chickpeas, yogurt, ice cream, apples, and baked beans.

DIARRHEA

Try yogurt, with live cultures (especially if the diarrhea is caused by prescription antibiotics, such as penicillin). Also blueberries, black currants, honey (not for infants, however, because of a botulism danger).

For youngsters, more *whole* milk may be a cure. Too little fat in the children's diets promote diarrhea and other intestinal infections. Soy milk or soybeans also may help fight diarrhea-producing bacteria.

DIVERTICULAR DISEASE

Number one choice: wheat bran. Also other foods high in fiber that give the stool bulk, such as legumes, oats, cabbage, carrots, and apples. If you already have the disease, check with a physician before loading up on high fiber.

EMPHYSEMA AND CHRONIC BRONCHITIS

Chili peppers, pungent garlic, onions, mustard, horseradish—all kinds of hot, spicy foods. These help keep the lungs healthy by keeping mucus flowing and the bronchial tubes open. Drinking milk has also been tied to lower rates of chronic bronchitis.

ENERGY (MENTAL)

Caffeine drinks rev up mental performance. Coffee is the most potent. Also tea, colas, cocoa. Also boosting mental-energy brain chemicals are high-protein, low-fat foods such as shellfish, lean fish, no-fat milk, and yogurt.

HEMORRHOIDS

Eat foods that produce a soft, bulky stool, reducing strain in bowel movements. Best: wheat bran. Other high fiber fruits and vegetables.

HIGH BLOOD PRESSURE

Mackerel—a couple of cans a week—can depress blood pressure. Also oat bran and high fiber fruits and vegetables of all types help. Shown also to push down blood pressure: olive oil, garlic, seaweed (kelp), yogurt, green tea, legumes, and milk. Surprisingly, coffee drinking does not cause or aggravate high blood pressure except, apparently, among smokers.

INFECTIONS (GENERAL)

Yogurt and garlic are recognized antibiotic superstars. Also potent in thwarting viruses and bacteria are orange juice, apples, tea, grape juice, apple juice, honey, wine, blueberries, cranberries, grapes, plums, raspberries, strawberries, peaches, and figs.

INSOMNIA

A sure bet: sugar or honey.

Myth: milk does not put you to sleep; just the opposite, it wakes you up.

MIGRAINE HEADACHE

Oils in fish (omega-3's) can prevent the onset and severity of migraines in some cases.

MOTION SICKNESS

Take ginger root, about half a teaspoon powdered in capsules, in tea or another beverage about a half hour before exposure to motion.

OSTEOPOROSIS

Drinking milk when you are young makes stronger bones, less susceptible to osteoporosis in later years. Milk itself is more effective than pure calcium.

PSORIASIS AND SKIN INFLAMMATION

Seafood high in omega-3 fatty acids: salmon, sardines, herring, mackerel, etc., may relieve psoriasis. Also oatmeal packs reduce skin inflammation.

STROKE

Fresh fruits and vegetables—even an extra serving a day, according to one study—may cut the risk of stroke-associated death by forty percent. In animal studies, compounds from black currants and blueberries helped prevent disease of blood vessels in the brain. Brown seaweed has prevented strokes in rodents.

ULCER

Plantains (unripe, large and green, especially in concentrated powder form) combat ulcers. Whole milk and yogurt, which contain drug-like protective prostaglandins in the fat may prevent, but not heal ulcers. Fresh cabbage juice heals or wards off ulcers in some people.

URINARY TRACT PROBLEMS

Cranberries, including juice, cocktail, and whole cranberries can prevent cystitis, help deodorize the urine, and help prevent kidney stones. Effective dose: half a cup to two cups of cocktail per day. Omega-3 type fish oils may help prevent kidney disease. Rice bran—about two thirds of an ounce a day—can prevent kidney stones.

REFERENCES

To list all the thousands of scientific references that went into this book would require impossible space. For those who wish further details, here are some of the most critical scientific papers from which further references can be obtained. Some of the papers, notably on anticancer foods, refer to several vegetables or fruits. In this listing, such papers are mentioned only once under the food section in which they first appear.

The abbreviations given are standard for medical libraries where the journals are found.

In many cases, the research has not yet been published and was obtained through personal interviews or papers delivered at scientific conferences.

APPLES

Konowalchuk, J., et al. "Antiviral Effect of Apple Beverages." *Applied and Environmental Microbiology* (December 1978) 36(6):798–801.

Reiser, S. "Metabolic Effects of Dietary Pectins Related to Human Health." *Food Technology* (February 1987) 91–99.

Sablé-Amplis, R., et al. "Further Studies on the Cholesterol-Lowering Effect of Apple in Humans: Biochemical Mechanisms Involved. *Nutr. Res.* (1983) 3:325–328.

APRICOTS

Mahmud, S.A., et al. "Apricot in the Diet of Hunza Population." *Hamdard* (January–June 1984) 27:166.

BANANA AND PLANTAIN

Best, R., et al. "The Anti-ulcerogenic Activity of the Unripe Plantain Banana (Musa Species)." *British Journal of Pharmacology* (1984) 82:107–116.

Goel, R.K., et al. "Anti-Ulcerogenic Effect of Banana Powder (Musa Sapientum Var. Paradisiaca) and Its Effect on Mucosal Resistance." *Journal of Ethno-Pharmacology* (1986) 18:33–44.

Usha, V., et al. "Effect of Dietary Fiber from Banana (Musa Paradisiaca) on Cholesterol Metabolism." *Indian Journal of Experimental Biology* (October 1984) 22:550–554.

BARLEY

Odes, H.S., et al. "Pilot Study of the Efficacy of Spent Grain Dietary Fiber in the Treatment of Constipation." *Israel Journal of Medical Science* (January 1986) 22(1):12–15.

Qureshi, A.A., et al. "Suppression of Cholesterogenesis by Plant Constituents; Review of Wisconsin Contributions to NC-167." *Lipids* (November 1985) 20(11):817–824.

BEANS

Anderson, J.W., et al. "Dietary Fiber: Hyperlipidemia, Hypertension, and Coronary Heart Disease." *American Journal of Gastroenterology* (1986) 81(10):907–919.

Anderson, J.W., et al. "Hypocholesterolemic Effects of Oat-Bran and Bean Intake for Hypercholesterolemic Men." *American Journal of Clinical Nutrition* (December 1984) 40:1146–1155.

Correa, P. "Epidemiological Correlations Between Diet and Cancer Frequency." *Cancer Research* (1981) 41:3685–3690.

Fleming, S.E., et al. "Influence of Frequent and Long-Term Bean Consumption on Colonic Function and Fermentation." *American Journal of Clinical Nutrition* (May 1985) 41:909–918.

Troll, W., et al. "Protease Inhibitors: Possible Anticarcinogens in Edible Seeds." *Prostate* (1983) 4:345–349.

BEER

Burr, M.L., et al. "Alcohol and High-Density-Lipoprotein Cholesterol: A Randomized Controlled Trial." *British Journal of Nutrition* (1986) 56:81–86.

Hennekens, C.H., et al. "Daily Alcohol Consumption and Fatal Coronary Heart Disease." *American Journal of Epidemiology* (1978) 107:196–200.

Kune, S., et al. "Case-Control Study of Alcoholic Beverages as Etiological Factors: The Melbourne Colorectal Cancer Study." *Nutrition and Cancer* (1987) 9(1):43–56.

Le, M.G., et al. "Alcoholic Beverage Consumption and Breast Cancer in a French Case-Control Study." *American Journal of Epidemiology* (September 1986) 120(3):244–247.

Nanji, A.A. "Alcohol and Ischemic Heart Disease: Wine, Beer or Both?" *International Journal of Cardiology* (August 1985) 8(4):487–489.

BLUEBERRY

Konowalchuk, J., et al. "Antiviral Activity of Fruit Extracts." *Journal of Food Science* (1976) 41:1013–1017.

Miskulin, M., et al. "Effect of Experimental Hypertension and Cholesterol-Induced Atheroma on the Permeability and Biochemical Composition of Brain Microvessels. Protective Effect of Anthocyanosides." International Symposium on Patholophysiology and Pharmacotherapy of Cerebrovascular Disorders, 1980.

BROCCOLI

Colditz, G.A., et al. "Increased Green and Yellow Vegetable Intake and Lowered Cancer Deaths in an Elderly Population." *American Journal of Clinical Nutrition* (January 1985) 41(1):32–36.

Graham, S., et al. "Diet in the Epidemiology of Cancer of the Colon and Rectum." *Journal of the National Cancer Institute* (September 1978) 61(3):709–714.

Wattenberg, L.W. "Inhibition of Carcinogenic Effects of Polycyclic Hydrocarbons by Benzyl Isothiocyanate and Related Compounds." *Journal of the National Cancer Institute* (February 1977) 58(2):395–398.

Wattenberg, L.W., et al. "Inhibition of Polycyclic Aromatic Hydrocarbon-Induced Neoplasia by Naturally Occurring Indoles." *Cancer Research* (May 1978) 38(5):1410–1413.

BRUSSELS SPROUTS

Bradfield, C.A., et al. "Effect of Dietary Indole-3-Carbinol on Intestinal and Hepatic Monooxygenase, Glutathione S-Transferase and Epoxide Hydrolase Activities in the Rat." *Food Chemistry Toxicology* (December 1984) 22(12):977–982.

Godlewski, C.E., et al. "Hepatic Glutathione S-Transferase Activity and Aflatoxin B1-Induced Enzyme Altered Foci in Rats Fed Fractions of Brussels Sprouts." *Cancer Letter* (September 15, 1985) 28(2):151–157.

Wattenberg, L.W. "Studies of Polycyclic Hydrocarbon Hydroxylases of the Intestine Possibly Related to Cancer." *Cancer* (July 1971) 28:99–102.

CABBAGE

Albert-Puleo, M. "Physiological Effects of Cabbage with Reference to Its Potential as a Dietary Cancer-Inhibitor and Its Use in Ancient Medicine." *Journal of Ethnopharmacology* (December 1983) 9(2):261–272.

Ansher, S.S., et al. "Biochemical Effects of Dithiolthiones." *Food Chem. Toxicol.* (May 1986) 24(5):405–415.

Barker, D.J.P., et al. "Vegetable Consumption and Acute Appendicitis in 59 Areas in England and Wales." *British Medical Journal* (April 5, 1986) 292:927–930.

Boyd, J.N., et al. "Modification of Beet and Cabbage Diets of Aflatoxin B1-induced Rat Plasma Alpha-foetoprotein Elevation, Hepatic Tumorigenesis, and Mutagenicity of Urine." *Food Chem. Toxicol.* (February 1982) 20(1):47–52.

Cheney, G., et al. "Anti-Peptic Ulcer Dietary Factor. (Vitamin "U") in the Treatment of Peptic Ulcer." *Journal of the American Dietetic Association* (1950) 26:668–672.

Graham, S., et al. "Diet and Colon Cancer." *American Journal of Epidemiology* (January 1979) 109(1):1–20.

Haenszel, W., et al. "A Case-Control Study of Large Bowel Cancer in Japan." *Journal of the National Cancer Institute* (January 1980) 64(1):17–22.

Hoff, G., et al. "Epidemiology of Polyps in the Rectum and Sigmoid Colon. Evaluation of Nutritional Factors." *Scandinavian Journal of Gastroenterology* (1986) 21:199–204.

Manousos, O., et al. "Diet and Colorectal Cancer: A Case-Control Study in Greece." *International Journal of Cancer* (July 15, 1983) 32(1):1–5.

Singh, G.B., et al. "Effect of Brassica Oleracea Var. Capitata in the Prevention and Healing of Experimental Peptic Ulceration." *Ind. Jour. Med. Res.* (September 1962) 50(5):741–749.

Spector, H., et al. "Reduction of X-Radiation Mortality by Cabbage and Broccoli." *Proceedings of the Society of Experimental Biology and Medicine* (1959) 100:405–407.

Tajima, K., et al. "Dietary Habits and Gastro-intestinal Cancers: A Comparative Case-Control Study of Stomach and Large Intestinal Cancers in Nagoya, Japan." *Japanese Journal of Cancer Research* (August 1985) 76(8):705–716.

Wattenberg, L.W. "Inhibition of Neoplasia by Minor Dietary Constituents." *Cancer Research* (Suppl.) (May 1983) 43:2488s–2453s.

CARROT

Colditz, G.A., et al. "Diet and Lung Cancer—A Review of the Epidemiologic Evidence in Humans." *Archives of Internal Medicine* (January 1987) 147:157–160.

Menkes, M.S., et al. "Serum Beta-Carotene, Vitamins A and E, Selenium, and the Risk of Lung Cancer." *New England Journal of Medicine* (November 13, 1986) 315(20)1250–1254.

Norell, S.E., et al. "Diet and Pancreatic Cancer: A Case-Control Study." *American Journal of Epidemiology* (1986) 124(6):894–902.

Peto, R., et al. "Can Dietary Beta-Carotene Materially Reduce Human Cancer Rates?" *Nature* (March 19, 1981) 290:201–208.

Robertson, J., et al. "The Effect of Raw Carrot on Serum Lipids and Colon Function." *American Journal of Clinical Nutrition* (September 1979) 32(9):1889–1892.

Shekelle, R.B., et al. "Dietary Vitamin A and Risk of Cancer in the Western Electric Study." *Lancet* (November 28, 1981) 1185–1189.

Ziegler, R.G., et al. "Carotenoid Intake, Vegetables, and the Risk of Lung Cancer Among White Men in New Jersey." *American Journal of Epidemiology* (1986) 123(6):1080–1093.

CHILI PEPPER

Henry, C.J.K., et al. "Effect of Spiced Food on Metabolic Rate." *Human Nutrition: Clinical Nutrition* (March 1986) 40(2):165–168.

"Hot Peppers and Substance P." *Lancet* (May 28, 1983) 1198.

Lundberg, J.M., et al. "Cigarette Smoke-Induced Airway Oedema Due to Activation of Capsaicin-Sensitive Vagal Afferents and Substance P. Release." *Neuroscience* (December 1983) 10(4):1361–1368.

Sambaiah, K., et al. "Hypocholesterolemic Effect of Red Pepper & Capsaicin." *Indian Journal of Experimental Biology* (August 1980) 18:898–899.

Visudhiphan, S., et al. "The Relationship Between High Fibrinolytic Activity and Daily Capsicum Ingestion in Thais." *American Journal of Clinical Nutrition* (June 1982) 35(6):1452–1458.

Ziment, I. (ed.). *Practical Pulmonary Disease.* John Wiley and Sons: New York, 1983.

Ziment, I. *Respiratory Pharmacology and Therapeutics.* W. B. Saunders Company: Philadelphia, 1978.

COFFEE

Becker, A.B., et al. "The Bronchodilator Effects and Pharmacokinetics of Caffeine in Asthma." *New England Journal of Medicine* (March 22, 1984) 310(12):743–746.

Boulenger, J.P., et al. "Increased Sensitivity to Caffeine in Patients with Panic Disorders. Preliminary Evidence." *Archives of General Psychiatry* (November 1984) 41(11):1067–1071.

Costill, D.L., et al. "Effects of Caffeine Ingestion on Metabolism and Exercise Performance." *Medicine and Science in Sports* (1978) 10(3):155–158.

Curb, J.D., et al. "Coffee, Caffeine, and Serum Cholesterol in Japanese Men in Hawaii." *American Journal of Epidemiology* (April 1986) 123(4):648–655.

Gong, H., Jr., et al. "Bronchodilator Effects of Caffeine in Coffee. A Dose-Response Study of Asthmatic Subjects." *Chest* (March 1986) 89(3):335–342.

Kashket, S., et al. "In-Vitro Inhibition of Glucosyltransferase from the Dental Plaque Bacterium Streptococcus Mutans by Common Beverages and Food Extracts." *Archives of Oral Biology* (1985) 30(11–12):821–826.

Nomura, A., et al. "Prospective Study of Coffee Consumption and the Risk of Cancer." *Journal of the National Cancer Institute* (April 1986) 76(4):587–590.

Shirlow, M.J., et al. "A Study of Caffeine Consumption and Symptoms; Indigestion, Palpitations, Tremor, Headache and Insomnia." *Int. J. Epidemiol.* (June 1985) 14(2):239–248.

Wattenberg, L.W. "Inhibition of Neoplasia by Minor Dietary Constituents." *Cancer Research* (Suppl.) (May 1983) 43:2488s–2453s.

CRANBERRY

Der Marderosian, A.H. "Cranberry Juice." *Drug Therapy* (November 1977) 151–160.

Moen, D.V. "Observations on the Effectiveness of Cranberry Juice in Urinary Infections." *Wisconsin Medical Journal* (1962) 61:282–283.

Papas, P.N., et al. "Cranberry Juice in the Treatment of Urinary Tract Infections." *Southwestern Medicine* (January 1966) 47(1):17–20.

Sobota, A.E. "Inhibition of Bacterial Adherence by Cranberry Juice: Potential Use for the Treatment of Urinary Tract Infections." *Journal of Urology* (May 1984) 131:1013–1016.

CURRANT

Jones, E., et al. "Quercetin, Flavonoids and the Life-Span of Mice." *Experimental Gerontology* (1982) 17(3):213–217.

Kyerematen, G., et al. "Preliminary Pharmacological Studies of Pecarin, a New Preparation from Ribes Nigrum Fruits." *Acta Pharm. Suececa* (1986) 23(2):101–106.

Millet, J., et al. "Improvement of Blood Filtrability with a Purified Extract of Black Currant Anthocyanosides in Cynomologus Monkeys on a Fat Diet." *Journal of Pharmacology* (October–December 1984) 15(4):439–445.

EGGPLANT

Ibuki, F., et al. "An Improved Method for the Purification of Eggplant Trypsin Inhibitor." *Journal of Nutri. Sci. and Vitaminology* (1977) 23(2):133–143.

Mitschek, G.H. "Effect of Solanum Melongena on Experimental Atheromatosis. VI. Enzyme Histochemical, Physiopathological and Chemical Studies on Cholesterol-Induced Atheromatosis in Rabbits. Conclusions" (author's transl). *Experimentelle Pathologie* (1975) 10(3–4):167–179.

FIG

Kochi, M., et al. "Antitumor Activity of a Benzaldehyde Derivative." *Cancer Treat. Rep.* (May 1985) 69(5):533–537.

Takeuchi, S., et al. "Benzaldehyde as a Carcinostatic Principle in Figs." *Agric. Biol. Chem.* (1978) 42(7):1449–1551.

FISH

Altschule, M.D. "A Tale of Two Lipids. Cholesterol and Eicosapentaneoic Acid." *Chest* (1986) 89(4):601–602.

Carroll, K.K. "Biological Effects of Fish Oils in Relation to Chronic Diseases." *Lipids* (1986) 21(12):731–732.

Cartwright, I.J., et al. "The Effects of Dietary Omega-3 Polyunsaturated Fatty Acids on Erythrocyte Membrane Phospholipids, Erythrocyte Deformability and Blood Viscosity in Healthy Volunteers." *Atherosclerosis* (June 1985) 55(3):267–281.

Chanmugam, P., et al. "Differences in the W3 Fatty Acid Contents in Pond-Reared and Wild Fish and Shellfish." *Journal of Food Science* (1986) 51(6):1556–1557.

Harris, W.S. "Health Effects of Omega-3 Fatty Acids." *Contemporary Nutrition* (August 1985) 10(8).

Herold, P.M., et al. "Fish Oil Consumption and Decreased Risk of Cardiovascular Disease: A Comparison of Findings from Animal and Human Feeding Trials." *American Journal of Clinical Nutrition* (April 1986) 43(4):566–598.

Kagawa, Y., et al. "Eicosapolenoic Acid of Serum of Japanese Islanders with Low Cardiovascular Disease." *J. Nutr. Sci. Vit.* (1982) 24:441.

Kinsella, J.E. "Food Components with Potential Therapeutic Benefits: The n-3 Polyunsaturated Fatty Acids of Fish Oils." *Food Technology* (February 1986) 89–97.

Kragballe, K., et al. "Arachidonic Acid in Psoriasis. Pathogenic Role and Pharmacological Regulation." *Acta. Derm. Venereol.* (Suppl.) (1985) 120:12–17.

Kromhout, D., et al. "The Inverse Relation between Fish Consumption and 20-Year Mortality from Coronary Heart Disease." *New England Journal of Medicine* (May 9, 1985) 312(19):1205–1254.

Lands, W.E.M. *Fish and Human Health.* Orlando, Fla.: Academic Press, Inc., 1983.

Podell, R.N. "Nutritional Treatment of Rheumatoid Arthritis. Can Alterations in Fat Intake Affect Disease Course?" *Postgraduate Medicine* (May 15, 1985) 77(7):68–69, 72.

Robinson, D.R., et al. "The Protective Effect of Dietary Fish Oil on Murine Lupus." *Prostaglandins* (July 1985) 30(1):51–75.

Singer, P., et al. "Long-Term Effect of Mackerel Diet on Blood Pressure, Serum Lipids and Thromboxane Formation in Patients with Mild Essential Hypertension." *Atherosclerosis* (1986) 62:259–265.

Weber, P.C. "Dietary Supplementation of Eicosapentaenoic Acid (C20:5 Omega-2; EPA), Platelet Function and Blood Pressure Regulation." *Br. J. Clin. Pract.* (Symp. Suppl.) (1984) 31:122–125.

Woodcock, B.E., et al. "Beneficial Effect of Fish Oil on Blood Viscosity in Peripheral Vascular Disease." *Br. Med. J.* (Clin. Res.) (February 25, 1984) 288(6417):592–594.

GARLIC

Apitz-Castro, R., et al. "Ajoene, the Antiplatelet Principle of Garlic, Synergistically Potentiates the Antiaggregatory Action of Prostacyclin, Forskolin, Indomethacin and Dypiridamole on Human Platelets." *Thrombosis Research* (1986) 42(3):303–311.

Augusti, K.T. "Hypercholesteraemic Effect of Garlic (Allium sativum Linn.)." *Ind. J. Exp. Biol.* (1977) 15:489.

Block, E. "The Chemistry of Garlic and Onions." *Scientific American* (March 1985) 114–119.

Bordia, A.K., et al. "Effect of the Essential Oil (Active Principle) of Garlic on Serum Cholesterol, Plasma Fibrinogen Whole Blood Coagulation Time and Fibrinolytic Activity in Alimentary Lipaemia." *J. Assoc. Phys. Ind.* (1974) 22:267.

Bordia, A. K., et al. "Effect of the Essential Oils of Garlic and Onion on Alimentary Hyperlipemia." *Atherosclerosis* (1975) 21:15–19.

Bordia, A. K. "Effect of Garlic on Blood Lipids in Patients with Coronary Heart Disease." *American Journal of Clinical Nutrition* (1981) 34:2100.

Bordia, A.K., et al. "Essential Oil of Garlic on Blood Lipids and Fibrinolytic Activity in Patients with Coronary Artery Disease." *Atherosclerosis* (1977) 28:155.

Chutani, S.K., et al. "The Effect of Fried vs. Raw Garlic on Fibrinolytic Activity in Man." *Atherosclerosis* (1981) 38:417.

Delaha, E.C., et al. "Inhibition of Mycobacteria by Garlic Extract (Allium sativum)." *Antimicrobial Agents and Chemotherapy* (April 1985) 27(4):485–486.

Departments of Neurology and Traditional Chinese Medicine and Pharmacology of the First Affiliated Hospital and Departments of Microbiology, Hunan Medical College, Changsha. "Garlic in Cryptococcal Meningitis: A Preliminary Report of 21 Cases." *Chinese Medical Journal* (1980) 93(2):123;126.

Fenwick, G.R. "The Genus Allium–Part 3." *CRC Crit. Rev. Food Sci. Nutri.* (1985) 23(1):1–73.

Lau, B.H.S., et al. "Allium Sativum (Garlic) and Atherosclerosis: A Review." *Nutrition Research* (1983) 3:119–128.

Sainani, G.S., et al. "Effect of Dietary Garlic and Onion on Serum Lipid Profile in Jain Community." *Ind. J. Med. Res.* (1979) 69:776.

Srivastava, K.C. "Evidence for the Mechanism by Which Garlic Inhibits Platelet Aggregation." *Prostaglandins, Leukotrienes, and Medicine* (1986) 22:313–321.

Sucur, M. "Effect of Garlic on Serum Lipids and Lipoproteins in Patients Suffering from Hyperlipoproteinemia." *Diabetol. Croatica* (1980) 9:323.

Tsai, Y., et al. "Antiviral Properties of Garlic: In Vitro Effects on Influenza B, Herpes Simplex and Coxsackie Viruses." *Planta Medica* (October 1985) 5:460–461.

GINGER

Dorso, Charles R., et al. "Correspondence." *New England Journal of Medicine* (September 25, 1980) 303(13):756–757.

Giri, J., et al. "Effect of Ginger on Serum Cholesterol Levels." *Ind. J. Nutr. Dietet.* (October 1984) 21:433–436.

Srivastava, K.C. "Effects of Aqueous Extracts of Onion, Garlic and Ginger on Platelet Aggregation and Metabolism of Arachidonic Acid in the Blood Vascular System: In Vitro Study. *Prostaglandins, Leukotrienes, and Medicine* (1984) 13:227–235.

GRAPE

Konowalchuk, J., et al. "Virus Inactivation by Grapes and Wines." *Applied Environmental Microbiology* (December 1976) 32(6):757–763.

Masquelier, J. "The Bactericidal Action of Certain Phenolics of Grapes and Wine." *The Pharmacology of Plant Phenolics.* New York: Academic Press, 1959.

Shackleton, B. *The Grape Cure: A Living Testament,* London: Thorsons Publishers Limited, 1964, pp. 111–128.

GRAPEFRUIT

Baig, M.M., et al. "Citrus, Pectic Polysaccharides—Their In Vitro Interaction with Low Density Serum Lipoproteins." *ACS Symposium Series* (1983) 214:185–190.

Baig, M.M., et al. "Studies on the Role of Citrus in Health and Disease." *ACS Symposium Series* (1980) 143:25–41.

Kroyer, G. "The Antioxidant Activity of Citrus Fruit Peels." *Z. Ernahrungswiss* (March 1986) 25(1):63–69.

HONEY

Armon, P.J. "The Use of Honey in the Treatment of Infected Wounds." *Tropical Doctor* (April 1980) 10(2):91.

Bergman, A., et al. "Acceleration of Wound Healing by Topical Application of Honey: An Animal Model." *American Journal of Surgery* (March 1983) 145(3):374–376.

Haffejee, I.E., et al. "Honey in the Treatment of Infantile Gastroenteritis." *British Medical Journal* (June 1985) 290:1866–1867.

Jeddar, A., et al. "The Antibacterial Action of Honey." *South African Medical Journal* (February 1985) 67(7):257–258.

Majno, G. *The Healing Hand: Man and Wound in the Ancient World.* Cambridge, Mass.: Harvard University Press, 1975.

KALE

Khachik, F., et al. "Separation, Identification, and Quantification of the Major Carotenoid and Chlorophyll Constituents in Extracts of Several Green Vegetables by Liquid Chromatography." *Journal of Agricultural & Food Chemistry* (July–August 1986) 34(4):603–616.

MacLennan, R., et al. "Risk Factors for Lung Cancer in Singapore Chinese, a Population with High Female Incidence Rates." *Int. J. Cancer* (1977) 20:854–860.

LEMON AND LIME

Kroyer, G. "The Antioxidant Activity of Citrus Fruit Peels." *Z. Ernahrungswiss* (March 1986) 25(1):63–69.

Risch, H.A., et al. "Dietary Factors and the Incidence of Cancer of the Stomach." *American Journal of Epidemiology* (1985) 122(6):947–957.

MELON

Altman, R., et al. "Identification of Platelet Inhibitor Present in the Melon (Cucurbitacea Cucumis Melo)." *Thrombosis and Haemostatis* (1985) 53(3):312–313.

MILK

Bellanti, J.A. (ed.). *Acute Diarrhea: Its Nutritional Consequences in Children.* New York: Raven Press, 1983.

Editorial. "Milk Fat, Diarrhoea, and the Ileal Brake." *Lancet* (March 22, 1986).

Garland, C., et al. "Dairy Vitamin D and Calcium and Risk of Colorectal Cancer: A 19-Year Prospective Study in Men." *Lancet* (February 9, 1985) 307–309.

Kiyosawa, H., et al. "Effects of Skim Milk and Yogurt on Serum Lipids, Development of Atherosclerosis and Excretion of Fecal Sterols in Cholesterol–Fed Rabbits." *Sapporo Medical Journal* (1984) 53(5):493–504.

Koopman, J.S. "Milk Fat and Gastrointestinal Illness." *American Journal of Public Health* (December 1984) 74:1371–1373.

Kumar, N. "Effect of Milk on Patients with Duodenal Ulcers." *British Medical Journal* (September 13, 1986) 293:666.

Materia, A., et al. "Prostaglandins in Commercial Milk Preparations: Their Effect in the Prevention of Stress-Induced Gastric Ulcer." *Archives of Surgery* (March 1984) 119:290–292.

Mietens, C., et al. "Treatment of Infantile E. coli Gastroenteritis with Specific Bovine Anti-E. coli Milk Immunoglobulins." *European Journal of Pediatrics* (1979) 132:239–252.

Paffenberger, R.S., Jr. "Chronic Disease Among Former College Students." *American Journal of Epidemiology* (1974) 100:307–315.

Tockman, M.S., et al. "Milk-Drinking and Possible Protection of the Respiratory Epithelium." *Journal of Chronic Diseases* (1986) 39(3):207–209.

Yolken, R.H. "Antibody to Human Rotavirus in Cow's Milk." *New England Journal of Medicine* (March 7, 1985) 312:605–610.

MUSHROOM

Cheng, T.O. "Changing Prevalence of Heart Diseases in People's Republic of China." *Annals of Internal Medicine* (1974) 80:108–109.

Chibata, I., et al. "Lentinan: A New Hypocholesterolemic Substance in Lentinus Edodes." *Experientia* (1969) 25:1237.

Chihara, G. "Experimental Studies on Growth Inhibition and Regression of Cancer Metastases." *Gan to Kagaju Ryoho* (June 1985) 12(6):1196–1209.

Hammerschmidt, D.E. "Szechuan Purpura." *New England Journal of Medicine* (May 22, 1980) 302(21):1191–1193.

Makheja, A.N., et al. "Identification of the Antiplatelet Substance in Chinese Black Tree Fungus." *New England Journal of Medicine* (1981) 304(3):175.

Sugano, N., et al. "Anticarcinogenic Actions of Water-Soluble and Alcohol-Insoluble Fractions from Culture Medium of Lentinus Edodes Mycelia." *Cancer Letters* (1982) 17:109–114.

Takehara, M., et al. "Isolation and Antiviral Activities of the Double-Strained RNA from Lentinus Edodes (Shiitake)." *Kobe Journal of Medical Science* (August 1984) 30(3–4):25–34.

Tam, S.C., et al. "Hypotensive and Renal Effects of an Extract of the Edible Mushroom Pleurotus Sajor-caju." *Life Sci.* (March 1986) 38(13): 1155–1161.

NUTS

Senter, S.D., et al. "Comparative GLC-MS Analysis of Phenolic Acids of Selected Tree Nuts." *Journal of Food Science* (1983) 48:798–800.

Wood, A.W., et al. "Inhibition of the Mutagenicity of Bay-Region Diol Epoxides of Polycyclic Aromatic Hydrocarbons by Naturally Occurring Plant Phenols: Exceptional Activity of Ellagic Acid." *Proceedings of the National Academy of Science* USA (September 1982) 79:5513–5517.

OATS

Anderson, J.W. "Physiological and Metabolic Effects of Dietary Fiber." *Fed. Proc.* (November 1985) 44(14):2902–2906.

Degroot, A.P., et al. "Cholesterol-Lowering Effect of Rolled Oats." *Lancet* (1983) 2:203–204.

Judd, P.A., et al. "The Effect of Rolled Oats on Blood Lipids and Fecal Steroid Excretion in Man." *American Journal of Clinical Nutrition* (1981) 34:2061.

Kirby, R.W., et al. "Oat-Bran Intake Selectively Lowers Serum Low-Density Lipoprotein Cholesterol Concentrations of Hypercholesterolemic Men." *American Journal of Clinical Nutrition* (May 1981) 34:824–829.

Roth, G., et al. "Long-Term Influence of Breakfast Cereals Rich in Dietary Fibers on Human Blood Lipid Values." *Aktuel Ernarh* (1985) 10:106–109.

Saeed, S.A., et al. "Inhibitor(s) of Prostaglandin Biosynthesis in Extracts of Oat (Avena sativa) Seeds." *Biochem. Soc. Trans.* (1981) 9:444.

Valle-Jones, J.C. "An Open Study of Oat-Bran Meal Biscuits ('Lejfibre') in the Treatment of Constipation in the Elderly." *Curr. Med. Res. Opin.* (1985) 9(10):716–720.

Van Horn, L.V., et al. "Serum Lipid Response to Oat Product Intake with a Fat-Modified Diet." *Journal of the American Dietetic Association* (June 1986) 86(6):759–764.

OLIVE OIL

Ferro-Luzzi, A., et al. "Changing the Mediterranean Diet: Effects on Blood Lipids." *American Journal of Clinical Nutrition* (November 1984) 40:1027–1037.

Grundy, S.M. "Comparison of Monounsaturated Fatty Acids and Carbohydrates for Lowering Plasma Cholesterol." *New England Journal of Medicine* (March 20, 1986) 314(12):745–748.

Keys, A., et al. "The Diet and 15-Year Death Rate in the Seven Countries Study." *American Journal of Epidemiology* (December 1986) 124(6): 903–915.

Sirtori, C.R., et al. "Controlled Evaluation of Fat Intake in the Mediterranean Diet: Comparative Activities of Olive Oil and Corn Oil on Plasma Lipids and Platelets in High-Risk Patients." *American Journal of Clinical Nutrition* (1986) 44:635–642.

Zoppi, S., et al. "Effectiveness and Reliability of Medium Term Treatment with a Diet Rich in Olive Oil of Patients with Vascular Diseases." *Acta Vitaminol. Enzymol.* (Italy) (1985) 7(1–2):3–8.

ONION

Attrep, K.A., et al. "Separation and Identification of Prostaglandin A1 in Onion." *Lipids* (1980) 15:292.

Augusti, K.T., et al. "Partial Identification of the Fibrinolytic Activators in Onion." *Atherosclerosis* (1975) 21:409–416.

Bordia, A., et al. "The Effect of Active Principle of Garlic and Onion on Blood Lipids and Experimental Atherosclerosis in Rabbits and Their Comparison with Clofibrate." *J. Assoc. Phys. Ind.* (1977) 25:509.

Gupta, N.N., et al. "Effect of Onion on Serum Cholesterol, Blood Coagulation Factors and Fibrinolytic Activity in Alimentary Lipaemia." *Ind. J. Med. Res.* (1966) 54(1):48–53.

Jain, R.C., et al. "Onion and Blood Fibrinolytic Activity." *British Medical Journal* (1969) 258:514.

Sharma, K.K., et al. "Antihyperglycaemic Effect of Onion: Effect on Fasting Blood Sugar and Induced Hyperglycemia in Man." *Ind. J. Med.* (1977) 65:422.

Sudhakaran Menon, I. "Onions and Blood Fibrinolysis." *British Medical Journal* (1970) 421.

ORANGE

Baig, M.M., et al. "Studies on the Role of Citrus in Health and Disease." *ACS Symposium Series* (1980) 143:25–41.

Ganguly, R., et al. "Effect of Orange Juice on Attenuated Rubella Virus Infection." *Indian J. Med. Res.* (September 1977) 66(3):359–363.

Kroyer, G. "The Antioxidant Activity of Citrus Fruit Peels." *Z. Ernahrungswiss* (March 1986) 25(1):63–69.

PEA

Barker, D.J.P., et al. "Vegetable Consumption and Acute Appendicitis in 59 Areas in England and Wales." *British Medical Journal* (April 5, 1986) 292:927–930.

Beiler, J.M., et al. "Anti-Fertility Activity of Pisum Sativum." *Experimental Medicine and Surgery* (1953) 11:179–185.

Sanyal, S.N. "Ten Years of Research on an Oral Contraceptive from Pisum Sativum." *Science and Culture* (June 1960) 25 (12):661–665.

POTATO

Brandl, W., et al. "Occurrence of Chlorogenic Acids in Potatoes." *Z. Lebensm Unters Porsch* (1984) 178(3):192–194.

Kantorovich-Prokudina, E.N., et al. "Effects of Protease Inhibitors on Influenza Virus Reproduction." *Vopr. Virusol* (July–August 1982) 27(4):452–456.

PRUNE

Hull, C., et al. "Alleviation of Constipation in the Elderly by Dietary Fiber Supplementation." *Journal of the American Geriatrics Society* (September 1980) 28(9):410–414.

RICE

Kempner, W., et al. "Treatment of Massive Obesity with Rice/Reduction Diet Program." *Archives of Internal Medicine* (December 1975) 135:1575–1584.

Khin-Maung-U, et al. "Effect of Boiled-Rice Feeding in Childhood Cholera on Clinical Outcome." *Human Nutrition: Clinical Nutrition* (1986) 40C:249–254.

Newborg, B. "Disappearance of Psoriatic Lesions on the Rice Diet." *North Carolina Medical Journal* (January 1986) 47(1):253–255.

Ohkawa, T., et al. "Rice Bran Treatment for Patients with Hypercalciuric Stones: Experimental and Clinical Studies." *Journal of Urology* (December 1984) 132:1140–1145.

Rahman, A.S.M.M. "Mothers Can Prepare and Use Rice-Salt Oral Rehydration Solution in Rural Bangladesh." *Lancet* (September 7, 1985) 539–540.

SEAWEED, OR KELP

Fujihara, M., et al. "Purification and Chemical and Physical Characterization of an Antitumor Polysaccharide from the Brown Seaweed Sargassum fulvellum." *Carbohyd. Res.* (1984) 125:97–106.

Funayama, S., et al. "Hypotensive Principle of Laminaria and Allied Seaweeds." *Journal of Medicinal Plant Research* (January 1981) 41(1):29–33.

Furusawa, E., et al. "Anticancer Activity of a Natural Product, Viva-Natural, Extracted from Undaria pinnantifida on Intraperitoneally Implanted Lewis Lung Carcinoma." *Oncology* (1985) 42(6):364–369.

Hopps, H.A., et al. (eds.). *Marine Algae in Pharmaceutical Science.* New York: DeGruyter, 1982, xi (309):111.

Shimada, A. "Regional Differences in Gastric Cancer Mortality and Eating Habits of People." *Gan. No. Rinsho* (May 1986) 32(6):692–698.

Teas, J. "The Consumption of Seaweed as a Protective Factor in the Etiology of Breast Cancer." *Medical Hypotheses* (1981) 7:(5)601–613.

Teas, J. "The Dietary Intake of Laminaria, a Brown Seaweed, and Breast Cancer Prevention." *Nutrition Cancer* (1983) 4(3):217–222.

Teas, J., et al. "Dietary Seaweed (Laminaria) and Mammary Carcinogenesis in Rats." *Cancer Research* (July 1984) 44(7):2758–2761.

Yamamoto, I., et al. "Antitumor Activity of Edible Marine Algae: Effect of Crude Fucoidan Fractions Prepared from Edible Brown Seaweeds against L-1210 Leukemia." *Hydrobiologia* (1984) 116/117:145–148.

Yamori, Y., et al. "Dietary Prevention of Stroke and Its Mechanisms in Stroke-Prone Spontaneously Hypertensive Rats—Preventive Effect of Dietary Fibre and Palmitoleic Acid." *J. Hypertens* (Suppl.) (October 1986) 4(3):S449–S452.

SHELLFISH

Childs, M.T., et al. "Effect of Shellfish Consumption on Cholesterol Absorption in Normolipidemic Men." *Metabolism* (January 1987) 36(1): 31–35.

SOYBEAN

Grundy, S.M., et al. "Comparison of Actions of Soy Protein and Casein on Metabolism of Plasma Lipoproteins and Cholesterol in Humans." *American Journal of Clinical Nutrition* (August 1983) 38:245–252.

Lo, G.S., et al. "Soy Fiber Improves Lipid and Carbohydrate Metabolism in Primary Hyperlipidemic Subjects." *Atherosclerosis* (1986) 62:239–248.

Messadi, D.V., et al. "Inhibition of Oral Carcinogenesis by a Protease Inhibitor." *Journal of the National Cancer Institute* (March 1986) 76(3):447–452.

Sirtori, C.R., et al. *Studies on the Use of a Soybean Protein Diet for the Management of Human Hyperlipoproteinemias. Animal and Vegetable Proteins in Lipid Metabolism and Atherosclerosis.* New York: Alan R. Liss, Inc., 1983, pp. 135–148.

Takeshi, H. "Epidemiology of Human Carcinogenesis: A Review of Food-Related Diseases." Stich, H.F., *Carcinogens and Mutagens in the Environment*, Vol. I, 1982 ed., pp. 13–30.

Troll, W., et al. "Soybean Diet Lowers Breast Tumor Incidence in Irradiated Rats." *Carcinogenesis* (June 1980) 1:469–472.

SPINACH

Barale, R., et al. "Vegetables Inhibit, In Vivo, the Mutagenicity of Nitrite Combined with Nitrosable Compounds." *Mutation Research* (1983) 120:145–150.

Iritani, N., et al. "Effect of Spinach and Wakame on Cholesterol Turnover in the Rat." *Atherosclerosis* (1972) 15:87–92.

Lai, C-N., et al. "Antimutagenic Activities of Common Vegetables and Their Chlorophyll Content." *Mutation Research* (1980) 77:245–250.

Marshall, J.R., et al. "Diet and Smoking in the Epidemiology of Cancer of the Cervix." *Journal of the National Cancer Institute* (May 1983) 70(5):847–851.

SQUASH (INCLUDING PUMPKIN)

Wieczorek, M., et al. "The Squash Family of Serine Proteinase Inhibitors. Amino Acid Sequences and Association Equilibrium Constants of Inhibitors from Squash, Summer Squash, Zucchini, and Cucumber Seeds." *Biochemical and Biophysical Research Communications* (January 31, 1985) 126(2):646–652.

SUGAR

Bollenback, G.N. "The Sweet Story of Sugar's Amazing Healing Powers." *Nutrition Today* (January-February 1986) 25–27.

Brewerton, T.D., et al. "Psychiatric Aspects of the Relationship Between Eating and Mood." *Nutrition Reviews* (Suppl.) (May 1986) 44:78–88.

Fernstrom, J.D. "Acute and Chronic Effects of Protein and Carbohydrate Ingestion on Brain Tryptophan Levels and Serotonin Synthesis." *Nutrition Reviews* (Suppl.) (May 1986) 44:25–36.

Kruesi, M.J.P. "Carbohydrate Intake and Children's Behavior." *Food Technology* (January 1986) 150–152.

Kruesi, M.J.P. "Diet and Human Behavior: How Much Do They Affect Each Other?" *Ann. Rev. Nutr.* (1986) 6:113–130.

Spring, B.J., et al. "Effects of Carbohydrates on Mood and Behavior." *Nutrition Reviews* (Suppl.) (May 1986) 44:51–60.

Wurtman, J.J. *Managing Your Mind and Mood Through Food.* New York: Rawson Associates, 1986.

Wurtman, J.J. "Ways That Foods Can Affect the Brain." *Nutrition Reviews* (Suppl.) (May 1986) 44:2–6.

TEA

Bokuchava, M.A., et al. "The Biochemistry and Technology of Tea Manufacture." *CRC Crit. Rev. Food Sci. Nutr.* (1980) 12(4):303–370.

Dubey, P., et al. "Effect of Tea on Gastric Acid Secretions." *Digestive Diseases and Sciences* (March 1984) 29(3):202–206.

Friedman, M., et al. "Fluoride Concentrations in Tea. Its Uptake by Hydroxyapatite and Effect on Dissolution Rate." *Clinical Preventive Dentistry* (January–February 1984) 6(1):20–22.

Henry, J.P., et al. "Reduction of Chronic Psychosocial Hypertension in Mice by Decaffeinated Tea." *Hypertension* (May–June 1981) 6(3):437–444.

John, T.J., et al. "Virus Inhibition by Tea, Caffeine and Tannic Acid." *Indian J. Med. Res.* (April 1979) 69:542–545.

Kada, T. "Desmutagens: An Overview." Stich, H.F. (ed.), *Carcinogens and Mutagens in the Environment*, Vol. II. Boca Raton, Florida: CRC Press, Inc., 1983, pp. 63–83.

Kada, T., et al. "Detection and Chemical Identification of Natural Bio-Antimutagens. A Case of the Green Tea Factor." *Mutation Research* (1985) 150:127–132.

Kashket, S., et al. "In-Vitro Inhibition of Glucosyltransferase from the Dental Plaque Bacterium Streptococcus Mutans by Common Beverages and Food Extracts." *Archs Oral Biol.* (1985) 30(11–12):821–826.

Oguni, I.K., et al. "On the Regional Differences in the Mortality of Cancer for Cities, Towns and Villages of Shizuoka Prefecture (1972–1978)." *Annual Report of Shizuoka Women's College*, No. 29 (1981) 49–93.

Onisi, M., et al. "Epidemiological Evidence about the Caries Preventive Effect of Drinking Tea." *Journal of Preventive Dentistry* (1980) 6:321–325.

Rosen, S., et al. "Anticariogenic Effects of Tea in Rats." *J. Dent. Res.* (May 1984) 63(5):658–660.

Stich, H.F., et al. "Inhibition of Mutagenicity of a Model Nitrosation Reaction by Naturally Occurring Phenolics, Coffee and Tea." *Mutat. Res.* (August 1982) 95(2–3):119–128.

Stich, H.F., et al. "Inhibitory Effects of Phenolics, Teas and Saliva on the Formation of Mutagenic Nitrosation Products of Salted Fish." *Int. J. Cancer* (December 15, 1982) 30(6):719–724.

Tanizawa, H., et al. "Natural Antioxidants. I. Antioxidative Components of Tea Leaf (Thea sinensis L.)." *Chem. Pharm. Bull.* (1984) 32(5): 2011–2014.

Young, W., et al. "Tea and Atherosclerosis." *Nature* (December 9, 1967) 216:1015–1016.

TOMATO

Taberner, P.V. *Aphrodisiacs: The Science and the Myth*. Philadelphia: University of Pennsylvania, 1985, p. 60.

WHEAT BRAN

Benson, J.A., Jr., et al. "Simple Chronic Constipation." *Postgraduate Medicine* (1975) 57:55.

Burkitt, D.P., et al. "How to Manage Constipation with High-Fiber Diet." *Geriatrics* (February 1979) 33–40.

Burkitt, D.P., et al. *Refined Carbohydrate Foods and Disease*. London and New York: Academic Press, Inc., 1975.

Cummings, J.H., et al. "Colonic Response to Dietary Fibre from Carrot, Cabbage, Apple, Bran and Guar Gum." *Lancet* (January 7, 1978) 5–8.

Cummings, J.H. "Short Chain Fatty Acids in the Human Colon." *Gut* (1981) 22:763–779.

Talbot, J.M. "Role of Dietary Fiber in Diverticular Disease and Colon Cancer." *Federation Proceedings* (Federation of American Societies for Experimental Biology) (July 1981) 40(9):2337–2342.

WINE

Masquelier, J. "The Bactericidal Action of Certain Phenolics of Grapes and Wine." *The Pharmacology of Plant Phenolics*. New York: Academic Press, 1959.

YOGURT

Alm, L. "Survival Rate of Salmonella and Shigella in Fermented Milk Products with and without Added Human Gastric Juice: An In Vitro Study." *Prog. Food Nutr. Sci.* (1983) 7(3–4):19–28.

Friend, B.A., et al. "Nutritional and Therapeutic Aspects of Lactobacilli." *Journal of Applied Nutrition* (1984) 36(2):125–153.

Goldin, B.R., et al. "The Effect of Milk and Lactobacillus Feeding on Human Intestinal Bacterial Enzyme Activity." *American Journal of Clinical Nutrition* (1984) 39:756–761.

Hamdan, I.Y., et al. "Acidolin: An Antibiotic Produced by Lactobacillus Acidophilus." *Journal of Antibiotics* (August 1974) 27(8):631–636.

Hepner, G., et al. "Hypocholesterolemic Effect of Yogurt and Milk." *American Journal of Clinical Nutrition* (January 1979) 32:19–24.

Kiyosawa, H., et al. "Effect of Skim Milk and Yogurt on Serum Lipids and Development of Sudanophilic Lesions in Cholesterol-Fed Rabbits." *American Journal of Clinical Nutrition* (September 1984) 40(3):479–484.

Le, M.G., et al. "Consumption of Dairy Produce and Alcohol in a Case-Control Study of Breast Cancer." *Journal of the National Cancer Institute* (September 1986) 77(3):633–636.

Lankester, E.R. "Elias Metchnikoff." *Nature* (July 27, 1916) 97(2439): 443–446.

Mann, G.V. "Factor in Yogurt Which Lowers Cholesteremia in Man." *Atherosclerosis* (1977) 26(3):335–340.

Metchnikoff, Elias. *The Prolongation of Life. Optimistic Studies.* London: William Heinemann, 1907.

Niv, M., et al. "Yogurt—In the Treatment of Infantile Diarrhea." *Clinical Pediatrics* (July 1963) 2(7):407–411.

Reddy, G.V., et al. "Antitumor Activity of Yogurt Components." *J. Food Prot.* (1983) 46:8–11.

Savaiano, D.A., et al. "Nutritional and Therapeutic Aspects of Fermented Dairy Products." *Contemporary Nutrition* (June 1984) 9(6).

Shahani, K.M., et al. "Properties of and Prospects for Cultured Dairy Foods." *Soc. Appl. Bacteriol. Symp. Ser.* (1983) 11:257–269.

Vesely, R., et al. "Influence of a Diet Additioned with Yogurt on the Mouse Immune System." *EOS—Journal of Immunology and Immunopharmacology* (1985) 5(1):30–35.

INDEX

A

Abdominal cancer, 211
Abdullah, Tarig, 200–201, 205
Abortion, 224
Acetaminophen, 153
Acidophilin, 95
Acidophilus. *See* Yogurt
Acquired immune deficiency syndrome.
    See AIDS
Actifed, 47
Adenosine, 27, 32, 33, 225
Aflatoxin, 61, 149, 238
Aging, 17–18
    See also Elderly; Longevity
Agoraphobia, 175
Agriculture Department. *See* United
    States Department
    of Agriculture
AIDS (acquired immune deficiency
    syndrome), 5, 200–201
Ajoene, 202
Alcoholic beverages. *See* Beer; Wine
Allergy, 218, 318
Allicin, 5, 6, 14, 47, 199–200, 203
Alliin, 47
Allyl isothiocyanate, 47
American Health Foundation, 265, 268
American Journal of Epidemiology, 58
American Medicine, 114, 151, 278
American Psychiatric Association, 176
Ampicillin, 80
Amygdalin, 119

Anderson, James, 38–42, 133, 135,
    137–38, 240, 241
Anemia, 294–95
Anthocyanoside, 144–45, 184–85
Antibiotic (antibacterial), 82–83, 326
    cabbage as, 153
    cranberry as, 79–83, 182–83, 326
    eggs as, 105–107
    fruit as, 84–88, 90
    garlic as, 3–7, 199–200, 326
    honey as, 217–18, 326
    milk as, 101–107, 325
    onion as, 249–50
    seaweed as, 266
    tea as, 290–91, 323
    wine as, 306–307
    yogurt as, 95–99, 315–16, 325, 326
Anticoagulant
    aspirin as, 34, 202, 225
    Chinese mushroom as, 26, 236
    garlic as, 13, 26–27, 34, 202–203
    ginger as, 208–209
    melon as, 224–25
    olive oil as, 244
    onion as, 13, 27, 32–33, 34, 247
    seaweed as, 267
    tea as, 89
Anticonvulsant, 187
Antidepressant, 170, 285
Antiinflammatory agent, 89
    artichoke as, 121
    blueberry as, 185
    fish as, 193
    oats as, 241

Antioxidant
  beta carotene as, 76, 77
  lemon as, 223
  olive oil as, 244
  polyphenols as, 87
  potato as, 257, 312
  squash/pumpkin as, 281
  strawberry as, 283
  tea as, 292, 293, 295
  yam as, 312
Antiseptic, 306–307
Anxiety, 175
Aphrodisiac, 9, 297, 298
Aphrodisiacs: The Science and the
  Myth (Taberner), 297
Appendicitis, 255, 321
Apple, 85–86, 90, 114–17
Apricot, 118–19, 259
Arachidonic acid, 52, 54, 193
Argentina, 224
Armon, P.J., 217
Arthritis
  chili pepper and, 166
  fish and, 191, 193
  guide to, 321
  mushroom and, 235
  tomato and, 298
Artichoke, 120–21
Ascorbic acid. *See* Vitamin C
Aspirin
  as anticoagulant, 34, 202, 225
  effect on stomach, 124
  heart disease and, 34
  mechanism of, 53
  melon studies and, 225
  prostaglandins and, 34, 53
Asthma
  chili pepper and, 165
  coffee and, 170, 172–73, 174
  garlic and, 194
  guide to, 321
  honey and, 218
Astringent, 184
Atherosclerosis, 17
  blueberry and, 144
  eggplant and, 187
  grapefruit and, 214
  milk and, 228

soybean and, 275
tea and, 89, 292–93
Athletic performance, 171–72, 174
Australia
  bean studies in, 135
  coffee studies in, 176
  milk studies in, 227, 233

B

Bacteria. *See* Antibiotic (antibacterial)
Bailey, John Martyn, 27, 34
Banana, 122–25, 129–30
Bang, Hans Olaf, 53
Barefoot Doctor's Manual, A, 26
Barley, 36–38, 42, 126–31, 138
Bean, 12, 70, 116, 132–38
  See also Soybean
Beaumont, William, 38
Beer, 82, 88, 128–29, 139–42, 168
Benzaldehyde, 189
Benzoic acid, 11
Berra, Bruno, 244, 245
Best, Ralph, 123
Beta carotene, 14, 72–77
  as additive, 104
  in apricot, 119
  in carrot, 157–58
  in kale, 220, 221
  in melon, 225
  -polyphenol comparison, 88
  in spinach, 279
  in squash/pumpkin, 281
  in yam, 311, 313
Beta glucans, 127, 128
Bioflavonoids, 293
Birth defects, 175
Birth of twins, 312
Black currant, 144–45, 184–85
Bladder cancer
  coffee and, 173–74
  garlic and, 204
  guide to, 322
  kale and, 221
  milk and, 233
  squash/pumpkin and, 281
Bladder infection, 79–83, 180–83
Blau, Ludwig, 162

Block, Eric, 202
Blood clotting
  apple and, 117
  chili pepper and, 166–67
  Chinese mushroom and, 24–29,
    234–35, 236
  fish and, 54, 191–92
  garlic and, 5, 13, 26–27, 34, 201–202
  ginger and, 208–209
  mechanism of, 16, 32
  melon and, 225
  olive oil and, 242
  onion and, 13, 27, 32–34, 246–48, 247
  seaweed and, 267
  seeds and, 67–68
  shellfish and, 270
  tea and, 89
  See also Anticoagulant
Blood pressure
  apple and, 114, 116
  bean and, 134
  beer and, 141
  coffee and, 173, 174–75
  fiber and, 39
  fish and, 194–95
  garlic and, 5, 202–203
  milk and, 228–29, 233
  olive oil and, 242, 244
  onion and, 32, 249
  peas and, 254
  rice and, 261–62
  seaweed and, 267
  tea and, 88, 89, 292–93, 295–96
  wine and, 309
Blood sugar
  apple and, 114, 116
  bean and, 133–34, 135
  fiber and, 12, 38, 39
  fish and, 197
  nuts and, 238
  oats and, 239
  onion and, 249
  peas and, 254
  rice and, 261
  soybean and, 274–75
  table sugar and, 287
  tea and, 296
Blood thinners. *See* Anticoagulant

Blueberry, 143–45, 185
Bokuchava, Mikhail, 89, 292
Bordia, Arun K., 201
Bowel cancer, 221, 233
Brain function, 325
  blueberry and, 144–45
  coffee and, 170–71
  fish and, 190, 191, 195, 271
  milk and, 231–233
  shellfish and, 271–72
  sugar and, 285–86
  yogurt and, 317
Bran, 12
  oat, 39–42, 241
  rice, 262, 263
  wheat, 39, 90, 241, 301–304
Brandt, Johanna, 211
Breast cancer
  beer and, 141–42
  cabbage and, 59
  fiber and, 41
  guide to, 322
  milk and, 233
  rice and, 262
  seaweed and, 265–66
  soybean and, 67, 134, 276
  wine and, 309
  yogurt and, 97, 317
Breast disease, cystic, 175, 294
Breast milk, 12, 101
Brekhman, I.I., 295
Britain
  banana studies in, 123
  beer studies in, 140, 141
  bran studies in, 38, 41, 302–303, 304
  bronchitis in, 43
  carrot studies in, 72–73, 158
  fish studies in, 192
  onion studies in, 33, 247
  pea studies in, 255
  tea use in, 295
  wine studies in, 309
British Medical Journal, 35, 168
Broccoli, 56–63, 77, 146–47
Bronchitis, 43–47, 165, 203, 228, 250,
  325
Brown, Michael S., 16
Brussels sprouts, 56–63, 147–49

Bulgaria
  garlic studies in, 202–203
  yogurt studies in, 92, 97
Bulgarican. *See* Yogurt
Burger, Warren C., 37
Burkitt, Denis, 38, 302
Burks, Thomas, 166
Burr, Aaron, 188

C

Cabbage, 56–63, 147, 149, 150–55
Caffeic acid, 87, 88, 117, 212
Caffeine, 170–77, 294
Calcium, 227, 228, 232, 263
California State Department of Health, 229
Canada
  apple studies in, 116
  coffee studies in, 172
  fruit studies in, 84–86
  grape studies in, 211–212
  tea studies in, 291–92
  vitamin C studies in, 12
Cancer
  apple and, 117
  apricot and, 119
  barley and, 127
  bean and, 134–35
  beer and, 141–42
  bran and, 40–41, 42, 303–304
  broccoli and, 56–63, 146–47
  brussels sprouts and, 56–63, 148–49
  cabbage and, 56–63, 147, 149, 150–53, 155
  carrot and, 71–76, 156–59
  cauliflower and, 160–61
  chili pepper and, 107, 168
  Chinese mushroom and, 234–35, 236
  coffee and, 88, 173–74
  corn and, 178, 179
  eggplant and, 187
  fig and, 189
  garlic and, 203–204, 209, 250
  ginger and, 209
  grape and, 211, 212
  grapefruit and, 215

  guide to, 322
  heart disease link, 17–18
  kale and, 220–21
  meat and, 87–88
  melon and, 225
  milk and, 227–28, 233
  nuts and, 64–70, 237–38
  oats and, 241
  olive oil and, 244
  onion and, 250
  orange and, 251–52
  peas and, 254
  potato and, 256–57, 311–12
  rice and, 262, 263
  seaweed and, 265–66
  seeds and, 64–70, 127, 134
  soybean and, 64, 66–68, 275–76
  spinach and, 278–79
  squash/pumpkin and, 280–81
  strawberry and, 283
  tea and, 8, 87–90, 291–92, 294, 295
  tomato and, 297–98
  turnip and, 299–300
  wine and, 308, 309
  vitamin C and, 12, 215
  yam and, 311–12
  yogurt and, 97–98, 316–17
  See also specific type, e.g., Colon cancer
Cancer Research, 59
Cantaloupe, 224–25
Canthaxanthin, 76
Capillary function, 89, 292
Capsaicin, 46, 47, 107, 165–68
Carbenoxolone, 123
Carbohydrate, 285–87
Cardiovascular system, 322
  See also Heart disease
Carotenoids, 71–78
  in kale, 220, 221
  in melon, 225
  in spinach, 279
  in squash/pumpkin, 281
  in turnip, 300
Carroll, Kenneth, 179
Carrot, 71–78, 156–59, 278, 281
Catechin, 88–89, 90, 292, 294
Cato the Censor, 150

Cauliflower, 160–61
Cavallito, Chester J., 199
Cavities, 323
    See also Tooth decay
Celery, 154
Cerda, James, 214
Cervical cancer, 147, 279
Cheese, 232, 233
Cheney, Garnett, 153–55
Cherry, 162–63
Chicken soup, 44, 45, 48
Chick peas, 64–65, 70
Childs, Marian, 270–71
Chili pepper, 43–48, 107, 164–68
China
    garlic use in, 4, 6, 200, 202, 204
    ginseng use in, 9
    heart disease in, 26
    mushroom use in, 26, 235
Chinese mushroom, 24–29, 234–36
Chinese Vegetarian Cookbook (Lin), 26
Chive, 249
Chlorogenic acid, 90, 117, 257, 312
Chlorophyll, 279
Cholesterol, 16
    apple and, 114, 115, 117
    artichoke and, 120–21
    banana and, 124
    barley and, 36–38, 127–30
    bean and, 133
    beer and, 139–41
    blueberry and, 144–45, 185
    cancer link, 17
    carrot and, 158
    chili pepper and, 167
    Chinese mushroom and, 235
    coffee and, 175
    corn and, 179
    drugs for, 34, 121, 214, 312
    eggplant and, 186–87
    fiber and, 12, 37, 38–42
    fish and, 50, 53, 54, 192, 196
    garlic and, 13, 201–202, 204,
        248–49, 250
    grapefruit and, 12, 214–15
    guide to, 323
    lemon and, 223
    liver function and, 36–37

-lowering flour, 19
    milk and, 228, 233
    Nobel prize for, 16
    nuts and, 238
    oats and, 39–42, 112, 239–41
    olive oil and, 242–44, 245
    onion and, 13, 30–34, 112, 246–48
    orange and, 252
    rice and, 261
    seaweed and, 267
    shellfish and, 269–71
    soybean and, 275
    spinach and, 279
    strawberry and, 283
    tea and, 293
    in vegetarians, 35–38
    wine and, 307
    yam and, 312
    yogurt and, 317, 318
Cholestyramine, 41, 214, 312
Cimetidine, 123, 230
Cinnamic acid, 90
Circulation, 13
    See also Anticoagulant; Blood clotting
Citrus fruit, 12, 111, 215
    See also Grapefruit; Lemon; Lime
Cochran, Kenneth, 235
Cod liver oil, 191, 196
Coffee, 88, 90, 169–77, 292
Colds
    apple and, 116
    black currant and, 184
    chili pepper and, 43–48, 165–66
    garlic and, 203
    onion and, 246, 250
Cold sore, 87, 309
Colon cancer, 107
    bean and, 134–35
    beer and, 141
    bran and, 40–41, 302, 303–304
    broccoli and, 57–58, 61–62, 147
    brussels sprouts and, 57–58, 61–62,
        147–49
    cabbage and, 57–58, 61–62,
        147–153, 155
    carrot and, 159
    cauliflower and, 160
    coffee and, 173–74

Colon cancer (*continued*)
  garlic and, 204
  guide to, 322
  kale and, 221
  milk and, 227, 233
  oats and, 241
  rice and, 262
  seaweed and, 266, 268
  soybean and, 67–68, 276
  spinach and, 279
  wine and, 309
  yogurt and, 97, 316–17
Conjunctivitis, 166
Constipation
  barley and, 128
  bean and, 135
  bran and, 41, 301–304
  carrot and, 158–59
  guide to, 323
  oats and, 241
  prunes and, 258–60
  tea and, 295
Contraceptives, 11, 253–54, 255, 276
Corn, 178–79
Cornell University, 149, 228–29
Coronary heart disease. *See* Heart disease
Correa, Pelayo, 67–68, 178
Corse, Joseph, 259
Cough, 133, 217
  See also Expectorant
Cranberry, 79–83, 180–83
CRC Critical Review in Food Science and Nutrition, 205
Cremer, Peter, 140–41
Crohn's disease, 304
Cummings, John H., 41, 302, 304
Currant, 144–45, 184–85
Cycloalliin, 33
Cynarin, 121
Cytotec, 229

D

Decongestant, 42–48, 165, 203
Delaha, Edward C., 3, 5
Denmark, 53, 54, 208
Depression, 133, 170, 285

Der Marderosian, Ara H., 182
DeSimone, Claudio, 96
Diabetes
  apple and, 116
  bean and, 133–34, 135
  corn and, 178
  drugs for, 249
  fiber and, 38, 39
  guide to, 325
  heart disease link, 17
  nuts and, 238
  onion and, 246
  potato and, 257
  rice and, 261
  soybean and, 274–75
Diarrhea
  apple and, 117
  black currant and, 184–85
  blueberry and, 143–44
  bran and, 304
  coffee and, 176
  egg and, 105–106
  drugs for, 144
  guide to, 325
  honey and, 218, 219
  milk and, 100–106, 230–31
  olive oil and, 245
  rice and, 262
  soybean and, 68–69
  yogurt and, 93, 314–16
Digestion, 189
Dithiolthiones, 60, 61, 152
Diuretic, 120, 178, 224
Diverticulitis, 241, 276, 325
Doctrine of Signatures, 8, 10
Dorso, Charles R., 209
Dramamine, 208
Duke, Jim, 153, 210
Duke University, 276
Dyerberg, Jorn, 53
Dysentery, 89, 94, 178, 290, 316
Dysmenorrhea, 26

E

Eczema, 241
Edinburgh Medical Journal, 170
Edinburgh New Dispensatory, 216

Egg, 105–107
Eggplant, 70, 186–87
Egypt, 249, 254
Ehret, Charles F., 177
Elderly
  coffee and, 173
  cranberry and, 181
  green/yellow vegetables and, 221
  raisins and, 212
  strawberry and, 283
  tomato and, 297
  wine and, 308
Ellagic acid, 87, 88, 90
Elson, Charles, 127
Emetic, 46, 47
Emphysema, 44, 47, 165, 325
*Encyclopedia of Natural Home
  Remedies* (Rodale), 143
  Endometrial cancer, 276, 279
Endorphin, 167
Energy (mental), 325
  See also Brain function
England. *See* Britain
Enoki, 236
Enzymes, 16
Epilepsy, 162, 187
Epsom salt, 259
Eskimos, 50–53, 192, 193
Esophageal cancer
  chili pepper and, 168
  guide to, 322
  kale and, 221
  peas and, 252
  spinach and, 279
  tea and, 294, 295
Essex County Geriatric Center (N.J.),
  259
Estrogen, 41, 276
Expectorant, 44, 46–47, 165, 203, 250
Experimental Gerontology, 185

F

Farnsworth, Norman, 10–12, 107, 254,
  295
Fat, dietary
  danger of, 49

fiber and, 39
fish and, 51–55, 196
in milk, 230–31, 233
olive oil and, 243–44, 245
onion and, 33, 247–48
seeds and, 68
in vegetables, 51–52
See also Cholesterol
Fertility, 11, 253–54, 255, 276
Ferulic acid, 87, 88, 90
Fiber
  in bananas, 124, 125
  cholesterol and, 12, 37, 38–42
  diabetes and, 38, 39
  in peas, 254
  physiology of, 40–41
  in prunes, 259
  in soybeans, 274
  See also Bran; Pectin
Fibrinogen, 32–33, 167, 202
Fibrinolytic system, 32–33, 166, 201,
  247
  See also Blood clotting
Fig, 188–89
Finland, 97, 231
Fish, 49–55, 190–97, 269–72
Fish oil capsules, 196–97
Fleming, Sharon, 135
Fluoride, 290, 295
Folk Medicine (Jarvis), 217
Food and Drink in History (Leclant),
  177
Forsyth Dental Center, 163, 173
Framingham Heart Study, 32
France
  apple studies in, 115, 117
  cabbage studies in, 151
  milk studies in, 233
  oat studies in, 241
  wine studies in, 306
  yogurt studies in, 97, 317
Free radicals, 18, 47, 65, 257, 293, 312
Fruit
  as antibiotic, 84–88, 90
  citrus, 12, 111
  sugar in, 287
  See also specific types
Fucoidan, 266

Fungal infection
  garlic and, 5–6, 200
  lemon and, 223
  orange and, 252

G

Galacturonic acid, 215
Galen, 45
Gall bladder, 162
Gallic acid, 90, 308
Gallotannic acid, 87
Gallstone, 275
Garagusi, Vincent F., 3–7, 10
Garland, Cedric, 227
Garlic, 3–7, 198–206, 248–49
  as antibiotic, 3–7, 199–200
  as anticoagulant, 13, 26–27, 34,
    208–209
  cancer and, 203–204, 209, 250
  chicken soup recipe, 48
  as expectorant, 44, 133
  heart disease and, 201–202
  historical use, 5, 198–99
  respiratory illness and, 44–45,
    47–48, 203
  vitamin C combination, 47
Garte, Seymour, 66
Gastric cancer, 204, 221
Gastrointestinal illness
  banana and, 122–24
  black currant and, 185
  egg and, 105–107
  milk and, 101–107, 230–31, 233
  soybean and, 68–69
  yogurt and, 94–95, 315–16
Gefarnate, 154
Gemfibrozil, 34
Georgetown University School of
    Medicine, 3
George Washington University, 5,
    26–27, 33–34
Germany
  beer studies in, 140–41
  blueberry studies in, 145
  cabbage studies in, 151, 154
  chili pepper studies in, 166

fish studies in, 194–95
lemon studies in, 223
melon studies in, 224
milk studies in, 105
Gillette, Marianne, 168
Ginger, 207–209
Gingerol, 209
Ginseng, 9, 295
Glucosinolates, 299–300
Glutathione, 60–61
Glycemic index, 116, 238, 257, 275
Goiter, 149, 155
Goldberg, Andrew P., 274
Goldin, Barry R., 98
Goldstein, Joseph L., 16
Gorbach, Sherwood L., 98
Gordon, Benjamin Lee, 8
Gout, 141, 162, 191, 282, 309
Graham, Saxon, 57–59, 147, 148, 152
Graham, Sylvester, 38–39, 301
Grains
  as antibiotic, 82
  cancer and, 70
  cholesterol and, 36–37
  See also specific types
Grape, 85, 86, 90, 211–212
Grape Cure, The (Brandt), 211
Grapefruit, 12, 213–15
Great Britain. *See* Britain
Green tea, 8, 87–90, 289–95
Grieve, Maud, 122, 184, 282, 310
Grundy, William, 243
Guaifenesin, 46
Gupta, N.N., 33, 248
Gurewich, Victor, 30–32, 247

H

Haffejee, I.E., 218
Hall, John, 111
Hammerschmidt, Dale, 24–29,
    209
Harvard School of Dental Medicine,
    250
Harvard Unversity, 229, 276
Hay fever, 218
HDL cholesterol. *See* Cholesterol

Headache
  Chinese mushroom and, 26, 234
  coffee and, 176
  fish and, 193–94
  guide to, 326
  tea and, 292
  wine and, 309
Healing Hand, The (Manjo), 217
Heart disease
  apple and, 115
  aspirin and, 34
  banana and, 124, 125
  barley and, 36–38, 127
  bean and, 133
  beer and, 139–42
  blueberry and, 144–45
  cancer link, 17
  carrot and, 158
  chili pepper and, 166–67
  Chinese mushroom and, 26, 234,
    236
  coffee and, 175
  corn and, 178, 179
  death rate from, 50
  drugs for, 36
  fiber and, 38–42
  fish and, 49–55, 191–92
  garlic and, 201–202
  grapefruit and, 214, 215
  guide to, 322
  melon and, 225
  milk and, 228
  nuts and, 238
  oats and, 240
  olive oil and, 242–44, 245
  onion and, 30–34, 247–48
  seeds and, 67–68
  shellfish and, 269–70
  soybean and, 274–75
  tea and, 292–93
  in vegetarians, 35–42
  wine and, 307, 309
Hemorrhage, 88
Hemorrhoids, 168, 241, 276, 325
Henkin, Robert I., 219
Hennekens, Charles, 74
Henry, James P., 293
Heparin, 267

Hepatitis, 89, 224, 290
Herbal tea, 294
Herberden, 45
Herpes simplex virus, 86, 212, 290
Herszage, Leon, 286
Hezekiah, 188, 189
Hippocrates, 7, 45, 199, 216, 301
Hippuric acid, 80, 181
Historia Naturalis (Pliny), 199
Hoff, Geir, 62
Holland. *See* Netherlands
Honest Herbal, The (Varro), 265
Honey, 216–219
Horseradish, 44, 45, 46
Hungary, 154
Hyperactivity, 286
Hypertension. *See* Blood pressure

I

Immunity
  cabbage and, 153
  Chinese mushroom and, 234–35
  corn and, 179
  egg and, 106
  fish and, 191
  garlic and, 200–201, 205
  milk and, 101, 104, 106, 230
  seaweed and, 266
  yogurt and, 95–98, 316
India
  banana studies in, 122–24
  cabbage studies in, 154
  chili pepper studies in, 167, 168
  garlic studies in, 201–202
  ginger studies in, 209
  lemon use in, 222
  milk studies in, 230
  onion studies in, 247–48, 249
  pea studies in, 253–54
  rice studies in, 262
  tea studies in, 89, 290
Indoles, 59, 60, 152
Infant formula, 102
Infection (general), 326
  See also Antibiotic; Virus
Influenza, 316

Insomnia, 176, 231–32, 287, 326
Insulin. *See* Blood sugar
Interferon, 96, 235
International Centre for Diarrhoeal
 Disease Research (Bangladesh), 262
Intestinal cancer, 266
Ipecac, 46
Ireland, 115
Irritable bowel syndrome, 233
Ismail, Amr Abdel–Fattah, 143
Israel, 128
Italy, 115, 283
 apple studies in, 115
 olive oil studies in, 243, 244
 soybean studies in, 274
 strawberry studies in, 283
 yogurt studies in, 94, 95, 96–97, 316

J

Jaloproctitis, 168
Japan
 artichoke studies in, 120
 beta carotene studies in, 76, 152, 155
 cabbage studies in, 151–52, 155
 cancer studies in, 18–19
 coffee studies in, 173
 eggplant studies in, 187
 fig studies in, 189
 fish use in, 51, 54, 192, 193, 196
 garlic studies in, 200, 202, 203
 ginger studies in, 209
 grapefruit studies in, 215
 heart disease in, 51, 54, 192
 milk studies in, 105, 228
 mushroom studies in, 235–36
 rice studies in, 262–63
 seaweed studies in, 265–67
 soybean studies in, 64, 275–76
 spinach studies in, 279
 tea studies in, 8, 87, 290–91, 293
 yam studies in, 311, 312
 yogurt studies in, 94, 95, 96, 316
Jarvis, D.C., 217
Jenkins, David, 19, 275
Jet lag, 177
Jewish Memorial Hospital (New York
 City), 94

John A. Burns School of Medicine
 (Hawaii), 266
Johns Hopkins University
 coffee studies at, 171, 175
 egg studies at, 105–106
 milk studies at, 228, 230
 soybean studies at, 68–69
 spinach studies at, 279
*Journal of the American Dietetic
 Association*, 13
*Journal of the National Cancer
 Institute*, 317

K

Kale, 76, 217–18
Kaopectate, 94
Karmali, Rashida, 193
Karolinska Institute (Stockholm), 171
Kashket, Shelby, 290
Kashket, Sidney, 173
Kefir. *See* Yogurt
Kelp, 264–66
Kempner, Walter, 262
Kennedy, Ann, 66–67, 134
Kensler, Thomas, 61, 107
Keys, Ancel, 243
Khachik, Frederick, 77
Kidney
 artichoke and, 121
 cherry and, 162
 cranberry and, 80, 181, 183
 fish and, 193–94
 rice and, 261–62
Kilbourn, J.P., 181, 182
Kinsella, John E., 197
Klurfeld, David, 275
Knutson, Richard A., 286
Kombu, 267
Konowalchuk, Jack, 84–87, 211, 307, 309
Koopman, James S., 230
Korea, 186
Kornhauser, Andrija, 74
Kourniss. *See* Yogurt
Kremer, Joel M., 193
Krinsky, Norman, 76
Kritchevsky, David, 275

Kromhout, Daan, 54, 192
Kyolic, 200, 201, 205

L

Lactobacilli, 94–99, 315
Lactose intolerance, 233, 318
Laetrile, 118, 119
Laminaria, 265–67
Lancet, 73, 202
Lands, William, 53–54, 55
Laragh, John, 228
Laryngeal cancer
  apricot and, 119
  carrot and, 75
  guide to, 322
  milk and, 233
  spinach and, 278–79
  squash/pumpkin and, 281
Lau, Benjamin, 201
Lawson, Terry, 168
Laxative
  barley as, 128
  black currant as, 184
  blueberry as, 145
  bran as, 41, 301–304
  oats as, 241
  olive oil as, 244
  prune as, 258–60
  soybean as, 276
  squash/pumpkin as, 280
LDL cholesterol. *See* Cholesterol
Leclant, Jean, 177
Legumes, 40, 70, 133–36, 254, 276
Lemon, 111, 222–23
Leukemia, 24–25, 235
Leukotrienes, 51, 53, 54, 191, 193, 194
Leung, Albert, 208
Levaelsole, 96
Lieberman, Harris, 170–71
Liebstein, A.M., 150, 211
Lime, 111, 222–23
Lin, Florence, 26
Lind, James, 111
Linnaeus, 282
Liver cancer, 67, 149, 238
Liver function, 72, 121, 149, 293
Longevity
  black currant and, 185

cabbage and, 151
Chinese mushroom and, 26, 234
olive oil and, 243–44
yogurt and, 13, 93, 97
Lovastatin, 36
Lung cancer
  apricot and, 119
  beer and, 141
  broccoli and, 146, 147
  carrot and, 73–75, 156–58
  guide to, 322
  kale and, 220, 221
  milk and, 228
  seaweed and, 266
  spinach and, 278–79
  squash/pumpkin and, 281
  tomato and, 297–98
  turnip and, 300
  wine and, 309
  yam and, 311, 322
Lung infection, 45–47, 165–66, 203, 250
Lupus erythematosis, 193
Lutein, 77
Lycopene, 298

M

Mackerras, Dorothy, 75
Magnesium, 259
Maimonides, 7, 45
Makheja, Amar N., 34
Manjo, Guido, 217, 306–307
Mann, George, 228
Mapo doufu, 24, 28–29
Marshall, James R., 147
Masquelier, J., 306
Masri, M. Sidney, 259
Materia Medica, 122
Mathews-Roth, Micheline, 74
M. avium, 5, 6
Mayo Clinic, 308
M.D. Anderson Hospital and Tumor
    Institute, 204, 250
Meat, 87–88
Medicine Throughout Antiquity
    (Gordon), 8
Melon, 224–25

Memorial Sloan Kettering
　　Cancer Center (New York),
　　97, 227
Meningitis, 4–5, 200
Menkes, Marilyn, 74–75, 157
Menopause, 232, 276
Menstruation, 26, 224
Merck Company, 95
Mertz, Walter, 12–13
Metchnikoff, Elias, 91–93,
　　314
Methylxanthines, 175
Mevacor (lovastatin), 36
Mevalonic acid, 37
Michigan State University, 116
Migraine headache, 309, 326
Milk, 12, 100–107, 226–33
　　See also Lactose intolerance;
　　Yogurt
Milk of magnesia, 259
Miller Brewing Company, 19
Minton, John, 175
Miso. See Soybean
Mithrydates, 188
Mitschek, G.H.A., 186–87
Mitsubishi-Kasei Institute of Life
　　Sciences (Tokyo), 189
Modern Herbal, A (Grieve), 184, 282,
　　310
Mo-er. See Chinese mushroom
Money, Samuel, 317
Monin, 177
Moore, Richard D., 139
Moosa, A., 218
Morphine, 11
Motion sickness, 208, 209, 326
Mouth disorders. See Cold sore; Oral
　　cancer
Mucodyne, 47
Mucokinetic agent, 45–46, 47
Mucus, 45–49
Multiple sclerosis, 235
Mushroom, 24–29, 234–36
Mushroom Research Institute of Japan,
　　236
Muskmelon, 224–25
Mustard, 45, 47
Mycobacteria, 5, 6

N

Nanji, Amin A., 307
Napralert, 11
National Cancer Institute
　　beta carotene studies at, 72
　　cabbage studies at, 59, 62
　　garlic studies at, 204
　　onion studies at, 250
　　orange studies at, 251
　　polyphenol studies at, 84
　　squash studies at, 281
　　yam studies at, 311
National Heart, Lung and Blood
　　Institute, 229
National Institute of Genetics (Japan),
　　291
National Institute of Mental Health,
　　175
National Institutes of Health, 55, 276,
　　280, 286
National Library of Medicine,
　　199
Natural History, 204
Nature, 73, 91, 92
Nature of Man, The (Metchnikoff),
　　91
Netherlands
　　fish studies in, 54, 192, 197
　　grapefruit studies in, 215
　　oats studies in, 39
New England Journal of Medicine, 26,
　　54
Newman, Rosemary K., 127, 128–29
Newmark, Harold, 87, 88
New York University Medical Center,
　　17
Nigeria, 186–87, 312
Nitrosamine, 87–88, 160, 251, 283,
　　291–92
Nori, 267
Norway
　　cabbage studies in, 61–62
　　cauliflower studies in, 160
　　coffee studies in, 173
　　fish studies in, 192
Nuts, 64–70, 237–38, 259
Nylander, Percy, 312

O

Oat bran muffins, 39, 42, 240
Oats, 39–42, 112, 239–41
Ocean Spray, 19, 82
Ohio State University, 291
Olive oil, 242–45
Omega-3 fatty acids, 51–55, 191–97, 270
Omega-6 fatty acids, 51–52
Oncogenes, 65–66, 134
Onion, 13, 27, 30–34, 112, 205–206, 246–250
Oral cancer, 88, 221, 233, 250, 292
Orange, 12, 251–52
Orinase, 249
Osteoporosis, 232, 326
Ovarian cancer, 68
Oyster, 8–10

P

Painkiller, 166, 167
Pakistan, 36
Pancreatic cancer, 119, 173, 215, 252, 322
Panic attacks, 175
Papas, Prodromos, 181
Pasteur, Louis, 5, 91, 249
Pasteur Institute, 91–92
Pea, 11, 253–255
Peach, 85, 259
Peanut, 238
Pecarin, 141, 184
Pectin
  in apple, 115, 117
  in banana, 124
  in grapefruit, 12, 214, 215
  in lemon, 223
  in orange, 252
  in strawberry, 283
Penicillin, 82, 199, 315
Penn, Arthur, 17
Pentose, 41, 304
Pepper, hot. See Chili pepper
Pepsin, 123, 124
Petkov, V., 202–203

Peto, Richard, 72
Pharyngeal cancer, 168, 279
Phenols. See Polyphenols
Phlegm, 162
Pick, Alois, 306
Plantain, 122–125
Pliny the Elder, 5, 188, 198, 213
Poland, 203, 316
Poliovirus, 85, 116, 144, 212, 290
Polyphenols, 84–90
  in coffee, 173–174
  in nuts, 237
  in strawberry, 283
  in wine, 85–86, 306
  in yam, 312
Potato, 70, 90 256–257
Prasad, Ananda A., 9
Pregnancy, 175, 197
Prevention magazine, 162
Prolongation of Life, The (Metchnikoff), 91
Propionate, 41
Prostaglandins
  aspirin and, 34, 53
  fish and, 52–55, 191–93, 196
  garlic and, 34
  mechanism of, 17, 33–34, 49, 51–52
  milk and, 229–30
  oats and, 241
  onion and, 34, 249
  yogurt and, 317
Prostate cancer
  corn and, 178
  guide to, 322
  kale and, 221
  peas and, 254
  rice and, 262
  seeds and, 67–68
  spinach and, 278–79
  squash/pumpkin and, 281
  tomato and, 297
Prostate infection, 181
Protease inhibitors, 64–70
  in barley, 127
  in beans, 134
  in corn, 178
  in eggplant, 187
  in nuts, 237

Protease inhibitors (*continued*)
  in oats, 241
  in peas, 254
  in potato, 257, 311
  in rice, 262
  in soybean, 276
  in squash/pumpkin, 280
  in yam, 311
Prune, 258–60
Psoriasis, 194, 241, 262, 326
Pumpkin, 280–81

Q

Quaker Oats Company, 39
Quinic acid, 80
Qureshi, Asaf, 36, 42

R

Raisin, 212
Ramses II, 242
Rectal cancer, 141, 147, 279, 309, 322
Reddy, B.S., 268
Respiratory illness
  apple and, 116
  chili pepper and, 43–48, 165–166
  coffee and, 172, 173
  garlic and, 203
  milk and, 228
Rheumatism, 89, 191, 256
Rice, 261–63
Robitussin, 44, 47, 165
Romania, 93
Rosenthal, Norman, 285
Rotavirus, 68, 101–106, 230
Roundworm, 223, 224
Rozin, Paul, 167
Rubella, 252
Ruhr University (Germany), 105
Russia
  garlic studies in, 200, 202, 203, 249
  ginseng studies in, 295

onion studies and, 249–50
  tea studies in, 89
Rutabaga, 299–300

S

Sablé-Amplis, R., 115
SAD. *See* Seasonal affective disorder
Salem, Norman, 196
Salmonella bacteria, 93, 94, 218, 249, 315
Salter, Hyde, 170
Sandberg, Finn, 144
Sandstead, Harold, 9
Sanyal, A.K., 123, 125
Sanyal, S.N., 253–54
Sauerkraut. *See* Cabbage
Scallion, 26
S. Carboxymethylcysteine, 47
Schwartz, Gary, 116
Schweitzer, Albert, 199
Scurvy, 111, 222–23
Seafood. *See* Fish
Searle, G.D., 229
Seasonal affective disorder (SAD), 285
Seaweed, 264–68
Sedative. *See* Tranquilizer
Seeds, 64–70, 127, 134
Seifter, Eli, 73
Semmelweis Medical University (Budapest), 144
Serotonin, 285–87
Sexuality, 9, 11
Shahani, Khem, 94–95, 315, 318
Shekelle, Richard, 73, 157, 227, 279
Shellfish, 269–72
Shigella bacteria, 94, 218
Shiitake, 234–35
Singh, G.B., 154
Sinuses, 46, 165
Sirtori, C.R., 274
Skin cancer, 67, 74, 119, 155, 311
Skin problems, 241, 282, 326
Sleep, 176, 219, 231–32, 287
Sleeper (film), 106
Sloan Kettering Institute for Cancer Research (New York), 97, 227

Smith Papyrus, 216
Smoking
  apricot and, 119
  broccoli and, 147
  carrot and, 73–75, 157–159
  chili pepper and, 43, 45, 47, 165
  coffee and, 175
  kale and, 220, 221
  milk and, 228, 229
  spinach and, 278–79
  squash/pumpkin and, 281
  yam and, 311
Sobota, Anthony, 79–82, 181–83
Sodium, 228, 267
Soviet Union. See Russia
Soybean, 64–70, 134, 273–77
Speirs, Joan I., 84, 211
Spicy foods, 43–48
Spinach, 76–77, 278–79
Squash, 280–81
Srivastava, K.C., 208
Stanford University, 308
State University of New York
  (Buffalo), 157
State University of New York Health
  Science Center, 229
Steinberg, Alfred D., 55, 193
Stich, Hans, 77, 88–89, 291–92, 308
Stomach cancer
  grapefruit and, 215
  guide to, 322
  kale and, 221
  milk and, 228
  orange and, 251
  rice and, 263
  soybean and, 276
  spinach and, 278–79
  squash/pumpkin and, 281
  tea and, 87
  tomato and, 297
  vitamin C and, 12
Stomach ulcer. See Ulcer
Strawberry, 84, 90, 282–83
Streptomycin, 218, 249
Stroke
  aspirin and, 34
  Chinese mushroom and, 236
  fish and, 53, 191–92

  grapefruit and, 214
  guide to, 327
  melon and, 225
  olive oil and, 243
  onion and, 32
  seaweed and, 267
  soybean and, 275
Stuart, Price, Jr., 80
Sucur, M., 202
Sugar, 231, 232, 284–88
Suicide, 285
Sweden
  barley studies in, 127
  black currant studies in, 184–85
  blueberry use in, 143–144
  capsaisin studies in, 165
  carrot studies in, 157
  fish studies in, 192
  grapefruit studies in, 215
  orange studies in, 252
  prostaglandin studies in, 52
  urinary tract infection studies in, 79
Sweet potato, 281, 310–13
Switzerland, 105, 120

T

Tabasco sauce, 44, 46
Taberner, Peter, 297
Tagamet, 123, 124, 230
Tannin, 84–86, 88, 144, 173, 212,
  290–295
Tapeworm, 280
Tea, 8, 85, 87–90, 289–96
Teas, Jane, 265–66
Tetracycline, 82, 199
Texas Reports on Biology and
  Medicine, 162
Thailand, 166–167
Theophrastus, 213
Thompson, Larry, 18
Throat cancer, 221
Thromboembolism, 166–167
Thrombophlebitis, 26
Thrombosis, 54, 89, 292
Thromboxane, 34, 53, 54
Tibet, 253

Tillotson, James, 19, 82
Tocotrienol, 37–38
Tofu. *See* Soybean
Tokin, B., 249
Tolbutamide, 249
Tomato, 71, 297–98
Toothache, 166
Tooth decay
  cherry and, 163
  coffee and, 173
  corn and, 179
  grape and, 212
  milk and, 232
  sugar and, 287
  tea and, 290–91
Toth, Bela, 236
Toxic shock syndrome, 103
Tranquilizer, 284–85, 287, 293
Tree ears. *See* Chinese mushroom
Triglycerides, 39
Troll, Walter, 64–70, 127, 134, 237
Tryptophan, 231, 285, 317
Tuberculosis, 5, 6, 249
Tumor. *See* Cancer
Turnip, 299–300
Twins, birth of, 312
Tyler, Varro, 264

U

Ulcer
  banana and, 122–124, 125
  cabbage and, 153–155
  chili pepper and, 168
  coffee and, 175
  drugs for, 154, 229
  guide to, 327
  milk and, 229–30
  seaweed and, 267
  tea and, 294, 295
United States Department of
  Agriculture (USDA), 36, 93,
  127, 259, 279, 296
University of California, 44, 230, 292
University of Connecticut, 117
University of Kentucky Medical
  College, 39, 244

University of Milan, 244
University of Newcastle upon Tyne
  (Britain), 33
University of Paris, 144
University of Texas, 183, 243
University of Wisconsin, 103, 127, 128
Urinary tract
  cancer, 141
  guide to, 327
  infection, 79–83, 180–83
Urine odor, 182
Uterine cancer, 68

V

Vanderbilt University School of
  Medicine, 173
Vanderhoek, Jack Y., 34
Vane, John, 53
Vegetables
  cancer and, 63, 70, 71–77, 88, 90
  cruciferous, 56–63, 149, 152
  dark green, 71–77, 147
  dark orange, 71–77, 147, 311
  fatty acids in, 51–52
  phenols in, 88, 90
  See also specific types
Vegetarians, 18–20, 35–42, 112, 134,
  273
Vinegar, 45
Virus, 17
  apple and, 116
  blueberry and, 144
  Chinese mushroom and, 235, 236
  cranberry and, 182
  egg and, 105–106
  fruit and, 84–85
  grape and, 212
  milk and, 100–107
  oats and, 241
  orange and, 252
  pea and, 254
  potato and, 256–57, 311
  soybean and, 67–70
  strawberry and, 282–83
  tea and, 290
  wine and, 306–307

Virus (*continued*)
  yam and, 311
  yogurt and, 93
Visudhiphan, Sukon, 166
Vitamin A, 72–76
  in apricot, 119
  in fish, 196
  in kale, 220
  in milk, 104, 228
Vitamin C
  as additive, 104
  in apples, 115
  capillary strength and, 89
  deficiency, 223
  garlic combination, 47
  meat processing and, 88
  in orange, 251–52
  respiratory illness and, 47
  scurvy and, 223
  stomach cancer and, 12
Vitamin D, 196, 227
Vitamin E, 88
Voltaire, 170

W

Wargovich, Michael J., 87
Washington Post, 18
Washington University School of
  Dentistry, 291
Wattenberg, Lee, 19
  brussels sprout studies by, 149
  cabbage studies by, 57–62, 152
  cauliflower studies by, 160

  coffee studies by, 173
  tea studies by, 87
Weight, 116, 287, 308
Weisburger, John, 303
Wheat bran, 39, 90, 240–241,
  301–304
White tree fungus, 26
Wine, 84–90, 140–142, 212, 305–309
Wisconsin Alumni Research Foundation
  (WARF), 38
Wound healing, 217, 284, 286, 287
Wurtman, Judith, 170–171, 174, 195,
  231, 271, 285–87
Wurtman, Richard, 231

Y

Yakult. *See* Yogurt
Yale University, 116
Yam, 281, 310–13
Yamamoto, Ichiro, 266
Yin-Yang therapy, 43
Yogurt 13, 91–99, 168, 227,
  314–318
Yolken, Robert H., 100–106, 230
Yugoslavia, 223

Z

Ziegler, Regina G., 158
Ziment, Irwin, 7, 43–48, 165–166,
  203, 250
Zinc, 9–10, 12